Podrid's Real-World ECGs

A Master's Approach to the Art and Practice of Clinical ECG Interpretation

Volume 1 The Basics

Podrid's Real-World ECGs

A Master's Approach to the Art and Practice of Clinical ECG Interpretation

Volume 1   The Basics

Philip Podrid, MD

Professor of Medicine
Professor of Pharmacology and Experimental Therapeutics
Boston University School of Medicine

Lecturer in Medicine
Harvard Medical School
Boston, Massachusetts

Attending Physician
West Roxbury VA Hospital
West Roxbury, Massachusetts

Rajeev Malhotra, MD, MS

Instructor in Medicine
Cardiology Division
Massachusetts General Hospital
Harvard Medical School
Boston, Massachusetts

Rahul Kakkar, MD

Cardiology Fellow
Massachusetts General Hospital
Harvard Medical School
Boston, Massachusetts

Peter A. Noseworthy, MD

Cardiology Fellow
Massachusetts General Hospital
Harvard Medical School
Boston, Massachusetts

cardiotext
PUBLISHING
Minneapolis, Minnesota

© 2013 Philip Podrid, Rajeev Malhotra, Rahul Kakkar, and Peter A. Noseworthy

Cardiotext Publishing, LLC
750 2nd St NE Suite 102
Hopkins, MN 55343
USA
www.cardiotextpublishing.com

Any updates to this book may be found at:
www.cardiotextpublishing.com/titles/detail/9781935395003

Comments, inquiries, and requests for bulk sales can be directed to the publisher at:
info@cardiotextpublishing.com

This book is intended for educational purposes and to further general scientific and medical knowledge, research, and understanding of the conditions and associated treatments discussed herein. This book is not intended to serve as and should not be relied upon as recommending or promoting any specific diagnosis or method of treatment for a particular condition or a particular patient. It is the reader's responsibility to determine the proper steps for diagnosis and the proper course of treatment for any condition or patient, including suitable and appropriate tests, medications or medical devices to be used for or in conjunction with any diagnosis or treatment.

Due to ongoing research, discoveries, modifications to medicines, equipment and devices, and changes in government regulations, the information contained in this book may not reflect the latest standards, developments, guidelines, regulations, products or devices in the field. Readers are responsible for keeping up to date with the latest developments and are urged to review the latest instructions and warnings for any medicine, equipment or medical device. Readers should consult with a specialist or contact the vendor of any medicine or medical device where appropriate.

Except for the publisher's website associated with this work, the publisher is not affiliated with and does not sponsor or endorse any websites, organizations or other sources of information referred to herein.

The publisher and the authors specifically disclaim any damage, liability, or loss incurred, directly or indirectly, from the use or application of any of the contents of this book.

Unless otherwise stated, all figures and tables in this book are used courtesy of the authors.

Cover design by Caitlin Crouchet and Elizabeth Edwards; interior design by Elizabeth Edwards

Library of Congress Control Number: 2012947870

ISBN: 978-1-935395-00-3

2 3 4 5 6

These workbooks are dedicated first to my wife Vivian and son Joshua, whose patience, tolerance, support, and love over the years have been limitless, exceptional, and inspirational. They are also dedicated to the many cardiology fellows, house staff, and medical students whom I have had the pleasure and honor of teaching over the past three decades and who have also taught me so very much.

Philip Podrid

To my wife Cindy and daughter Sapna, for all their love, support, and encouragement.

Rajeev Malhotra

To my darling daughters, Mia and Eila, whom I love to infinity.

Rahul Kakkar

For Katie and Jack

Peter A. Noseworthy

Contents

Foreword

The invention of the electrocardiogram (ECG) by Dr. Willem Einthoven, first reported in 1901, ranks as one of the all-time great discoveries in medicine. Einthoven's landmark achievement was duly recognized in 1924, when he was awarded the Nobel Prize in Medicine.

By the early 1940s, all of the components of the 12-lead ECG that we use today were in place. When I finished my cardiology training 50 years ago, the ECG was one of very few cardiodiagnostic tools available to us. As a result, we received an intensity of training in electrocardiography that is generally not encountered in many of today's cardiology fellowship programs, where the emphasis has shifted toward the newer high-tech diagnostic modalities. Yet the ECG remains a major pillar in the evaluation of disorders of the heart. In a patient with a cardiac arrhythmia, what diagnostic information does the treating physician want the most? Of course—the ECG. Although the medical world progresses rapidly and changes constantly, the body of knowledge surrounding the ECG is virtually timeless. What was true 50 years ago is largely true today, and will remain so 50 years from now.

This wonderful series of ECG workbooks, appropriately entitled "Real-World ECGs," by Dr. Philip Podrid and three outstanding young cardiologists from Massachusetts General Hospital—Dr. Rajeev Malhotra, Dr. Rahul Kakkar, and Dr. Peter Noseworthy—offers a splendid opportunity for self-education in electrocardiography (and a bit of fun at the same time). An esteemed academic cardiologist, Dr. Podrid has had a career-long interest in electrocardiography. Over many years he has collected and saved thousands of ECGs for teaching purposes, and it is a portion of his incredible collection that has been used to spawn these books.

There are scores of textbooks on electrocardiography, but what sets these volumes apart is that every ECG is tied directly to an actual clinical case. Each ECG is initially presented in a visually attractive and readable format accompanied by a clinical vignette. On the next page, the salient features of the ECGs are highlighted, dissected, and discussed in meticulous detail, followed by a summary of the patient's clinical problem and treatment, particularly as they relate to the ECG findings.

The first volume in this unique series covers electrocardiography basics. It is followed by five more volumes covering the entire spectrum of electrocardiography: myocardial abnormalities, conduction abnormalities, arrhythmias, narrow and wide complex tachycardias, and a sixth volume amalgamating a potpourri of paced rhythms, congenital abnormalities, and electrolyte disturbances. As I perused one of the workbooks, I truly enjoyed the experience. It is fun to try to guess the clinical problem from the ECG. In fact, on my teaching rounds, that is often exactly what I do. I will ask the trainee to present first just the ECG and with other trainees try to deduce from it what might be going on clinically. For example, in an adult with marked left ventricular hypertrophy and strain, one of three conditions is almost always present: severe aortic valve disease, hypertrophic cardiomyopathy, or hypertensive heart disease.

These books should prove to be valuable for the teaching and learning of electrocardiography at all levels—from nursing and medical students to residents to cardiology fellows to practicing internists and cardiologists. They should be especially helpful for those seeking board certification or recertification in cardiovascular diseases, where knowledge of electrocardiography still is given a very high priority.

There is one further important dividend for those who utilize this series. In addition to the six workbooks, hundreds of other ECGs handled in a similar format are available online. From clinical diagnoses to interactive questions to patient management, realworldECGs.com offers ECG-centric clinical cases for the viewer to further master the art of ECG interpretation.

Anyone who reads these books and views the auxiliary electronic material cannot help but be impressed by the prodigious amount of work that went into their preparation. Drs. Podrid, Malhotra, Kakkar, and Noseworthy should be justifiably proud of the final results of their Herculean efforts. I am confident that other readers will find these books and their electronic supplement as informative and enjoyable as I did.

Roman W. DeSanctis, MD
Physician and Director of Clinical Cardiology, Emeritus
Massachusetts General Hospital
James and Evelyn Jenks and Paul Dudley White Professor of Medicine
Harvard Medical School

Foreword

The electrocardiogram (ECG) was born in the Netherlands at the beginning of the 20th century when physiologist Willem Einthoven made the first recording of the spread of electrical activity in the beating heart from the surface of the body in a living human being. Since then, the ECG has become the indispensable "workhorse" in the management of patients suspected to have a cardiac problem.

The reasons are obvious. An ECG can be obtained anywhere. A recording is easily and quickly made, noninvasive, inexpensive, reproducible, and patient-friendly. The ECG gives instantaneous diagnostic information, is essential in selecting appropriate management, and allows documentation of the effect of treatment in cases of acute and chronic cardiac ischemia, rhythm and conduction disturbances, structural changes in the cardiac chambers, electrolyte and metabolic disorders, medication effects, and monogenic ECG patterns indicating the likelihood of cardiac abnormalities. The ECG is also a valuable tool for epidemiologic studies and risk stratification of the cardiac patient.

In the 110 years during which the ECG has been in use, we have seen continual improvements in its value in light of information gleaned from other invasive and noninvasive diagnostic techniques, such as coronary angiography, intracardiac localization of abnormal impulse formation and conduction disturbances, echocardiography, MRI, and genetic evaluation. This means that not only does the novice health care professional need to be informed about all the information currently available from the ECG, but the more senior physician also needs to stay up-do-date with ever-evolving new developments.

Dr. Philip Podrid is known worldwide as an expert in electrocardiography. He is also a superb teacher. When you combine his input with beautiful ECGs, not surprisingly, you will have a series of "Real-World ECGs" that demonstrate the art and practice of clinical ECG interpretation as only a real master can. I hope that many readers will profit from this exceptional educational exercise.

Hein J. Wellens, MD
Professor of Cardiology
Cardiovascular Research Institute Maastricht
Maastricht, The Netherlands

Preface

The electrocardiogram (ECG) is one of the oldest technologies used in medicine and remains one of the most frequently obtained tests in the physician's office, outpatient clinic, emergency department, and hospital. ECGs continue to play an essential role in the diagnosis of many cardiac diseases and in the evaluation of symptoms believed to be of cardiac origin. The ECG is also important in the diagnosis of many noncardiac medical conditions.

Like any other skill in medicine, the art of ECG interpretation requires frequent review of the essentials of ECG analysis and continual practice in reading actual ECGs. However, many health care providers who wish to augment their expertise in the interpretation of ECGs and develop the skills necessary to understand the underlying mechanisms of ECG abnormalities have realized that the currently available resources do not adequately meet their needs.

Teaching in medical schools and house staff programs does not typically emphasize ECG analysis. Consequently, many physicians do not feel adequately trained in interpreting the ECG. The currently available textbooks used for teaching ECG analysis are based on pattern recognition and memorization rather than on understanding the fundamental electrophysiologic properties and clinical concepts that can be applied to an individual ECG tracing, regardless of its complexity. The physician is not, therefore, trained in the identification of important waveforms and subtle abnormalities.

The workbooks and website of *Podrid's Real-World ECGs* aim to fill the gap in ECG education. These unique teaching aids prepare students and health care providers of all levels for the spectrum of routine to challenging ECGs they will encounter in their own clinical practice by providing a broad and in-depth understanding of ECG analysis and diagnosis, including discussion of relevant electrophysiologic properties of the heart, associated case scenarios, and clinical management.

The Workbooks

Each of the six volumes in *Podrid's Real-World ECGs* teaches the art of ECG interpretation by careful analysis of specific examples and identification of important waveforms. Each ECG is taken from a real clinical case and incorporates a discussion of important diagnostic findings and essential associated electrophysiologic mechanisms, as well as critical clinical management decisions. The purpose of the series is to provide readers from all fields of medicine with a systematic approach to ECG interpretation using a concise, case-based format.

Volume 1 provides an essential introduction to the basics of ECG reading, outlining the approaches and tools that are utilized in the interpretation of all ECGs. The subsequent volumes focus on particular disease entities for which the ECG is useful:

- Myocardial abnormalities, including infarction, hypertrophy, and inflammation

- Atrioventricular (AV) and intraventricular conduction disturbances and enhanced AV conduction

- Sinus, atrial, junctional, and ventricular arrhythmias

- Narrow and wide complex tachycardias and forms of aberration

- Recording methods and miscellaneous conditions, including pacemakers, electrolyte disorders, and acquired and congenital cardiac conditions

Each volume in the series starts with a didactic introduction that addresses the important ECG findings associated with each clinical category. This is followed by core illustrative case-based ECGs that lead the reader through identification of the important ECG findings associated with the specific abnormalities being discussed and provide informa-tion about the basic electrophysiologic mechanisms involved. This section is followed by a random assortment of topic-related ECGs and clinical scenarios to further enhance the student's skills at ECG analysis. Importantly, each case presentation is followed by an in-depth discussion of the ECG findings, with the important waveforms on the ECG highlighted.

Philip Podrid, MD
Rajeev Malhotra, MD, MS
Rahul Kakkar, MD
Peter A. Noseworthy, MD

Introduction
The Basics

This workbook presents the essentials of electrocardiogram (ECG) analysis: the heart's conduction system, the normal activation sequence, the lead system, a systematic approach for analysis of the ECG, the normal waveforms and intervals, and axis determination. The ECGs that follow the introduction demonstrate various abnormalities of atrioventricular (AV) and intraventricular conduction, features of myocardial abnormalities, and the common supraventricular and ventricular arrhythmias.

Components of the ECG

The ECG is a recording of the electrical activity of the heart. The waveforms that make up the ECG (P, QRS, and T) reflect depolarization and repolarization of the atrial and ventricular myocardium. The activity of the heart's electrical, or conduction, system (sinus node, AV node, and His-Purkinje system) is not transmitted to the surface of the body and hence is not recorded or manifested on the ECG. However, abnormalities of the conduction system can be established by careful analysis of the waveforms and intervals that are routinely measured on the ECG (PR interval, QRS duration, and QT interval).

The electrical system of the heart (FIGURE 1), which is responsible for generating an action potential and transmitting this action potential to all parts of the atrial and ventricular myocardium in a uniform

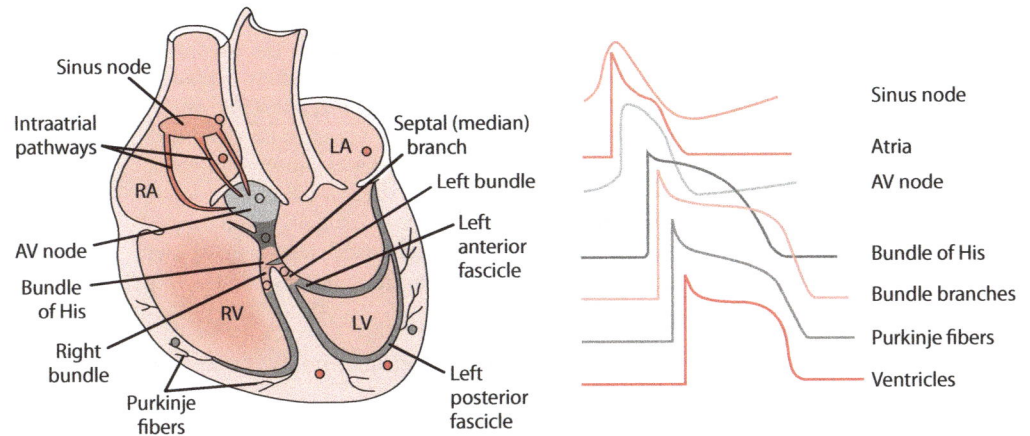

Figure 1: The electrical system of the heart and the action potentials associated with each structure. The electrical impulse is initiated in the sinoatrial or sinus node, which generates the impulse via a slow action potential. The impulse then spreads to the right atrium (RA) via intraatrial pathways and to the left atrium (LA) via an interatrial pathway. The atrial myocardium generates the impulse via a fast action potential. The impulse then arrives at the atrioventricular (AV) node, which generates an impulse via a slow action potential. From here the impulse enters the bundle of His and spreads to the right (RV) and left (LV) ventricles via a right bundle (to the RV) and left bundle (to the LV). The left bundle divides into two major fascicles (left anterior and left posterior) and one median fascicle (septal branch) to serve the LV, which has a greater muscle mass than the RV. The bundles and ventricular myocardium generate an impulse via a fast action potential.

and simultaneous fashion, includes the sinus or sinoatrial node (the dominant pacemaker of the heart as it generates an impulse with higher frequency than any other tissue), conduction pathways through the right and left atria, the AV node or junction, the bundle of His, the right bundle (which innervates the right ventricle), the left bundle (which innervates the left ventricle), and the Purkinje fibers (which bring the impulse to the individual myocardial cells). Since the muscle mass of the left ventricle is large, the left bundle splits into two major fascicles and one minor fascicle that result in simultaneous activation of the entire left ventricular myocardium. These fascicles include a minor septal branch or median fascicle (innervating the interventricular septum) and two major fascicles (the left anterior fascicle and left posterior fascicle).

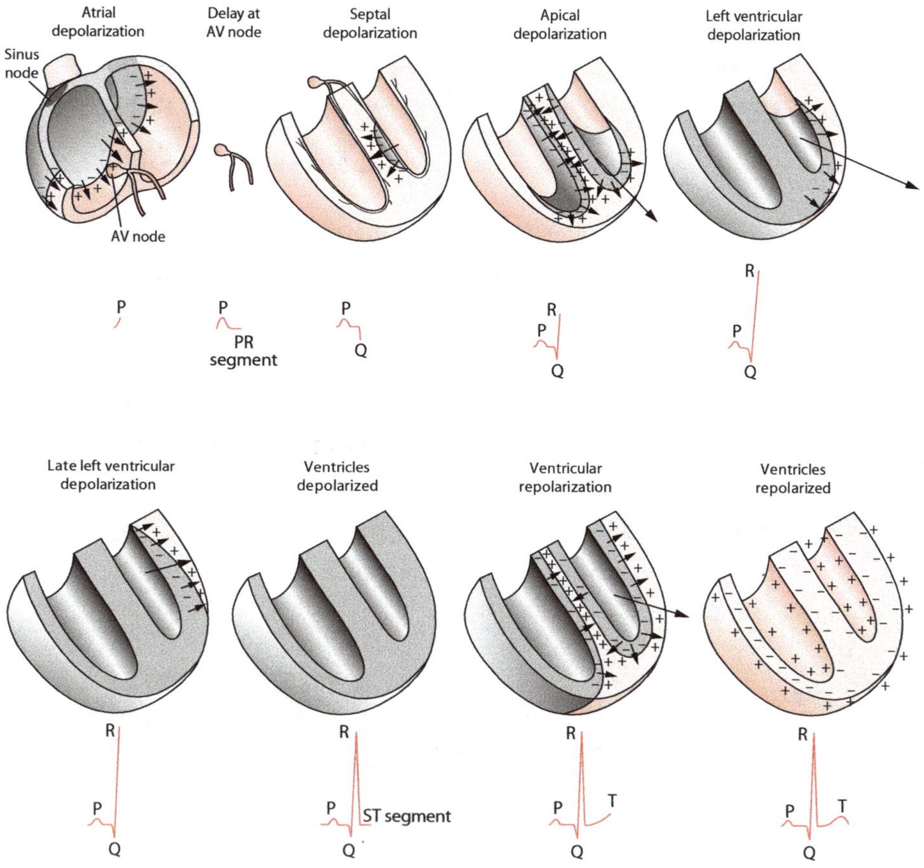

Normal Activation of the Atria and Ventricles

The normal activation sequence of the heart can be seen in **FIGURES 2 AND 3**. The initial impulse activating the heart is normally generated by the sinus node, which is located in the proximal portion of the right atrium. This impulse then spreads to depolarize the right and left atria. The activation sequence is from right to left and proximal to distal (up to down). Atrial depolarization generates a P wave on the surface ECG.

Figure 2: **Normal activation of the atria and ventricles and the ECG waveforms generated.** The dominant pacemaker is the sinus node. The impulse that originates in this structure conducts to the right and left atria, and depolarization or activation of these structures generates a P wave on the surface ECG. The impulse then conducts through the atrioventricular (AV) node and then the bundle of His and right and left bundles. These structures are too small to generate electrical activity that can be recorded. Hence on the ECG this is the PR segment, which is the time for conduction from the atrium to the ventricles via the AV node and His-Purkinje system. The first part of the ventricles to be depolarized or activated is the left side of the septum. As the impulse goes from left to right, there is a small negative deflection in most leads, termed a Q wave. The rest of the left and right ventricular myocardium becomes activated or depolarized in a right-to-left direction. This generates the entire QRS complex on the surface ECG. After the ventricles complete their depolarization, there is a period of electrical quiescence, which is the ST segment on the surface ECG. Repolarization of the ventricles follows this and generates a T wave on the ECG.

Based on the direction of activation, the P wave will be positive in the left-sided and inferior leads (*ie*, leads I, II, aVF, and V4-V6) and negative in the right-sided lead (*ie*, lead aVR). The impulse then reaches the AV node, which is the structure within the electrical system with the slowest conduction velocity. Hence there is a delay in impulse conduction through this structure. After passing through the AV node, the impulse reaches the His-Purkinje system and then enters the right and left bundles. Since these structures are small and generate very little electrical activity, no manifestation of their activation is seen at the surface of the body. The ECG does not record any electrical activity as the impulse travels through the AV node and His-Purkinje system. This accounts for the PR segment, which is at baseline or zero potential. Therefore, the PR segment represents AV conduction time and includes conduction through the AV node and His-Purkinje system.

The first part of the ventricle to be depolarized is the intraventricular septum, and the impulse arises from a septal (median) branch of the left bundle. Hence the direction of septal depolarization is from left to right, accounting for the small initial negative waveform (septal Q wave) of the QRS complex seen in left-sided leads and the small positive deflection (R wave) seen in right-sided leads. Thereafter, the rest of the right and left ventricles are depolarized simultaneously. Since the left ventricular muscle mass is much greater than that of the right ventricle, the QRS complex on the surface ECG primarily represents left ventricular depolarization; this occurs in a right-to-left direction, accounting for a tall positive deflection (R wave) in the left-sided leads

(*ie*, leads I and V4-V6) and a negative deflection (S wave) in the right-sided leads (*ie*, leads aVR and V1). The last part of the left ventricle to be depolarized is the lateral and posterior walls; this occurs in a left-to-right direction, accounting for the terminal negative deflection (S wave) in the left-sided leads. Once depolarization is completed, there is a brief period during which no electrical activity occurs (*ie*, the ST segment is at baseline or zero potential). This is followed by repolarization, which generates a T wave (see **FIGURE 3**).

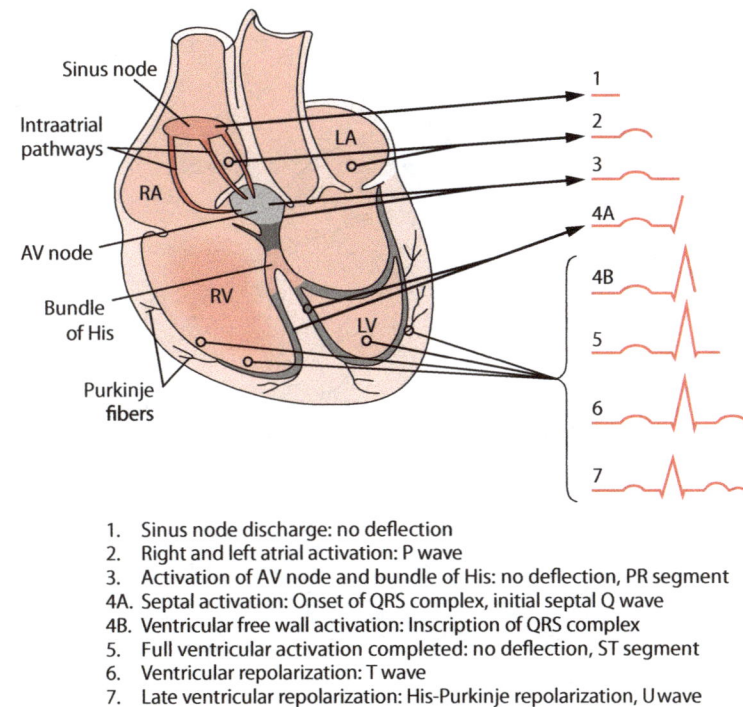

1. Sinus node discharge: no deflection
2. Right and left atrial activation: P wave
3. Activation of AV node and bundle of His: no deflection, PR segment
4A. Septal activation: Onset of QRS complex, initial septal Q wave
4B. Ventricular free wall activation: Inscription of QRS complex
5. Full ventricular activation completed: no deflection, ST segment
6. Ventricular repolarization: T wave
7. Late ventricular repolarization: His-Purkinje repolarization, U wave

Figure 3: Normal activation of the atria and ventricles and the waveforms generated.

Frequently seen following the T wave is a U wave, which is believed to represent late repolarization of the His-Purkinje system. Some believe that the U wave may represent late repolarization of the papillary muscles. This is a low-amplitude positive waveform after the T wave, best seen in the right precordial leads (*ie*, leads V1-V3).

Lead System

The standard ECG includes 12 leads: six limb leads (recording the electrical current in the frontal plane) and six precordial or chest leads (recording the electrical current in the horizontal plane).

The six limb leads include the following (**FIGURES 4 AND 5**):

- **Lead I** is a bipolar lead that records the impulse as it travels from right arm to left arm. Impulses going toward the left produce a positive waveform in this lead; impulses going toward the right produce a negative waveform. Therefore, in normal situations the P wave (due to atrial activation that goes from right to left) is positive in this lead. The QRS complex, which is due to impulse conduction in a right-to-left direction, is also positive, and there may be a small septal Q wave (representing septal depolarization that occurs in a left-to-right direction) before the tall positive waveform, or R wave, representing left ventricular depolarization.

- **Lead II** is a bipolar lead that records the impulse as it travels from the right arm to the left foot. Impulses going toward the foot generate a positive waveform in this lead; a negative waveform is generated if the impulse is directed away from the foot toward the right arm. Therefore, in normal situations the

Figure 4: Leads I, II, and III are bipolar leads. In lead I an impulse that travels toward the left arm generates a positive waveform, and an impulse that travels toward the right arm generates a negative waveform. In leads II and III, an impulse that travels toward the foot generates a positive waveform and an impulse that goes away from the foot toward the arms generates a negative waveform.

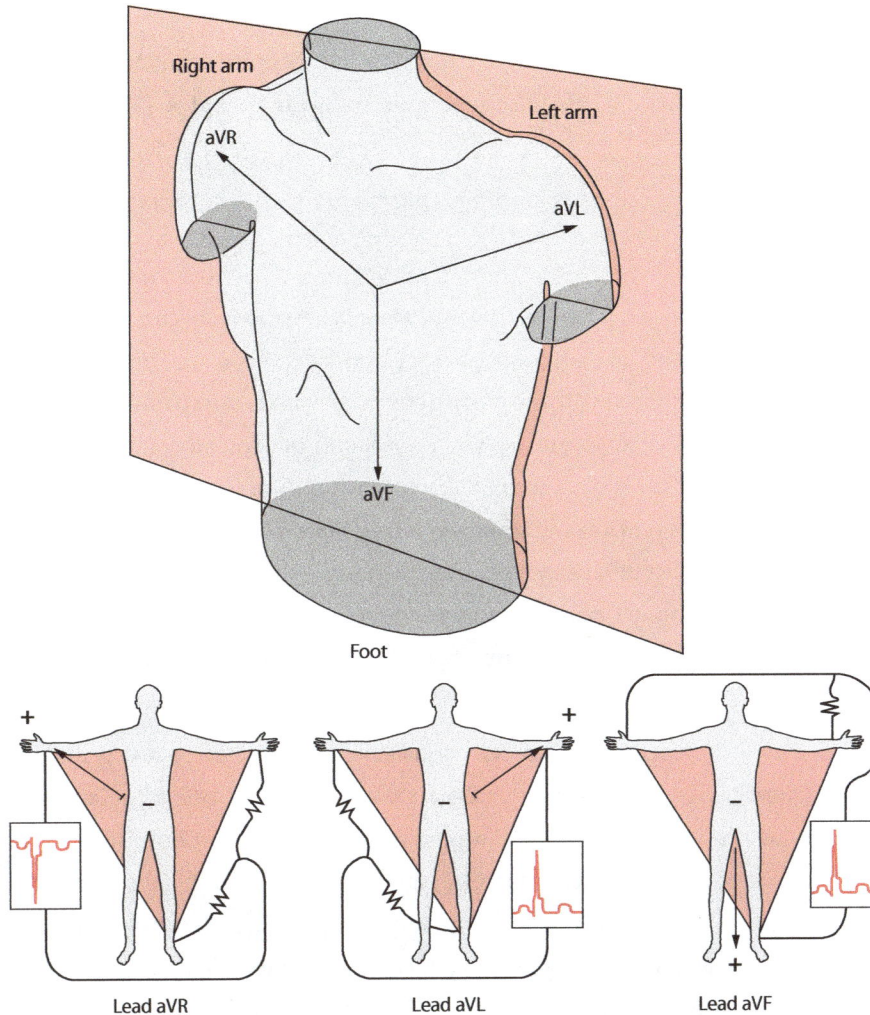

Figure 5: Leads aVR, aVL, and aVF are unipolar leads.
The impulse is imagined as originating from the middle of the heart. An impulse that goes toward any of these leads generates a positive waveform, and an impulse that goes away from these leads generates a negative waveform. Since the cardiac impulse goes primarily from right to left and up to down (superior to inferior), the waveforms are positive in leads aVL and aVF but negative in lead aVR.

P wave (representing atrial activation that occurs in a proximal-to-distal direction) is positive in this lead. The QRS complex (representing ventricular depolarization that occurs from proximal to distal) is also positive, and there may be a small septal Q wave before the tall positive waveform, or R wave, representing left ventricular depolarization.

- **Lead III** is a bipolar lead that records the impulse as it travels from the left arm to the left foot. Impulses going toward the foot generate a positive waveform in this lead; a negative waveform is generated if the impulse is directed away from the foot toward the left arm. Based on the angle of lead III in relation to the heart, the waveforms may be positive or negative depending on small changes in the direction of electrical activation. Hence lead III is an indeterminate lead and should not be evaluated by itself.

- **Lead aVR** is an augmented unipolar right arm lead, meaning that the impulse is recorded as if it originates from the center of the heart. An impulse that is directed toward the right arm produces a positive waveform in this lead; a negative waveform is generated if the impulse is directed away from the right arm. Hence lead aVR is the only limb lead that is right sided. Since the impulses in the heart are primarily directed from right to left (away from the right arm), the waveforms are normally negative in this lead (*ie*, they are mirror images of waveforms in other leads). Therefore, the P wave is normally negative and there is an initial septal R wave followed by a large negative waveform, or S wave, representing left ventricular depolarization.

5

- **Lead aVL** is an augmented unipolar left arm lead, meaning that the impulse is recorded as if it originates from the center of the heart. An impulse that is directed toward the left arm produces a positive waveform; the waveform is negative if the impulse is directed away from the left arm. Therefore, in normal situations the P wave (generated by an impulse that is directed from right to left) is positive in this lead. The QRS complex (due to impulse generation in a right-to-left direction) is also positive, and there may be a small septal Q wave before the tall positive waveform, or R wave, representing left ventricular depolarization.

- **Lead aVF** is an augmented unipolar left foot lead, meaning that the impulse is recorded as if it originates from the center of the heart. An impulse that is directed toward the left foot generates a positive waveform; an impulse directed away from the left foot produces a negative waveform. Therefore, in normal situations the P wave (due to impulse generation that travels proximally to distally) is positive in this lead. The QRS complex (resulting from an impulse that travels proximally to distally) is also positive, and there may be a small septal Q wave before the tall positive waveform, or R wave, representing left ventricular depolarization.

Precordial leads V1-V6 are placed on the chest wall in the following locations (FIGURE 6):

- **Lead V1** is placed at the second intercostal space below the clavicle to the right of the sternum.

- **Lead V2** is placed at the second intercostal space below the clavicle to the left of the sternum.

- **Lead V4** is placed at the fifth intercostal space below the clavicle at the midclavicular line.

- **Lead V3** is placed midway between leads V2 and V4.

- **Lead V5** is placed at the fifth intercostal space below the clavicle at the anterior axillary line.

- **Lead V6** is placed at the fifth intercostal space below the clavicle at the midaxillary line.

As with the augmented limb leads, leads V1-V6 are unipolar leads and the impulse is recorded as if it originates from the center of the heart. An impulse that is directed toward a precordial lead produces a positive deflection, and the deflection is negative if the impulse is directed away from a precordial lead (FIGURE 7). Lead V1 is mostly

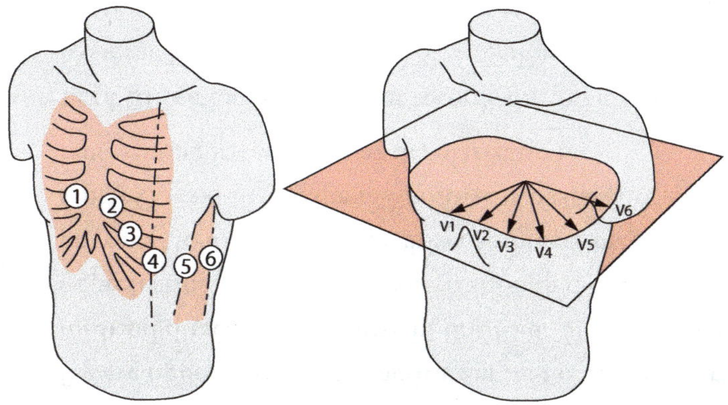

Figure 6: Placement of the precordial leads (V1-V6).

over the right ventricle and right atrium, while leads V2-V3 are primarily over the intraventricular septum toward the left ventricle and leads V4-V6 are over the left ventricle and left atrium. Therefore, in lead V1 (and occasionally in lead V2) the P wave is biphasic, as the initial depolarization is from the right atrium (going toward lead V1) and the second part of the P wave is from the left atrium, going away from lead V1. The P waves in leads V3-V6 are normally positive as these leads are primarily over the left atrium and reflect left atrial activation, which goes toward these leads.

Based on the location of the V leads, there is an initial small positive waveform (R wave) in lead V1, representing septal depolarization going from left to right and hence toward this lead. This is followed by a deep S wave representing left ventricular depolarization, which goes in a right-to-left direction (away from this lead). In contrast, lead V6 has an initial negative waveform (Q wave) representing initial septal activation going from left to right or away from this lead. This is followed by a tall positive deflection (R wave) representing left ventricular depolarization, which travels in a right-to-left direction and hence toward this lead. As one inspects leads V1-V6 (which go in a right-to-left direction across the chest), there is a gradual increase in the amplitude of the R wave (reflecting more left ventricular forces directed toward the lead) and a decrease in the depth of the S wave (which reflects left ventricular forces going away from the lead). Hence the gradual increase in the amplitude of the R wave (going from V1-V6) is called R-wave progression across the precordium (FIGURE 8). The transition (R/S ≥ 1) usually occurs between leads V3 and V4.

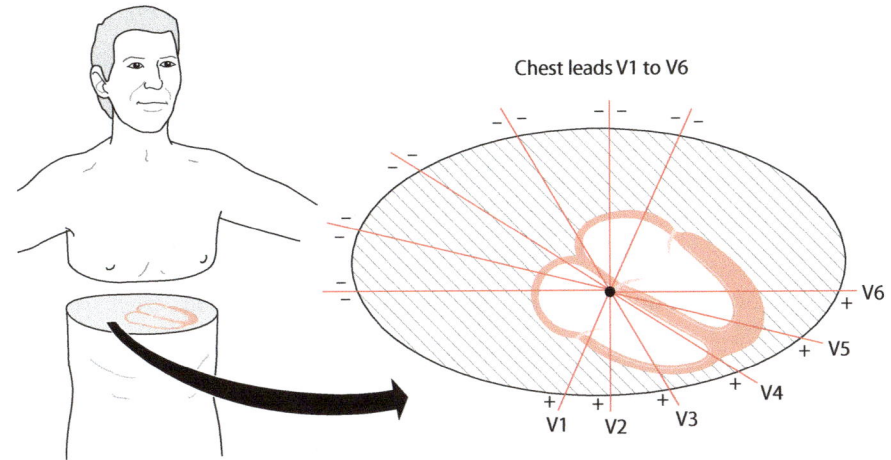

Chest leads V1 to V6

Figure 7: **Precordial chest leads in the horizontal plane.** An impulse directed toward a precordial lead produces a positive deflection, while an impulse directed away from a precordial lead produces a negative deflection.

Figure 8: **R-wave progression across the precordium.** Going from lead V1 (which sits over the right ventricle) to lead V6 (which is over the left ventricle), there is a gradual increase in the amplitude of the R wave and decrease in the depth of the S wave. In lead V1 the initial R wave represents a septal force, while the S wave is the left ventricular force. Going from leads V1 to V6 (*ie*, from right to left ventricles), the left ventricular forces become more prominent (*ie*, the R-wave amplitude increases and the S-wave depth decreases as the left ventricular forces are going toward the lead).

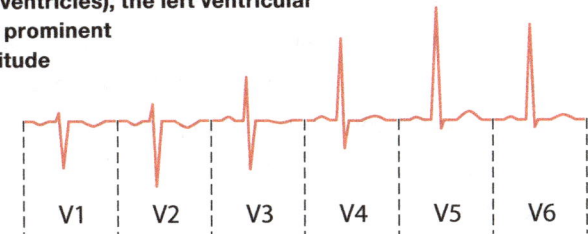

V1   V2   V3   V4   V5   V6

7

Approach to ECG Analysis

ECGs should be analyzed thoroughly and systematically while considering the patient's clinical history. By following a standardized sequence of steps, subtle abnormalities in the ECG will become evident.

1. Establish the heart rate. The normal heart rate ranges from 60 to 100 bpm; bradycardia is defined as a heart rate of 60 bpm or lower and tachycardia as a heart rate of 100 bpm or higher. Heart rate can be established in two ways:

   - Count the number of QRS complexes and multiply by 6 (as an ECG recording takes 10 seconds). This is the preferred method when the rhythm is irregular.

   - Use the grid on the ECG tracing. Heart rate = 300 ÷ the number of large boxes within one RR interval. If the RR interval duration is between two large boxes, the number of small boxes (five per large box) is then used to approximate the heart rate. For example, if the RR interval is between one and two large boxes (*ie*, the heart rate is between 300 and 150), each small box is 150 ÷ 5 or 30 bpm. If the RR interval is between two and three large boxes (*ie*, heart rate between 150 and 100 bpm), each small box is 50 ÷ 5 or 10 bpm. If the RR interval is between three and four large boxes (*ie*, heart rate between 100 and 75 bpm), each small box is 25 ÷ 5 or 5 bpm. If the RR interval is between four and five large boxes (*ie*, heart rate between 60 and 75 bpm), each small box is 15 ÷ 5 or 3 bpm.

2. Establish where the rhythm originates, that is, in which structure is the pacemaker that initiates the impulse. This is based on the presence or absence of a P wave, location of the P wave (before or after the QRS complex), and P-wave morphology. A sinus origin for the atrial activity is associated with a positive P wave in leads I, II, aVF, and V4-V6. The normal atrial impulse direction generates a positive waveform in these leads. If the P wave is negative in any of these leads, the impulse direction is not normal and hence the origin is not the sinus node but rather somewhere else in the atrium; therefore, this is an atrial rhythm. If there is no P wave before any QRS complex, the origin of the impulse is not sinus or atrial but is either the AV node or AV junction (if the QRS complex is narrow and normal) or the ventricular myocardium (if the QRS complex is wide with an unusual morphology).

3. Establish the regularity of the rhythm. Note whether the RR intervals are regular, regularly irregular (irregular but with a pattern often based on abnormalities in AV conduction or AV block), or irregularly irregular (no pattern to the RR intervals).

4. Determine the electrical axis in the frontal plane (*ie*, normal, leftward, rightward, or indeterminate).

5. Measure the PR interval, QRS complex duration, and QT interval.

6. Evaluate the R-wave progression across the precordium. This will also establish the electrical axis in the horizontal plane (*ie*, normal, clockwise, or counterclockwise rotation).

7. Evaluate the P-wave amplitude, duration, and morphology.

8. Establish the QRS complex duration, amplitude, and morphology.

9. Indicate the presence of pathologic Q waves (*ie*, longer than 0.04 sec in duration).

10. Evaluate the ST-segment (morphology and elevation or depression) and J-point changes.

11. Note T-wave abnormalities.

12. Indicate the presence of other waveforms (*eg*, U waves, pacemaker spikes, artifact).

Normal Waveforms and Intervals

Components of the normal waveform include the P wave, PR interval, QRS complex, QT interval, T wave, and U wave (FIGURE 9).

P Wave

The normal P wave, which should be positive in leads I, II, aVF, and V4-V6, represents right atrial followed by left atrial depolarization. The normal P-wave duration is 0.12 second or less, and the usual amplitude is less than 2.5 mV (2.5 small boxes).

PR Interval

The PR interval, which includes the P wave and PR segment, is a measure of AV conduction, or the time required for the impulse to go from atrium to ventricle (including conduction through the atrium, which is the P wave, and conduction through the AV node and His-Purkinje system, which is the PR segment). The PR interval is determined by measuring the duration from the beginning of P wave to the first wave of QRS complex (either a Q or R wave). The normal PR interval is between 0.14 and 0.20 second. The PR segment should be at baseline or zero potential as there is no electrical activity measured on the surface

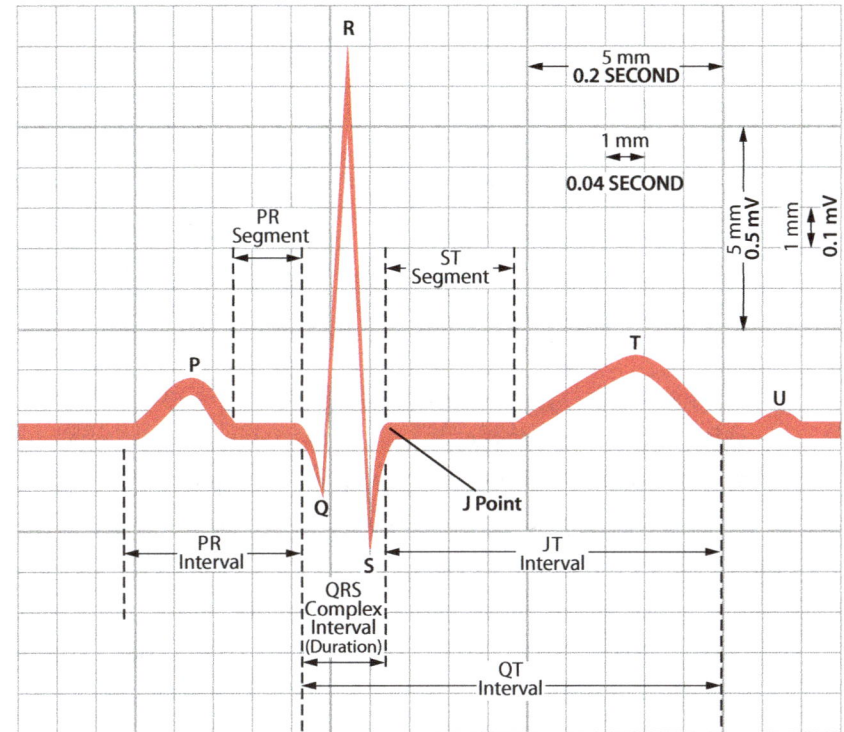

Figure 9: **Components of a typical waveform and the usual intervals that are measured.** The PR interval (time for AV conduction) is measured from the beginning of the P wave to the beginning of the QRS complex (either a Q or R wave). The PR interval includes the P wave and PR segment. The QRS complex duration or interval, which is the time for ventricular depolarization, is measured from the beginning of the QRS complex (either a Q or R wave) to the end of the QRS complex, which is the J point. The QT interval, which is the time for ventricular depolarization and repolarization, is measured from the beginning of the QRS complex (either a Q wave or R wave) to the end of the T wave. This interval includes the QRS complex, ST segment, and T wave.

ECG during this time, even though there is electrical activity occurring within the AV node and His-Purkinje system.

The PR interval changes with heart rate, primarily reflecting changes in AV nodal conduction time (which is the major determinant of the PR segment). Conduction through the His-Purkinje system is constant as there is no alteration of conduction velocity related to heart rate changes (*ie*, conduction through this part of the conduction system is all or none). At slower sinus rates (higher vagal tone and less sympathetic stimulation), conduction through the AV node slows and hence the PR interval (segment) lengthens. With fast sinus rates, reflecting less vagal tone and increased sympathetic stimulation, AV nodal conduction velocity increases and the PR interval (segment) shortens. There is, however, no method available to correct the PR interval for rate.

At a given heart rate, the PR interval should be constant. Any variability reflects an AV conduction abnormality. When there is no pattern to the variability, AV dissociation is present. The presence of progressive lengthening of the PR interval is seen with type 1 second-degree AV block (Mobitz I or Wenckebach).

QRS Complex

The QRS complex duration (or interval) represents time for ventricular depolarization. The duration is measured from the beginning of the QRS complex (either a Q or R wave) to the end of the QRS complex (which is defined as the J point and is located at the end of the QRS complex and the beginning of the ST segment). Right and left ventricular depolarization is simultaneous. However, since the left ventricular myocardial mass is much greater than the right ventricular mass, the QRS complex primarily reflects left ventricular depolarization. The normal QRS duration is between 0.06 and 0.10 second and does not change with heart rate (*ie*, His-Purkinje impulse conduction is all or none). A QRS complex duration that is 0.10 second or longer is called an intraventricular conduction delay (IVCD). If the QRS complex duration is 0.12 second or longer with a typical pattern, the IVCD may represent a bundle branch block.

QT Interval

The QT interval is a measure of the time for ventricular repolarization. It is measured from the beginning of QRS complex (either a Q or R wave) to the end of T wave. It must be remembered that since the QT interval measurement includes the QRS complex, it is not just a measure of left ventricular repolarization but also includes the time of left ventricular depolarization. It is also important to remember that a prolonged QRS duration (due to a bundle branch block or a nonspecific IVCD) may result in lengthening of the measured QT interval. In this situation, the prolonged QT interval is not due to prolongation of repolarization. As the normal QT interval measurements are based on a normal QRS duration (*ie*, 0.06 to 0.10 sec), any prolongation of the QRS duration above this value needs to be considered and the increased duration (in milliseconds) subtracted from the QT measurement.

The QT interval changes with heart rate, that is, it is prolonged at slower rates and shortens with faster rates. Therefore, the QT interval must be corrected for rate (*ie*, QTc), using Bazett's formula:

$$QTc = QT \div \sqrt{RR \text{ interval}} \text{ (in seconds)}$$

The normal QTc is less than 0.44 to 0.48 second.

T Wave

The T wave actually represents ventricular repolarization. The T-wave axis is usually the same as that of the QRS complex. That is, the T-wave direction (positive or negative) is the same direction as the major deflection of the QRS complex; if the QRS complex is positive the T wave is positive, and if the QRS complex is negative the T wave is negative. The normal T wave is asymmetric regardless of amplitude (*ie*, it has a slower upstroke than downstroke). Also, the normal T wave is smooth in both its upstroke and downstroke. Any notches, bumps, or other irregularities on the T wave may represent superimposed P waves.

U Wave

The U wave is a low-amplitude positive waveform that follows the T wave. The U wave is believed to represent delayed repolarization of the His-Purkinje system, although it has been suggested that it may represent delayed repolarization of the papillary muscles. It is most often seen in the right precordial leads (*ie*, leads V1-V3).

Normal ECG Recording

In most cases, 12 leads are recorded (*ie*, six limb leads and six precordial [chest] leads). The standard layout for the ECG is four columns with three leads in each column (I, II, III; aVR, aVL, aVF; V1, V2, V3; V4, V5, V6). Each column is simultaneously recorded while each line is continuously recorded. One or several rhythm strips (one lead continuously recorded over time) may be present at the bottom of ECG.

The paper speed for recording is usually 25 mm/sec (10 sec for a full 12-lead recording). Occasionally a paper speed of 50 mm/sec is used. In this situation, there are only six leads per sheet of paper; the PR, QRS, and QT intervals are very long (twice normal), and the heart rate is very slow (half of normal) (FIGURE 10).

Most often, normal standardization is used. Standardization indicates the amplitude covered by 1 mV of electric current. Normal standardization means that 1 mV = 10 mm (10 small boxes) in height. When QRS amplitude is high, half-standard may be used, or 1 mV = 5 mm (five small boxes). When QRS amplitude is small, double standard may be used, or 1 mV = 20 mm (20 small boxes) (see FIGURE 10).

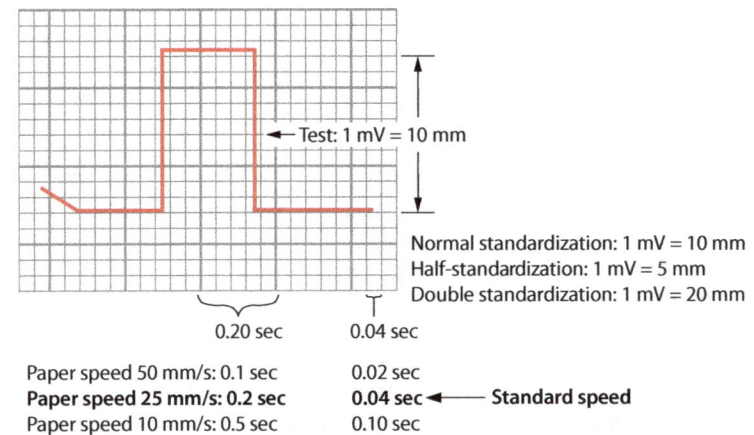

Test: 1 mV = 10 mm

Normal standardization: 1 mV = 10 mm
Half-standardization: 1 mV = 5 mm
Double standardization: 1 mV = 20 mm

0.20 sec   0.04 sec

Paper speed 50 mm/s: 0.1 sec	0.02 sec
Paper speed 25 mm/s: 0.2 sec	**0.04 sec** ◄── **Standard speed**
Paper speed 10 mm/s: 0.5 sec	0.10 sec

Figure 10: Paper speeds and standardizations used for recording an ECG. In a typical ECG, the normal paper speed is 25 mm/sec and normal standardization is used.

P Wave and PR Interval

Since the sinus node is located in the proximal portion of the right atrium and depolarization occurs in a right-to-left and up-to-down (proximal to distal) direction, the normal P wave is positive (upright) in leads I, II, aVF, and V4-V6. Atrial repolarization occurs during the time of the QRS complex and hence is not seen.

There is often a slight notching of the P wave, reflecting right followed by left atrial depolarization. A broad, notched P wave is seen with left atrial hypertrophy (or abnormality) and is called P mitrale (**FIGURE 11**). A narrow, peaked P wave is seen with right atrial hypertrophy (or abnormality) and is called P pulmonale (**FIGURE 12**). The P wave is negative in lead aVR.

The P wave is often biphasic (positive-negative) in lead V1, reflecting right atrial depolarization (impulse toward lead V1) followed by left atrial depolarization (impulse away from lead V1) (**FIGURE 13**). The P-wave duration is 0.12 second or less, and the amplitude is usually 0.25 mV or less.

P waves that are inverted or biphasic (negative-positive) in leads I, II, aVF, and V4-V6 are abnormal, reflecting an ectopic atrial focus. Negative P waves that follow a QRS complex are retrograde, due to retrograde (ventriculoatrial) conduction.

Every P wave should have an associated QRS complex, and every QRS complex should be preceded by a P wave. The PR interval should be stable. The normal PR interval is 0.14 to 0.20 second measured from the beginning of the P wave to the beginning of the QRS complex (either a Q or R wave). Inconsistent variability of PR interval is AV dissociation; gradual prolongation of the PR interval is seen with Wenckebach or second-degree AV block (Mobitz type I).

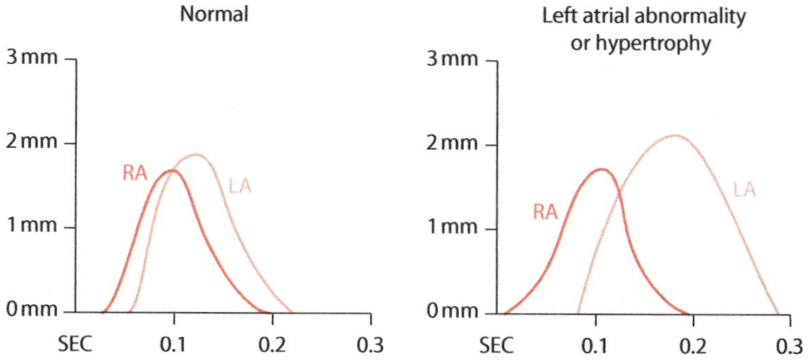

Figure 11: The P wave in left atrial hypertrophy (or abnormality) is broad and notched. This is termed P mitrale.

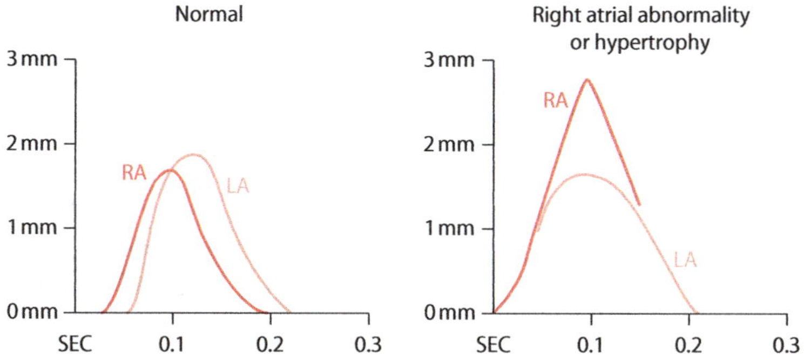

Figure 12: The P wave in right atrial hypertrophy (or abnormality) is tall, narrow, and peaked. This is termed P pulmonale.

QRS Complex

The direction of the waveforms or deflections of the QRS complex determine the letter applied to the components of the QRS complex (FIGURE 14). If the first deflection is negative it is called a Q wave. Any first positive deflection is called an R wave (there may or may not be a Q wave). Any negative deflection after the R wave is called an S wave. If there is a second positive deflection, it is termed an R' (R prime).

The first depolarization of the left ventricle occurs in the left septum (via the septal or median branch of the left bundle) in a left-to-right direction. Hence there is normally a small septal Q wave in leads I and V5-V6 and a small septal R wave in lead V1. The direction of the rest of ventricular activation is right to left and proximal to distal. Therefore, the normal QRS complex is positive in leads I, II, aVF, and V1-V6 and negative in lead aVR. There may be a small R' in lead V1, which is a normal variant reflecting a slight conduction delay in the right ventricle. The QRS complex may have notching, which is a normal variant.

Since the precordial leads reflect activation from the right to the left ventricle, the initial septal forces are directed toward lead V1 (small R wave) and away from lead V6 (small Q wave). The rest of the left ventricular forces are directed away from lead V1 (hence an S wave) and toward lead V6 (hence an R wave). Therefore, going from lead V1 to V6, the R-wave amplitude progressively increases and the S-wave depth decreases; that is, R/S becomes greater

	Lead II	Lead V1
Normal	RA ⌢ LA ⌢ Combined ⌢	⌢ ⌣ ∿
Right atrial hypertrophy or abnormality	RA ⌢ LA	RA ⌢ LA
Left atrial hypertrophy or abnormality	RA ⌢ LA	RA ⌣ LA

Figure 13: Appearance of the P wave in leads II and V1 in right and left atrial hypertrophy. The normal P wave in lead V1 is biphasic as the initial force (depolarization) is from the right atrium, going toward lead V1 (and hence a positive deflection), while left atrial depolarization is slightly later, going away from lead V1 and hence generating a negative waveform. With right atrial hypertrophy or abnormality, the depolarization is primarily toward lead V1, thereby generating a positive waveform. With left atrial hypertrophy or abnormality, the depolarization is primarily away from V1, thereby generating a negative waveform.

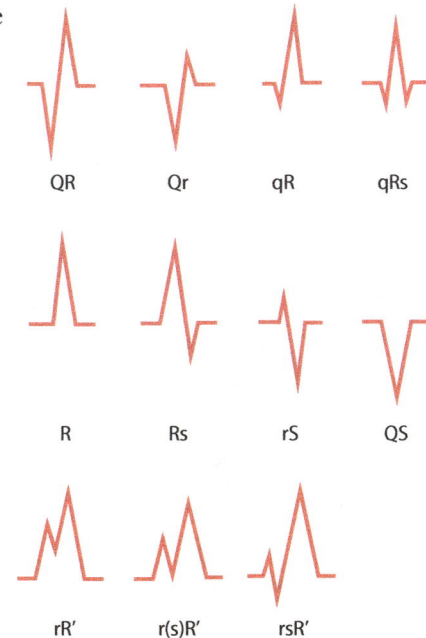

QR Qr qR qRs

R Rs rS QS

rR' r(s)R' rsR'

Figure 14: The direction of the waveforms or deflections of the QRS complex determine the letter applied. If the first deflection is negative it is termed a Q wave. Any first positive waveform (with or without a Q wave) is termed an R wave. A negative deflection after the R wave is termed an S wave. If there is a second positive deflection after the S wave it is called R'.

than 1 (*ie*, normal R-wave progression). The transition point at which R/S is 1 or greater is leads V3-V4. This is termed R-wave progression (see FIGURE 8).

An increased QRS amplitude in precordial and/or limb leads, which reflects increased voltage recorded at the body surface, is seen in young subjects, in those with thin chests and no lung disease, and in individuals with myocardial hypertrophy. Low QRS amplitude is defined as a QRS amplitude of 5 mm or less in each limb lead and/or less than 10 mm in each precordial lead. This may reflect a reduction in impulse conduction to the surface of the body, which may be due to lung disease, obesity, thick pericardium, pericardial effusion, or a reduction in myocardial muscle mass.

Small septal Q waves are often seen in limb leads and lateral precordial leads. Significant (pathologic) Q waves—that is, any Q wave in leads V1-V3 (although QS may normally be seen in leads V1-V2) or a Q wave more than 0.04 second in duration and more than 1 mm in depth in leads I, II, aVL, or aVF or in two consecutive leads V4-V6— are indicative of old myocardial infarction (MI). An isolated Q wave in lead III is of no significance as it may be normal. An infarction is diagnosed if there is also a significant Q wave in lead II and/or lead aVF.

The normal QRS complex duration is 0.06 to 0.10 second. A QRS complex duration longer than 0.10 second is considered an IVCD. When the QRS complex duration is 0.10 to 0.12 second, the IVCD is often called incomplete right bundle branch block (RBBB) or incomplete left bundle branch block (LBBB) if there is a morphology resembling either RBBB or LBBB. However, since His-Purkinje conduction is all or none and not incomplete, an IVCD (to either the right or left ventricle) is a more appropriate term. A QRS complex duration 0.12 second or

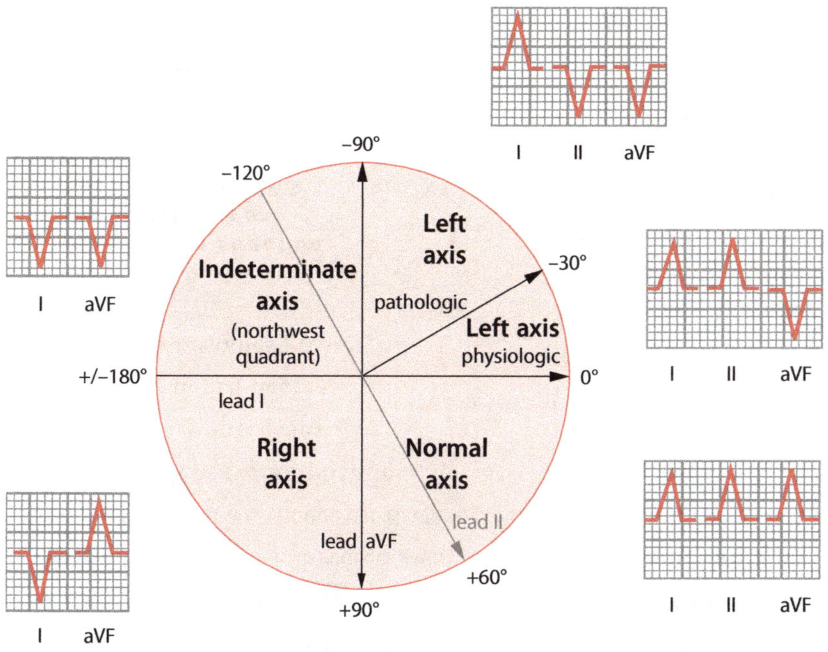

Figure 15: **The QRS axis in the frontal plane is determined by analyzing the direction of the QRS complex in the limb leads.** The heart is divided into four equal quadrants of 90° each (0° to +90°, +90° to +/-180°, 0° to -90° and -90° to +/-180°). The two leads that are perpendicular to each other and divide the heart in this fashion are leads I and aVF. Hence these two leads are looked at first. A normal axis is between 0° and +90°. A rightward axis, which is never normal, is between +90° and +180°. If the axis is leftward (*ie*, between 0° and -90°), it may be physiologic (and hence a normal leftward axis) if between 0° and -30° or pathologic (and hence abnormal) if between -30° and -90°. This is established by looking at lead II, which is perpendicular to -30°. If the QRS complex is positive in lead II, the axis is physiologically leftward; if the QRS complex is negative in lead II, the axis is pathologically leftward.

longer occurs with RBBB or LBBB; bundle branch blocks are associated with a specific QRS complex morphology. When the QRS complex morphology is without a specific pattern of a bundle branch block, it is an IVCD. A QRS complex duration of 0.16 to 0.22 second is often seen with severe cardiomyopathy, drug effect, or hyperkalemia. When the QRS complex duration is 0.24 second or longer, the cause is hyperkalemia.

QRS Axis

Frontal Plane

The QRS axis in the frontal plane is determined by analysis of the QRS complex direction in the limb leads (FIGURE 15). The axis may be normal, leftward, rightward, or indeterminate, as established by an initial analysis of leads I and aVF, which are perpendicular to each other and divide the heart into four equal quadrants (0° to +90°, +90° to ±180°, 0° to −90° and −90° to +/-180°). An impulse going toward the left (toward 0°) is positive in lead I, and an impulse going toward the right (toward +180°) is negative in lead I. An impulse directed toward the foot (toward +90°) is positive in lead aVF, and an impulse directed away from the foot (toward −90°) is negative in lead aVF.

A normal axis is 0° to +90°. In this situation the QRS complex is positive in leads I and aVF. A leftward axis is 0° to −90° (the QRS complex is positive in lead I and negative in lead aVF). However, a leftward axis may be physiologic (normal) when it is between 0° and −30° or pathologic (abnormal) when it is between −30° and −90°. In the presence of a left axis, therefore, lead II is evaluated, as it is perpendicular to −30°. An impulse that is directed toward the foot (less negative than −30°) is positive in lead II, and an impulse that is directed away from the foot (more negative than −30°) is negative in lead II.

A physiologic left axis is 0° to −30° (the QRS complex is positive in leads I and II and negative in lead aVF). An extreme or pathologic left axis is −30° to −90° (the QRS complex is positive in lead I and negative in leads II and aVF, ie, rS complex). This is referred to as a left anterior fascicular block (LAFB). However, it is important to exclude inferior wall MI as a cause for left axis (ie, Qr complex in leads II and aVF). An LAFB cannot be established in the presence of an inferior wall MI. Limb lead switch must also be excluded.

A right axis is between +90° and +180° (the QRS complex is negative in lead I, ie, rS complex, and positive in lead aVF). This is referred to as a left posterior fascicular block (LPFB). However, other causes for a right axis must be excluded, including a lateral MI (Qr complex in leads I and aVL), right ventricular hypertrophy (RVH), Wolff-Parkinson-White pattern, dextrocardia, or right-to-left arm lead switch. An indeterminate axis, between −90° and +/-180° (the QRS complex is negative in leads I and aVF), is either an extreme leftward axis or an extreme rightward axis. There is no conduction sequence through the normal His-Purkinje system that will be associated with an indeterminate axis. Hence an indeterminate axis is seen whenever two abnormalities co-exist. For example, RVH, which is associated with a right axis, may co-exist with an LAFB, which is associated with a marked left axis, resulting in an indeterminate axis. Other situations include a lateral wall MI (with deep Q waves in leads I and aVL), which will present as a right axis, associated with an LAFB; a lateral wall MI associated with an inferior wall MI (deep Q waves in leads II and aVF), which will have a left axis; or an inferior wall MI associated with an LPFB, which causes a right axis. An indeterminate axis is also seen when there is direct myocardial activation, such as with a ventricular complex, Wolff-Parkinson-White pattern, or a paced complex.

Horizontal Plane

The QRS axis in the horizontal plane is determined by analysis of the QRS complex direction in the precordial leads (FIGURE 16). This axis is established by imagining the heart as viewed from under the diaphragm (*ie*, the right ventricle is anterior and the left ventricle is to the left). Here, the normal QRS transition point (R/S > 1) occurs at leads V3-V4. Clockwise rotation is present when the left ventricular electrical forces are shifted to the back and seen late in the precordial leads. Therefore, there is poor R-wave progression with late transition. R-wave amplitude increases slowly across the precordium, and the transition (R/S > 1) is later, between leads V4 and V6. Counterclockwise rotation is present when the left ventricular electrical forces are shifted anteriorly and seen early in the precordial leads. There is early transition (R/S > 1 in lead V2) or a tall R wave in lead V2.

Beat-to-beat changes in the QRS axis and/or amplitude are called electrical (or QRS) alternans. There may also be beat-to-beat changes in T-wave amplitude/morphology, *ie*, T-wave alternans.

ST Segment

The ST segment begins at the J point (the point of transition at the end of the QRS complex and the beginning of the ST segment) and ends

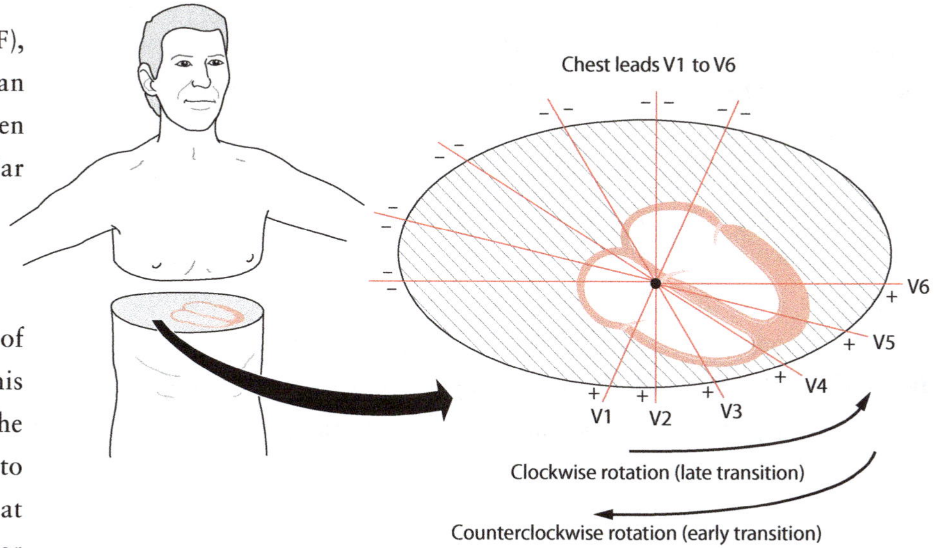

Figure 16: The QRS axis in the horizontal plane is determined by analyzing the direction of the QRS complex in the precordial leads. This is established by imagining the heart as viewed from under the diaphragm. With clockwise rotation, the left ventricular forces are seen later in the precordial leads. This presents with poor R-wave progression and late transition. With counterclockwise rotation, left ventricular forces develop earlier in the precordial leads. This presents with a tall R wave in lead V2, which is termed early transition.

at the onset of T wave (FIGURE 17). It represents the period of time between the end of depolarization and the beginning of repolarization. The normal ST segment is slightly concave. The J point and ST segment are usually isoelectric or at zero potential, which is established by the TP segment. If the TP segment cannot be identified, as with a tachycardia (when the T and P waves are on top of each other), the PR segment is used to establish the isoelectric baseline.

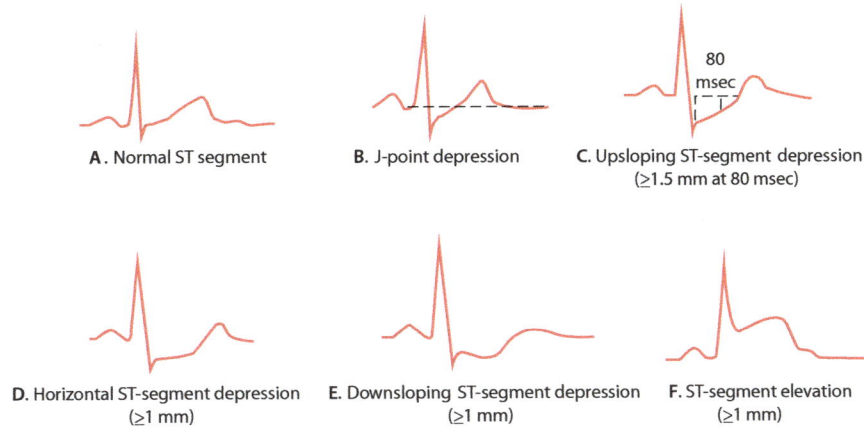

A. Normal ST segment

B. J-point depression

C. Upsloping ST-segment depression
(≥1.5 mm at 80 msec)

D. Horizontal ST-segment depression
(≥1 mm)

E. Downsloping ST-segment depression
(≥1 mm)

F. ST-segment elevation
(≥1 mm)

Figure 17: Types of ST segment shifts. (A) Normal ST segment. The normal J point and ST segment are at baseline, which is established by the TP segment (*ie*, from the T wave of the preceding complex to the P wave). (B) A depressed J point. (C) Upsloping ST-segment depression; the J point is depressed and the ST segment slopes upward toward baseline. (D) Horizontal ST-segment depression; the J point is depressed and the ST segment is flat or horizontal. (E) Downsloping ST-segment depression; the J point is depressed and the ST segment slopes downward. (F) ST-segment elevation; the J point and ST segment are above the baseline TP segment.

ST-segment flattening is a nonspecific change. J-point and ST-segment elevation are seen with various situations, including early repolarization (which may be seen when the QRS amplitude is increased as with young subjects or patients with left ventricular hypertrophy [LVH]), transmural ischemia (as may occur with coronary artery vasospasm), ST-segment elevation MI (STEMI, or transmural MI), or pericarditis.

J-point and ST-segment depression (upsloping, horizontal, or downsloping) are seen with subendocardial ischemia (LVH or

coronary disease) and non–ST-segment elevation MI (NSTEMI, or subendocardial MI). ST-segment depression is considered significant if it is more than 1 mm below the baseline (*ie*, the TP segment). J-point depression and upsloping ST-segment depression may be seen as a normal finding in sinus tachycardia. This is due to alteration or depression of the J point by the T wave of the P wave (*ie*, atrial repolarization), which results from the shortening of the PR interval (due to sympathetic enhancement of AV nodal conduction) and movement of the T wave of the P wave from out of the QRS complex and onto the J point. As J-point depression and upsloping ST-segment depression may be a normal variant, the ST segment should be evaluated 80 msec past the J point, accounting for the effect of the T wave of the P wave. If at this point the ST segment is back to baseline, the ST-segment depression is a normal variant. If the ST segment is still more than 1.5 mm below baseline, then myocardial ischemia can be diagnosed.

A normal J point with ST-segment depression (sagging, scoped out, hammock-like) is seen as an effect of digoxin (not digoxin toxicity). J-point elevation and a normal ST segment may be an Osborne (J) wave, as seen with hypothermia.

QT Interval

The QT interval, indicating the time for repolarization, is measured from the onset of the QRS complex (either a Q or R wave) to the end of the T wave (see **FIGURE 9**). The lead that has the best or sharpest T wave is used. As the QT interval includes the QRS complex, the presence of an increased QRS complex duration needs to be considered when measuring the QT interval, and any increase in QRS complex duration (msec) above normal (*ie*, 0.06 to 0.10 sec) needs to be subtracted from the QT-interval measurement. Thereafter, the QT interval needs to be corrected for heart rate. The normal QTC is 0.44 to 0.48 second or less.

A long QT interval may result from delayed or prolonged repolarization. With delayed repolarization, the ST-segment duration is long while the T-wave duration is normal. This is seen with metabolic abnormalities, particularly low calcium or low magnesium levels. In prolonged repolarization, the ST segment is normal in duration but the T wave is broad or prolonged. This is due to drugs (acquired QT prolongation) or a genetic abnormality producing a channelopathy (congenital long QT syndrome). Congenital QT prolongation may have a prominent U wave interrupting the T wave (QT-U wave).

A short QT interval is due to a metabolic abnormality (high calcium or high magnesium levels) or a congenital short QT syndrome.

T Waves / U Waves

Normal T waves are asymmetric, regardless of amplitude, with a slower upstroke than downstroke (**FIGURE 18**). The hyperacute T wave is tall, peaked, and symmetric, as can be seen with hyperkalemia (systemic or localized as in acute MI). The T-wave upstroke and downstroke are smooth. Any notches, bumps, or irregularities of the T wave suggest a superimposed P wave. T-wave abnormalities can be flat, biphasic, or inverted. They are very common and may be seen in many situations, including ischemia (inverted symmetric T waves usually associated with ST-segment changes), LVH, pericarditis/myocarditis, metabolic abnormalities, anemia, fever, lung disease, enhanced catecholamine state, pH

Normal T wave   Hyperacute T wave

Figure 18: **The normal T wave is asymmetric, with a slower upstroke and faster downstroke.** **A hyperacute T wave is tall, peaked and, most importantly, symmetric (upstroke and downstroke are equal).**

changes, use of certain drugs, central nervous system abnormalities, or even as a normal physiologic change. T-wave abnormalities may also be nonspecific when there is no clinical history to suggest a cause.

The U wave is an upright waveform following the T wave. It is normally seen in the right precordial leads. Increased U-wave amplitude and U waves that are present more diffusely in all precordial leads, and often in the limb leads as well, are seen with hypokalemia. A U wave may also be seen in congenital long QT syndrome, in which case the U wave interrupts the T wave (QT-U wave). Negative U waves, particularly during exercise testing, are suggestive of ischemia as a result of a stenosis of the left anterior descending artery. ◼

Core ECGs

A 32-year-old man presents to an outpatient clinic with complaints of a productive cough, headache, shortness of breath, and fever. A routine ECG is obtained.

Are there any abnormalities of concern on the ECG?

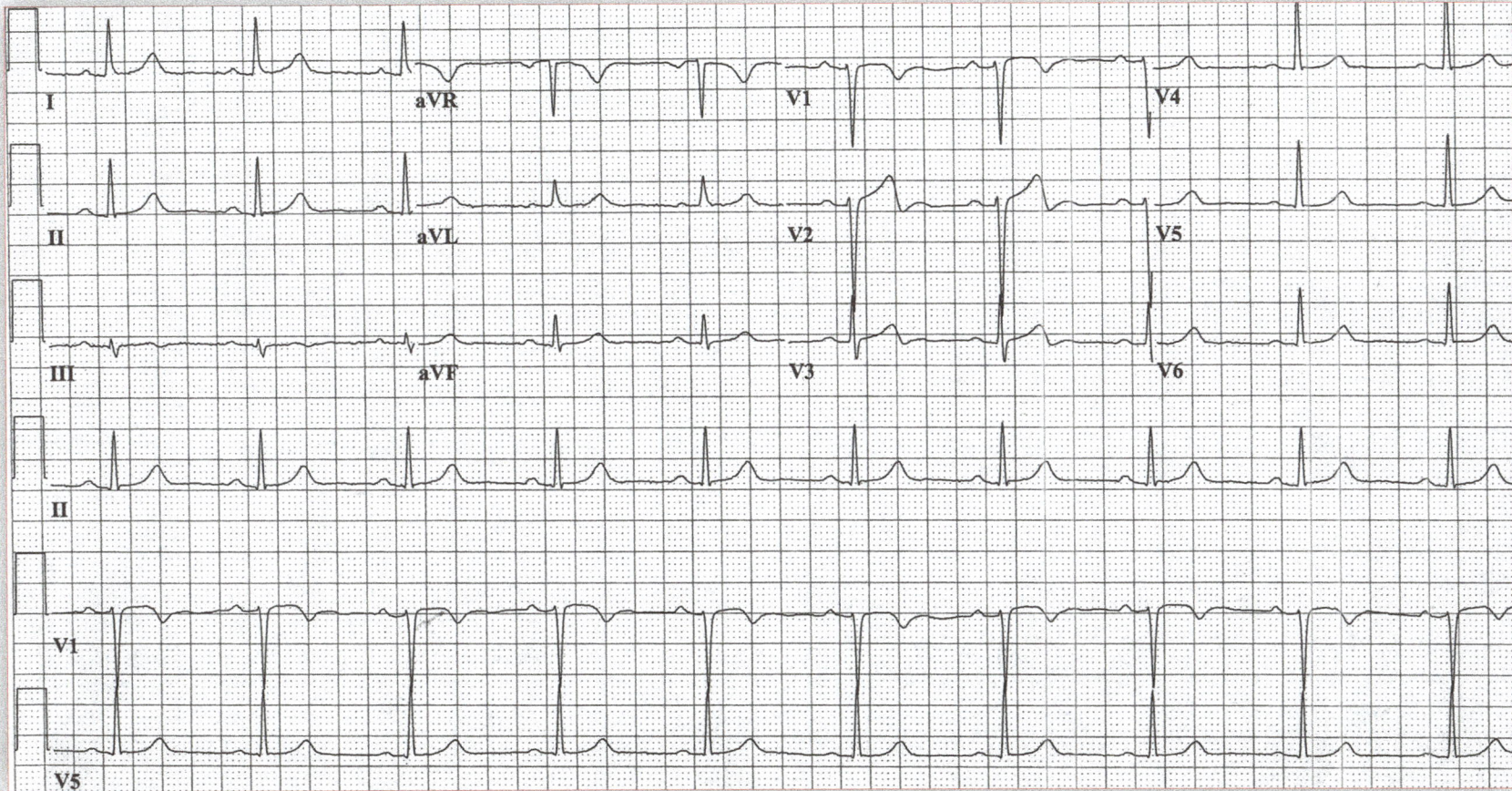

ECG 1 Analysis: Normal sinus rhythm, normal axis and interval

There is a regular rhythm at a rate of 60 bpm. There is a P wave (+) before each QRS complex, with a stable PR interval (0.18 sec). The P wave is positive in leads I, II, aVF, and V4-V6; it has a normal morphology and duration (0.12 sec). Hence this is a normal sinus rhythm.

The QRS complex duration is normal (0.08 sec), and it has a normal morphology. There is normal R-wave progression across the precordium, and the transition (R/S > 1) is at lead V3. The axis is normal, between 0° and +90° (positive QRS complex in leads I and aVF). The ST segment, which begins at the J point (▲) and ends at the beginning of the T wave, is at baseline (which is defined by the TP segment), and it has a normal concave morphology. The QT interval is 400 msec (QTc = 400 msec). The T wave (↓) has a normal morphology; it is asymmetric with a slower upstroke and more rapid downstroke. A low-amplitude waveform can be seen following the T wave in leads V2-V3; this is a U wave (↑). Hence this is a normal 12-lead ECG. ■

A 22-year-old woman with scleroderma presents to your office with progressive dyspnea on exertion. There is a loud P2 with a holosystolic murmur that exhibits respirophasic variation, heard best at the lower left sternal border. A routine ECG is obtained.

What is the most likely cause of the patient's symptoms?

What ECG findings support this diagnosis?

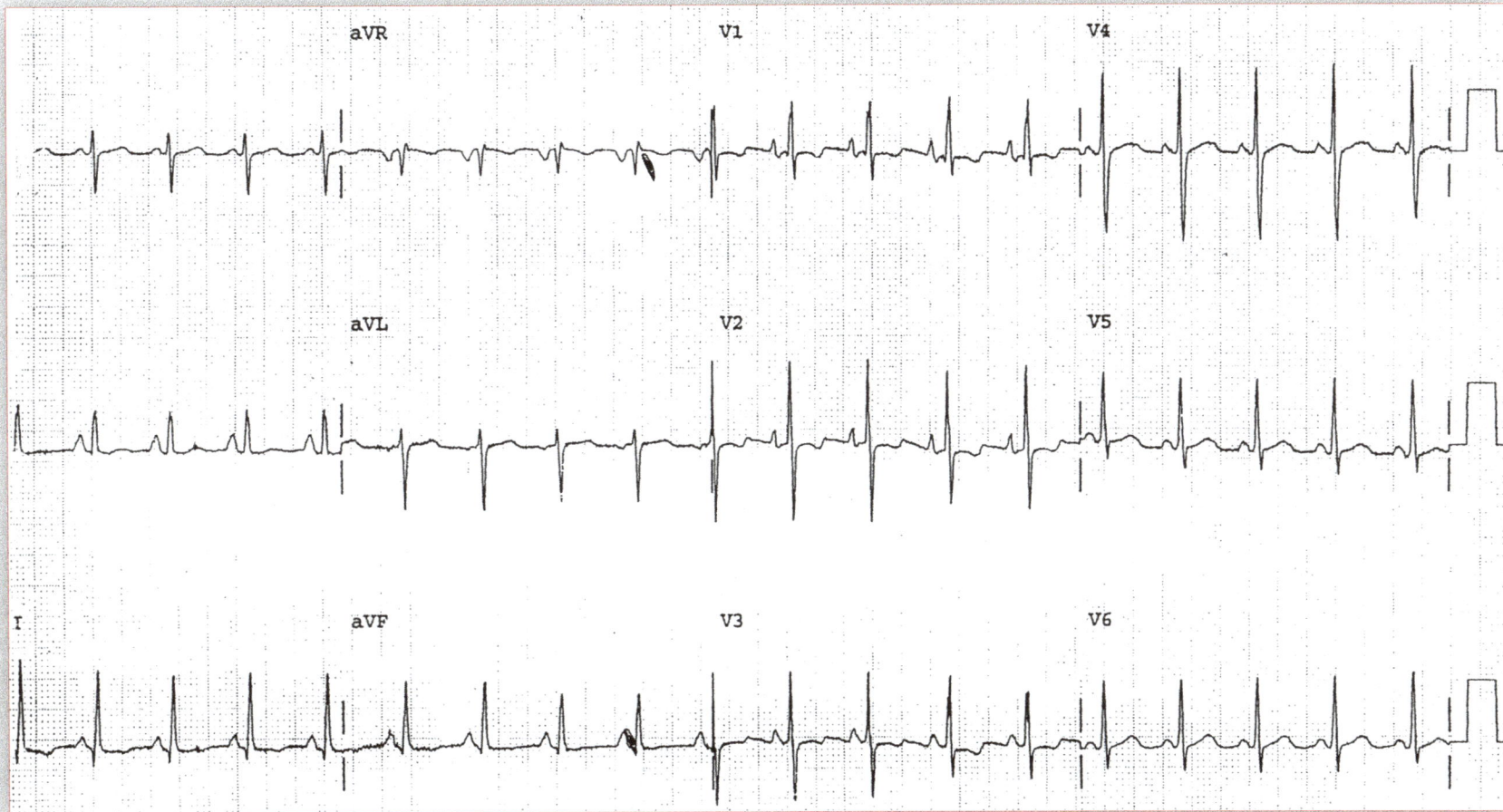

ECG 2 Analysis: Sinus tachycardia, right atrial hypertrophy, right ventricular hypertrophy (RVH), right axis deviation, counterclockwise rotation

The ECG shows a regular rhythm at a rate of 110 bpm. There is a P wave (+) before each QRS complex, with a stable PR interval (0.16 sec). The P wave is positive in leads I, II, aVF, and V4-V6, and it has a normal duration (0.10 sec). Hence this is a sinus tachycardia. The P waves are abnormal, and they are tall, narrow, and peaked in leads II, aVF, and V1-V2. The P-wave morphology is characteristic of a P pulmonale, a result of right atrial hypertrophy. This may also be termed a right atrial abnormality.

The QRS complex duration is normal (0.08 sec). The QT/QTc intervals are normal (300/410 msec). However, the QRS complex has an abnormal morphology. The axis is rightward, between +90° and +180° (negative QRS complex in lead I and positive QRS complex in lead aVF). The major finding is a tall R wave in lead V1 (←), defined as an R wave taller than 7 mm (seven small boxes) or an R/S > 1. The tall R wave in lead V1 along with the rightward axis and a P pulmonale (right atrial hypertrophy) are characteristic of right ventricular hypertrophy (RVH). In addition, there is a tall R wave in lead V2 (↓). Although this can be the result of RVH, it may also represent counterclockwise rotation of the electrical axis in the horizontal plane. This is established by imagining the heart as viewed from under the diaphragm; the right ventricle is in front and the left ventricle is to the left side. With counterclockwise rotation there is early transition, that is, left ventricular forces are shifted anteriorly and occur earlier in the precordial leads.

The diagnosis of RVH is often difficult to establish as the QRS complex primarily represents depolarization of the left ventricle, which has a far greater myocardial mass compared with the right ventricle. Hence the finding of RVH on the ECG implies a substantially thickened right ventricular myocardium.

The criteria for the diagnosis of RVH include:

- R-wave amplitude (in mm) in lead V1 > 7 mm
- R/S ratio in lead V1 > 1
- R/S ratio in lead V6 (or V5) < 1, indicating increased forces directed from the left to the right

Supporting criteria for RVH include:

- Right axis deviation (between +90° and +180°), which is diagnosed by a QRS complex that is negative in lead I and positive in lead aVF
- Right atrial hypertrophy (P pulmonale); the P wave is tall (> 0.25 mV), narrow (< 0.12 sec), and peaked in the limb leads and positive in lead V1
- Associated ST-segment depression and T-wave abnormalities in leads V1-V3

continues

The combination of RVH and right atrial hypertrophy on the ECG and a loud P2 on exam suggests the presence of elevated pulmonary pressures. Pulmonary arterial hypertension is clinically associated with scleroderma and is the most likely diagnosis.

It is important to note that there are other causes for a tall R wave in lead V1 that need to be excluded, although the presence of the other ECG features will generally establish RVH as the etiology. The other causes include a posterior wall myocardial infarction (MI) (which is usually associated with an inferior wall MI), Wolff-Parkinson-White pattern (with a short PR interval and a QRS complex that is widened as a result of a delta wave), hypertrophic cardiomyopathy with septal hypertrophy (often with prominent septal Q waves in the lateral leads), early transition (counterclockwise rotation), Duchenne muscular dystrophy (associated with a posterolateral MI pattern), dextrocardia (associated with reverse R-wave progression, right axis, and negative P wave in lead I), and lead switch (V1, V2, V3); it may also be a normal variant. ▪

A 72-year-old man who has not seen a physician in more than 20 years comes to your clinic with no specific complaints. Physical examination reveals a blood pressure of 185/100 mm Hg, equal in both arms, as well as a left ventricular heave and an S4. An ECG is obtained.

What are the pertinent findings on the ECG?
What is the clinical diagnosis?
What is the most likely etiology?

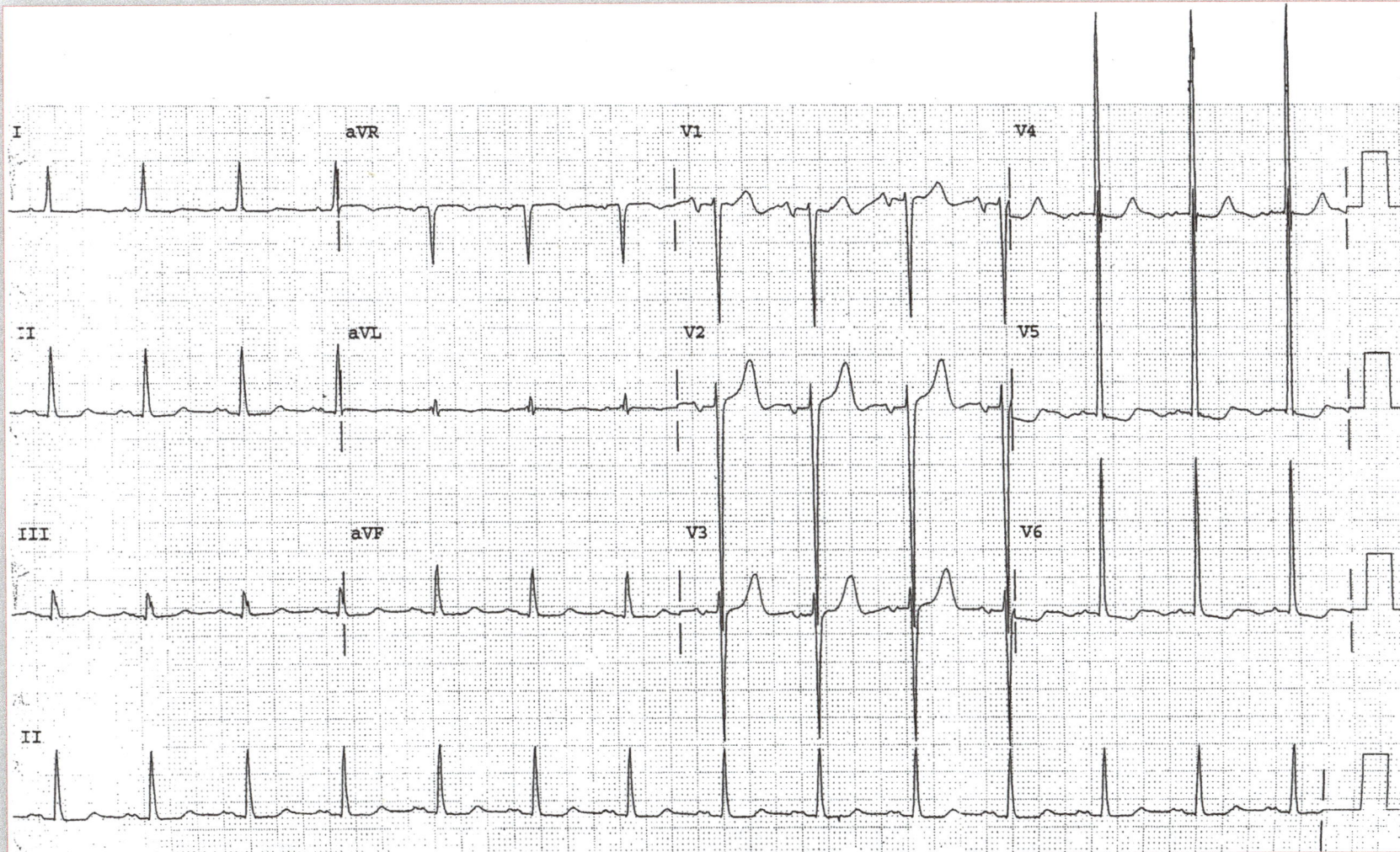

ECG 3 Analysis: Normal sinus rhythm, left atrial hypertrophy, left ventricular hypertrophy (LVH)

The ECG shows a regular rhythm at a rate of 88 bpm. There is a P wave (+) before each QRS complex, with a stable PR interval (0.20 sec). The P wave is positive in leads I, II, aVF, and V4-V6. Hence this is a normal sinus rhythm. The P wave is broad (> 0.12 sec), notched (*) in leads II and V4 (termed P mitrale), and negative (↑) in leads V1 and V2. This is characteristic of left atrial hypertrophy, also termed left atrial abnormality.

The QRS complex duration is normal (0.08 sec), and the axis is normal, between 0° and +90° (the QRS complex is positive in leads I and aVF). The QT/QTc intervals are normal (360/440 msec). The major finding is the marked increase in QRS voltage (R-wave amplitude or S-wave depth) seen in the precordial leads (S-wave depth in lead V2 = 39 mm [ ]] and R-wave amplitude in lead V5 = 40 mm [[ ] for a total of 79 mm), which is diagnostic for left ventricular hypertrophy (LVH) (ie, S-wave depth in lead V2 + R-wave amplitude in lead V5 ≥ 35 mm). Associated with LVH are ST-T wave changes or repolarization abnormalities seen in leads V4-V6 (↑). These ST-T wave changes, often referred to as a "strain pattern," actually reflect subendocardial ischemia. The last portion of the myocardium to receive blood supply is the subendocardium, and when LVH is present the oxygen supply to this territory is limited.

A number of criteria have been proposed for diagnosing LVH on the surface ECG. They are primarily related to QRS complex amplitude or voltage. However, an important limitation to the use of QRS complex voltage is related to factors that may influence the transmission of the electrical impulse to the surface of the body, including body habitus (especially obesity), pulmonary disease, and pericardial thickening or effusion. In these settings, the ECG may not reflect the presence of LVH. The proposed criteria for diagnosing LVH include:

- S-wave depth (in mm) in lead V1 or V2 + R-wave amplitude (in mm) in lead V5 or V6 ≥ 35 mm if over age 45 or ≥ 45 mm if under age 45 (Sokolow-Lyon criteria)

- Deepest S wave (in mm) + tallest R wave (in mm) in any two precordial leads ≥ 35 mm (or ≥ 45 mm if under age 45)

- S-wave depth (in mm) or R-wave amplitude (in mm) in any one precordial lead ≥ 25 mm

- R-wave amplitude (in mm) in lead aVL ≥ 11 mm (≥ 18 mm in presence of left axis) (Sokolow-Lyon criteria)

- R-wave amplitude (in mm) in any one limb lead ≥ 20 mm

- R-wave amplitude (in mm) in lead aVL + S-wave depth (in mm) in lead V3 ≥ 28 mm for men or ≥ 20 mm for women (Cornell criteria)

The voltage criteria are based on the ECG recorded at normal standard, where 1 mV = 10 mm or 10 small boxes in height.

continues

LVH may be associated with other changes on the ECG, including:

- Intraventricular conduction delay due to slow activation of the thickened myocardium.

- Often the upstroke of the QRS complex is prolonged (> 0.05 sec); this is termed a delayed intrinsicoid deflection (the intrinsicoid deflection is measured from the beginning of the QRS complex to the peak of the R wave)

- Physiologic left axis deviation, between 0° and −30° (positive QRS complex in leads I and II and negative QRS complex in lead aVF)

- Presence of left atrial hypertrophy (or abnormality), called a P mitrale, defined as a P wave that is broad (> 0.12 sec in duration) and notched (with a tall second component). Left atrial hypertrophy may also be present when the P wave in lead V1 (and V2) is primarily negative (rather than biphasic positive-negative, which is normal).

- Ischemic-type ST-T wave abnormalities (ie, due to subendocardial ischemia), most often seen in leads I, aVL, and V4-V6

- J-point and ST-segment elevation (early repolarization), most often seen in leads V4-V6

As indicated, QRS amplitude, as measured at the surface of the body, is affected by a number of conditions; therefore, LVH may be present even if QRS amplitude criteria are not. This is the basis for the Romhilt-Estes scoring system, which assigns a point score to various ECG abnormalities seen with LVH.

Romhilt-Estes Scoring System

Romhilt-Estes Criterion	Points
R-wave height or S-wave depth in any limb lead ≥20 mm	3
OR	
S-wave depth in lead V1 or V2 ≥ 30 mm	
OR	
R-wave height in lead V5 or V6 ≥ 30 mm	
ST-T wave changes typical of LVH	
Taking digoxin	1
Not taking digoxin	3
Left atrial hypertrophy	
(terminal force in lead V1 ≥ 1 mm in depth and > 0.04 sec in duration)	3
Left axis deviation (< −30°)	2
QRS duration ≥ 90 ms (ie, intraventricular conduction delay)	1
Intrinsicoid deflection in lead V5 or V6 > 0.05 sec	1

A score of 5 or more indicates definite LVH;
a score of 4 indicates probable LVH.

The patient has physical exam findings and ECG features all consistent with LVH, most likely from chronic untreated hypertension. Other etiologies of LVH include aortic stenosis, coarctation of the aorta, extreme athleticism, and hypertrophic cardiomyopathy from genetic mutations. The mainstay of treatment is adequate blood pressure control for hypertension, particularly with β-blockers, calcium-channel blockers, angiotensin-converting enzyme inhibitors, or angiotensin receptor blocking drugs; surgery for coarctation or aortic stenosis; and assessment of hemodynamic abnormalities and ventricular arrhythmia risk in patients with hypertrophic cardiomyopathy. ■

A 61-year-old woman with hypertension as her only known risk factor for coronary artery disease now presents with 3 days of persistent chest pressure. Sublingual nitroglycerin does not relieve her symptoms. An ECG is obtained, and an initial set of cardiac biomarkers reveals normal troponin, creatine kinase (CK), and CK-MB levels.

Based on the ECG, is this patient having an acute coronary syndrome?

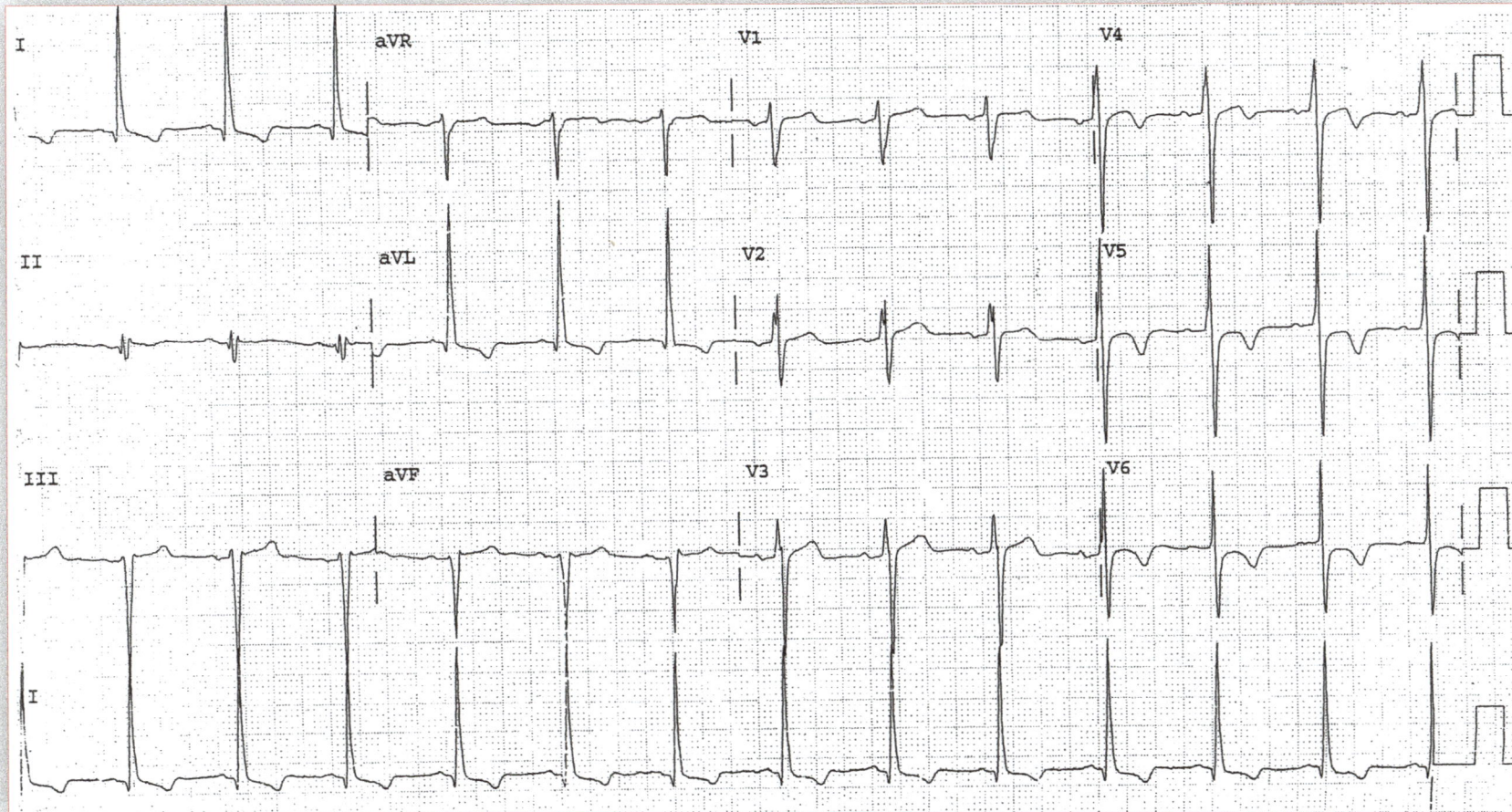

ECG 4 Analysis: Normal sinus rhythm, left ventricular hypertrophy (LVH) with ST-T wave changes

The ECG shows a regular rhythm at a rate of 76 bpm. There is a P wave (+) before each QRS complex, with a stable PR interval (0.16 sec). The P wave is positive in leads I, II, aVF, and V4-V6. Hence this is a normal sinus rhythm. The QRS complex duration is normal (0.10 sec), and the axis is leftward, between 0° and –30° (positive QRS complex in leads I and II and negative QRS complex in lead aVF). The QT/QTc intervals are normal (360/410 msec). The major finding is an increase in QRS voltage in lead I ( ]) (R-wave amplitude = 20 mm) and lead aVL ([ ) (R-wave amplitude = 24 mm), which is diagnostic for left ventricular hypertrophy (LVH) (*ie*, voltage in any limb lead > 20 mm or R-wave amplitude in lead aVL > 11 mm or > 18 mm in the presence of a left axis). Also noted is a delayed intrinsicoid deflection in leads V4-V6 (↑), an intraventricular conduction delay (*ie*, QRS width ≥ 0.10 sec), leftward axis, and the ST-T wave changes (^) associated with LVH as noted in leads I, aVL, and V4-V6.

Typically, the ST-T wave abnormalities associated with LVH consist of ST-segment depressions and deep, asymmetric T-wave inversions, as illustrated in this case. Therefore, in the presence of LVH with the associated ST-T wave abnormalities, which are due to chronic subendocardial ischemia, the ECG cannot definitively diagnose nor can it rule out acute ischemia or a non–ST-segment elevation myocardial infarction (NSTEMI) due to coronary artery disease. Although the clinical story is potentially concerning for an acute coronary syndrome, the ECG in this setting does not help to make the diagnosis. In contrast, the presence of ST-segment elevations is indicative of an acute ST-segment elevation myocardial infarction (STEMI) despite the presence of LVH. In this case, the LVH could be explained by the patient's chronic hypertension. ■

A 54-year-old woman presents to the emergency department after a syncopal episode. She has had three similar episodes in the past and has noted worsening chest pressure with exertion over the past many months. On physical examination, you hear a grade III/VI systolic murmur, loudest at the upper sternal border, that radiates to the carotids and does not increase with Valsalva. The murmur is mid to late peaking. S2 is heard but does not split. An ECG is obtained.

What is the most likely diagnosis?

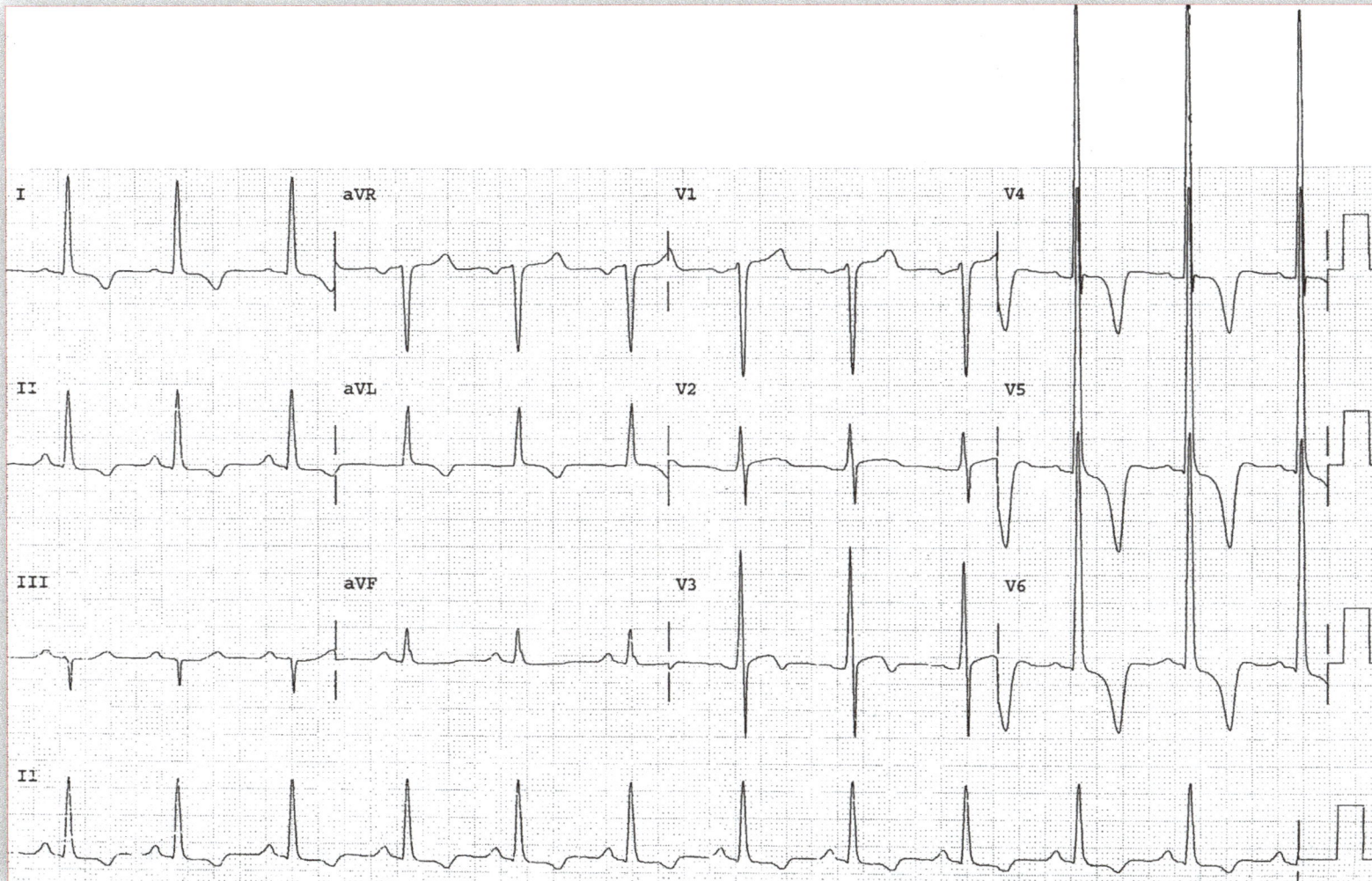

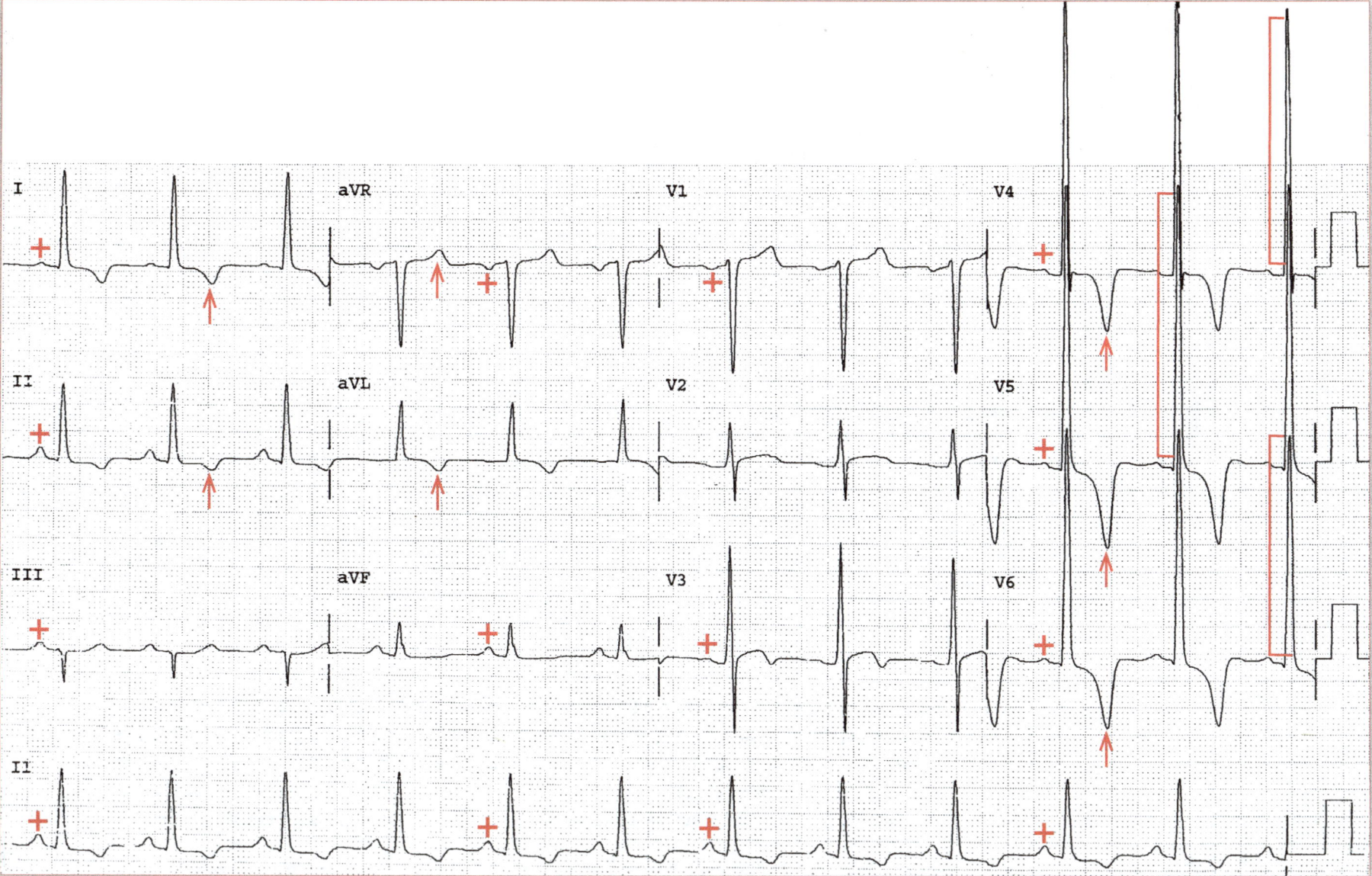

ECG 5 Analysis: Normal sinus rhythm, left ventricular hypertrophy (LVH) with ST-T wave changes

The ECG shows a regular rhythm at a rate of 70 bpm. There is a P wave (+) before each QRS complex, with a stable PR interval (0.18 sec). The P wave is positive in leads I, II, aVF, and V4-V6. Hence this is a normal sinus rhythm.

The QRS complex duration is normal (0.10 sec), and the axis is normal, between 0° and +90° (positive QRS complex in leads I and aVF). The QT/QTc intervals are normal (400/410 msec). The striking feature is the very markedly increased QRS voltage in leads V4-V6 (R-wave amplitude [[ ] = 40 to 50 mm), which meets one of the criteria for left ventricular hypertrophy (LVH) (S-wave depth or R-wave amplitude in any precordial lead > 25 mm). In addition, there are marked ST-T wave changes (↑) associated with the LVH (asymmetric and deeply inverted) in leads I, II, aVR (the positive T wave is actually inverted in this lead), and V4-V6.

Given the clinical history, physical exam, and ECG findings, the most likely diagnosis is valvular aortic stenosis. The classic triad of symptoms associated with severe aortic stenosis is angina, syncope, and heart failure. The murmur associated with aortic stenosis is a crescendo–decrescendo systolic (ejection type) murmur best heard at the right upper sternal border. The timing of the murmur (early, mid, or late) correlates with the severity of aortic stenosis. The quality of the carotid pulse also is an indicator of the severity of aortic stenosis (*ie*, parvus [low amplitude] and tardus [slow upstroke]). Physiologic splitting of S2 can also be lost due to delayed opening and closure of the aortic valve. When valvular stenosis is very severe, paradoxical splitting of S2 may be present. Aortic stenosis is associated with findings of LVH and occasionally a left bundle branch block on the ECG. The major etiologies of valvular aortic stenosis include calcific or senile changes (predominant in the over-70 age group), rheumatic heart disease, and congenital bicuspid aortic valve. ■

Notes

A 74-year-old man presents to his physician for a routine physical examination. He states that his only medical history is that of hypertension. A routine ECG is obtained.

Does this patient have left ventricular hypertrophy?

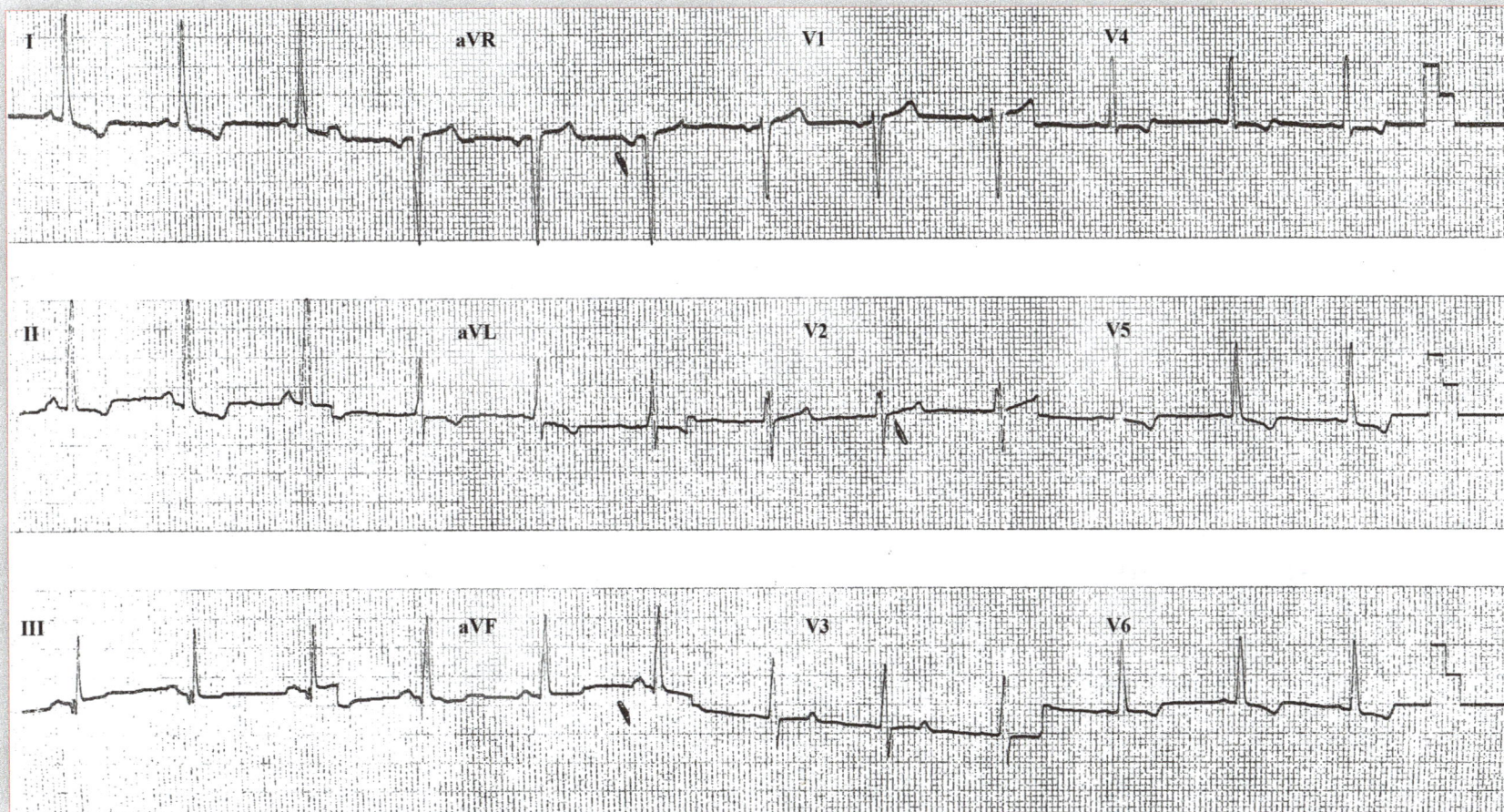

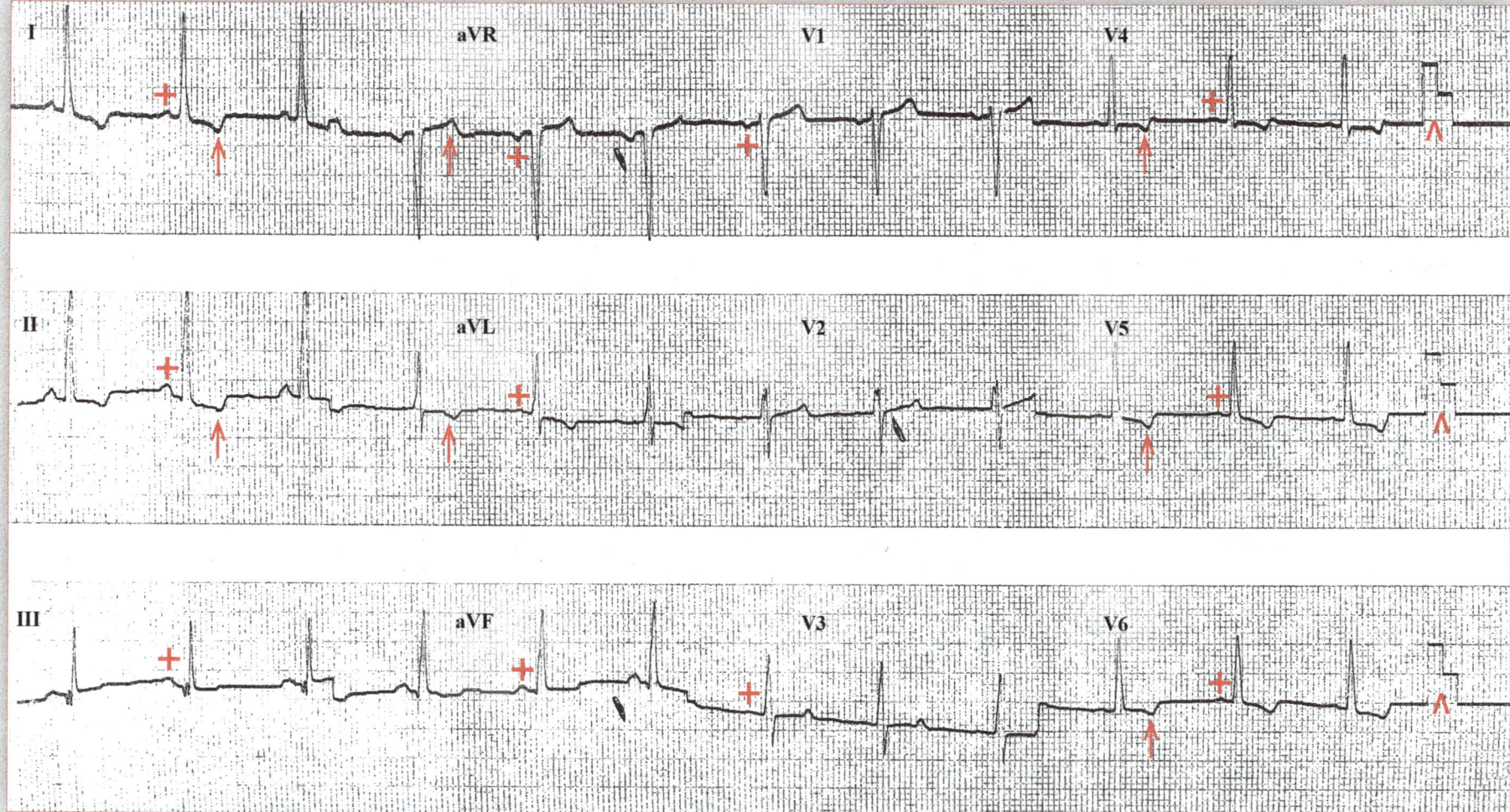

ECG 6 Analysis: Normal sinus rhythm, left ventricular hypertrophy, half-standard

The ECG shows a regular rhythm at a rate of 70 bpm. There is a P wave (+) before each QRS complex, with a stable PR interval (0.16 sec). The P wave is positive in leads I, II, aVF, and V4-V6. Hence this is a normal sinus rhythm.

The QRS complex duration is normal (0.08 sec), and the axis is normal, between 0° and +90° (positive QRS complex in leads I and aVF). The QRS complex has a normal morphology. The QT/QTc intervals are normal (360/390 msec). Although the voltage in all leads is normal as recorded, it is important to note the standardization (^) seen at the end of the ECG tracing, which indicates that the limb leads were recorded at normal standard (1 mV = 10 mm or 10 small boxes in height) while the precordial leads were recorded at half-standard (1 mV = 5 mm or five small boxes in height). Hence the QRS amplitude as measured in the precordial leads needs to be doubled. Therefore, the R-wave amplitude in lead V5 is 24 mm and the S-wave depth in leads V1 and V2 is 26 and 14 mm, respectively, for a total of 50 mm using S-wave depth in lead V1 + R-wave amplitude in lead V5 and 38 mm using S-wave depth in lead V2 + R-wave amplitude in lead in V5. This meets one of the criteria for left ventricular hypertrophy (S-wave depth in lead V1 or V2 + R-wave amplitude in lead V5 or V6 ≥ 35 mm). Also present are the typical ST-T wave changes associated with left ventricular hypertrophy (↑) seen in leads I, II, aVR (the positive T wave is actually inverted in this lead), and V4-V6. ■

A 45-year-old man with no past medical history presents with symptoms of "indigestion," with chest burning and throat tightness over the past 2 weeks occurring with activity. Over the past 2 days he experienced chest burning at rest. He has a 25 pack-year history of smoking, and his father died of a myocardial infarction at the age of 52. An ECG is obtained. Cardiac troponins are negative.

What is the diagnosis on ECG?

What is the next step in the management of this patient?

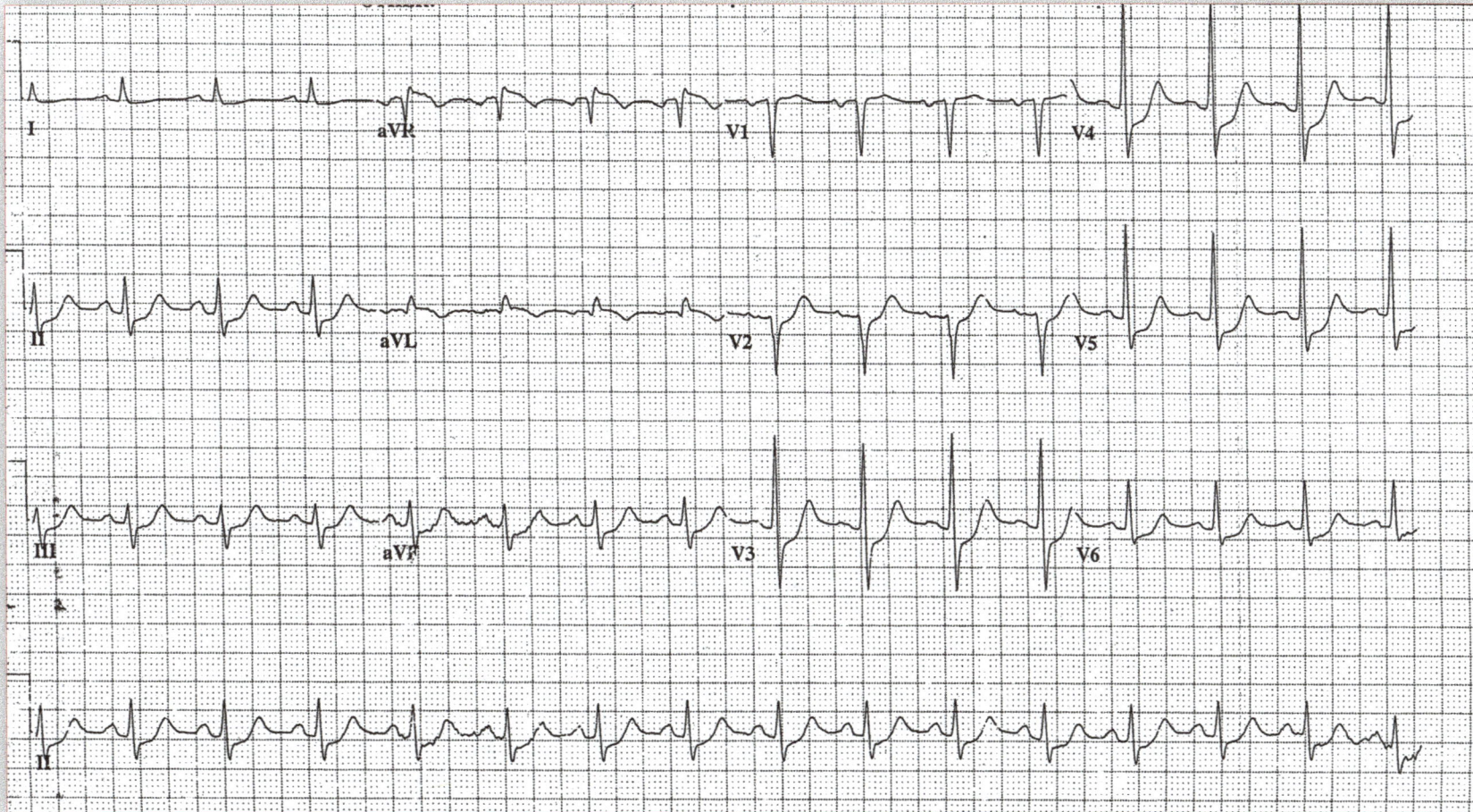

ECG 7 Analysis: Normal sinus rhythm, upsloping
ST-segment depression due to subendocardial ischemia

The ECG shows a regular rhythm at a rate of 92 bpm. There is a P wave (+) before each QRS complex, with a stable PR interval (0.18 sec). The P wave is positive in leads I, II, aVF, and V4-V6. Hence this is a normal sinus rhythm.

The QRS complex duration is normal (0.08 sec), and the axis is normal, between 0° and +90° (positive QRS complex in leads I and aVF). The QT/QTc intervals are normal (340/420 msec). The major finding is J-point depression (↓) with upsloping ST-segment depression (^) seen in leads II, III, aVF, and V2-V6 and ST-segment elevation (▼) in lead aVR (which is actually ST-segment depression). J-point and ST-segment depression is an indicator of subendocardial myocardial ischemia; the subendocardium of the myocardium is the last region to receive blood flow and hence is prone to ischemia. Ischemia usually occurs first in the subendocardial region before extending to the entire thickness of the myocardium.

The J point and ST segment should be at baseline, which is determined by the TP segment; the PR segment can be used to establish the baseline if there is no obvious TP segment. Three types of ST-segment depression (J point and ST segment below baseline) are indicative of myocardial ischemia: upsloping, horizontal, and downsloping. Upsloping ST-segment depression is the least specific for myocardial ischemia as it may occur with sinus tachycardia as a normal finding. In this situation, the J-point depression results from the atrial repolarization (the T wave of the P wave). Normally, the T wave of the P wave occurs during the QRS interval. During sinus tachycardia (which is the result of an augmented sympathetic state) and the shortening of the PR interval (due to enhanced AV nodal conduction), the T wave of the P wave moves out from the QRS complex and falls on the J point, depressing it. The ST segment therefore slopes back up toward baseline. As a result, when upsloping ST-segment depression is present, the amount of depression is determined by evaluating the degree of ST-segment depression at 80 msec past the J point. An ST segment that is more than 1.5 mm below baseline at this time is diagnostic for ischemia. The baseline is the TP segment, although with tachycardia the TP segment may be difficult to establish; hence the PR segment may be used. In this ECG, sinus tachycardia is not present and the ST segment is still depressed 2 mm below baseline at 80 msec beyond the J point, confirming that these are true ischemic ECG changes.

continues

The patient's symptoms and ECG findings are concerning for an acute coronary syndrome. The spectrum of acute coronary syndrome includes unstable angina, non–ST-segment elevation myocardial infarction (NSTEMI), and ST-segment elevation myocardial infarction (STEMI). Since cardiac biomarkers are negative, the patient would fall into the unstable angina category. His symptoms first began as chronic stable angina of effort but became worse and unstable as they also occurred at rest. The first step in the management of a patient with unstable angina includes administration of aspirin, oxygen, nitrates, and β-blockers. Anticoagulation with some form of heparin should also be initiated, and antiplatelet therapy with clopidogrel along with aspirin has been shown to have a mortality benefit. A high-dose statin is also recommended, regardless of the lipid levels, as these agents have been shown to stabilize unstable plaques, which are the cause of unstable angina. Once the patient's symptoms stabilize and the patient is free of angina, a noninvasive evaluation (exercise test) should be performed to determine whether there is any ongoing ischemia. If so, cardiac catheterization may be performed. ■

A 74-year-old veteran presents with symptoms of angina. The following ECG is obtained.

Which coronary arteries are likely to have significant stenoses?

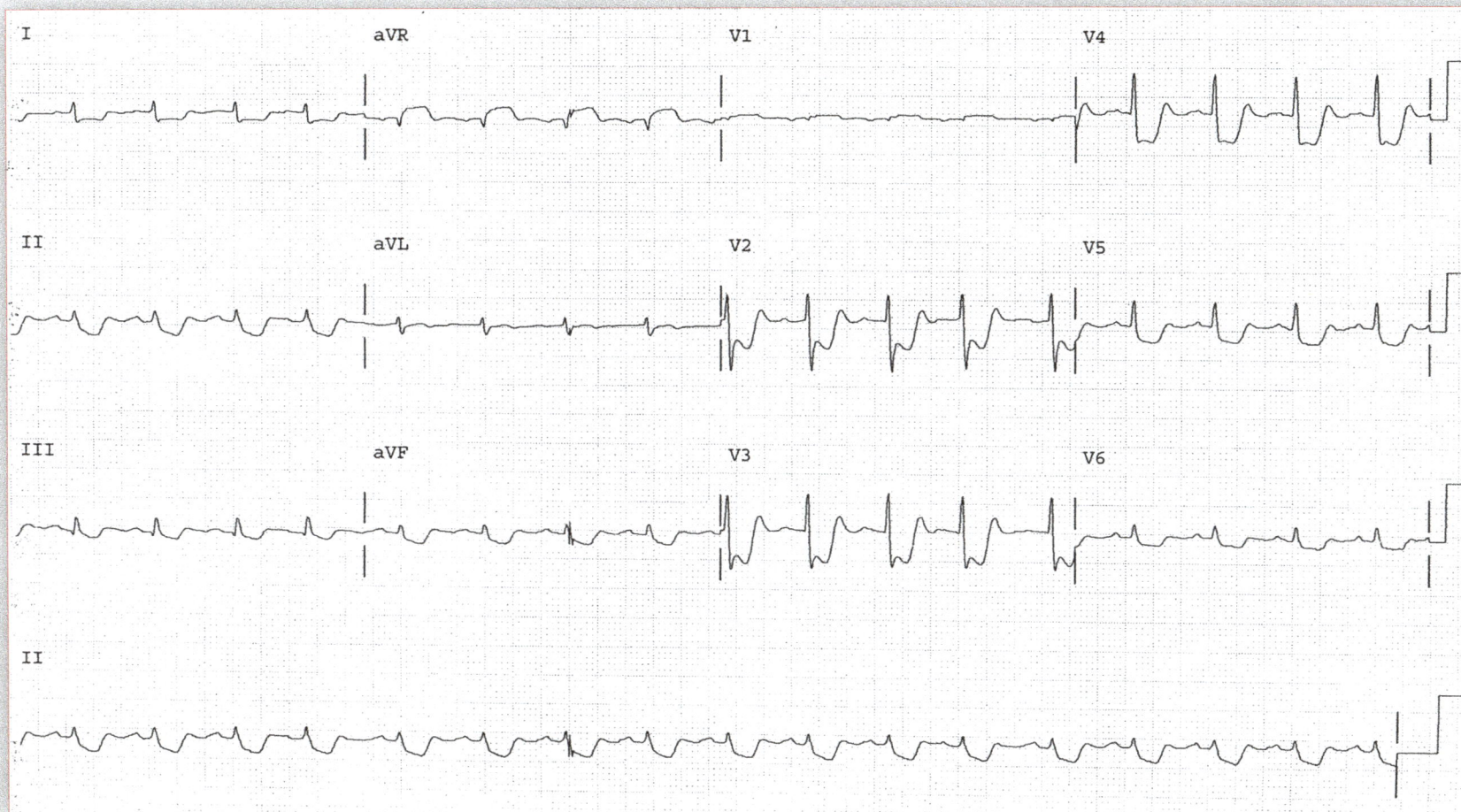

ECG 8 Analysis: Sinus tachycardia, horizontal
ST-segment depression due to subendocardial ischemia, low voltage

The ECG shows a regular rhythm at a rate of 110 bpm. There are P waves (+) before each QRS complex, with a stable PR interval (0.18 sec). The P wave is positive in leads I, II, aVF, and V4-V6. Hence this is a sinus tachycardia.

The QRS complex duration is normal (0.08 sec), and the axis is normal, between 0° and +90° (positive QRS complex in leads I and aVF). The QT/QTc intervals are normal (280/380 msec). There is low QRS voltage (< 5 mm in each limb lead and/or < 10 mm in each precordial lead). Diffuse ST-segment depressions (↑) can be seen in all leads (the ST-segment elevation in lead aVR [▼] is actually ST-segment depression). The ST-segment depression is horizontal in leads I and V3-V6, reaching a maximal depth in lead V3 of 5 mm below baseline, which is the TP segment (↓). The ST segments are downsloping in leads II, III, aVF, and V2. Although the leads in which ST-segment depression are seen do not generally indicate the location of subendocardial ischemia, the diffuse nature of the ST-segment depression in this case indicates widespread ischemia due to multivessel, likely three-vessel, coronary artery disease. ■

The patient is a 60-year-old man with hypertension and known coronary artery disease who underwent percutaneous coronary intervention (balloon angioplasty) of the right coronary artery and left anterior descending artery 3 years ago as therapy for angina. He presents with 2 months of recurrent angina. The baseline ECG following an exercise test showed left ventricular hypertrophy with 1-mm ST-segment depression in leads I, aVL, and V4-V6. This ECG was obtained 3 minutes into the recovery period.

Does this patient have ischemia?

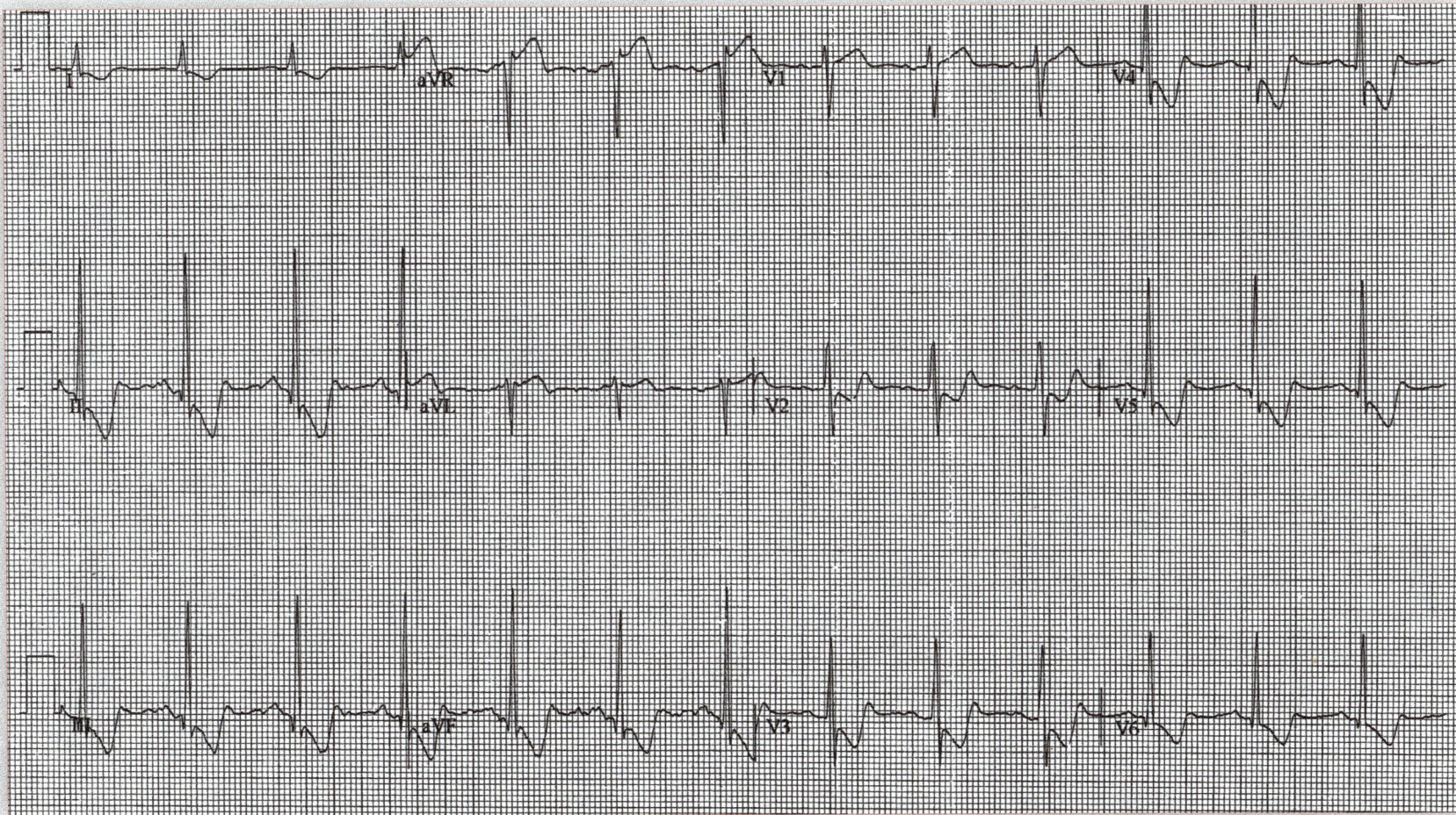

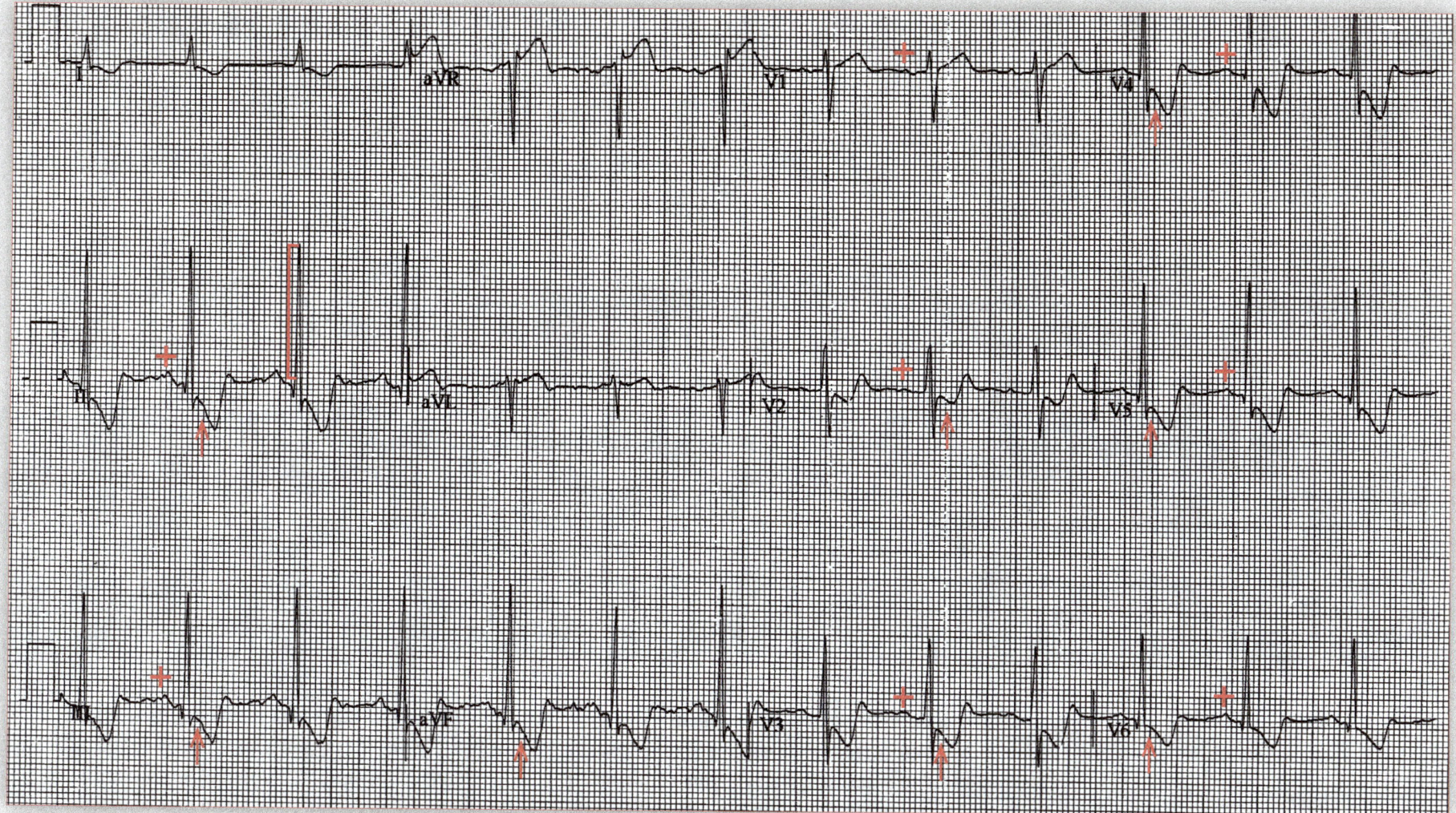

ECG 9 Analysis: Normal sinus rhythm, downsloping
ST-segment depression due to subendocardial ischemia

The ECG demonstrates a regular rhythm at a rate of 80 bpm. There is a P wave (+) before each QRS complex, with a stable PR interval (0.16 sec). The P wave is positive in leads I, II, aVF, and V4-V6. Hence this is a normal sinus rhythm.

The QRS complex duration is normal (0.08 sec) and the axis is normal, between 0° and +90° (positive QRS complex in leads I and aVF). The QT/QTc intervals are normal (360/420 msec). The major finding is significant ST-segment depression (↑), which is downsloping. Although there is voltage criteria for left ventricular hypertrophy (LVH) (*ie*, R-wave amplitude of 25 mm in lead II [[ ]), the ST segments are more depressed than is generally seen with LVH and are more depressed compared with baseline (*ie*, > 1 mm), reaching a maximum level of 5 mm below the baseline TP segment. Downsloping ST-segment

changes have the strongest correlation with ischemia and generally indicate more severe coronary artery disease, particularly when the changes are widespread.

However, ST-segment depression can be nondiagnostic for ischemia due to coronary artery disease if the patient has LVH (which is associated with subendocardial ischemia not due to coronary artery disease) or routinely takes digitalis. The ST-segment changes seen with digitalis drugs are different as the J point is usually at baseline while there is sagging depression of the ST segment (hammock-like or scooped). Nevertheless, significant ST-segment depression beyond that seen at baseline is indicative of ischemia despite the present of LVH or digitalis use. ◼

A 56-year-old diabetic man presents with acute-onset crushing substernal chest pressure over the past 2 hours. The following ECG is obtained.

What is the diagnosis?

What is the next step in management?

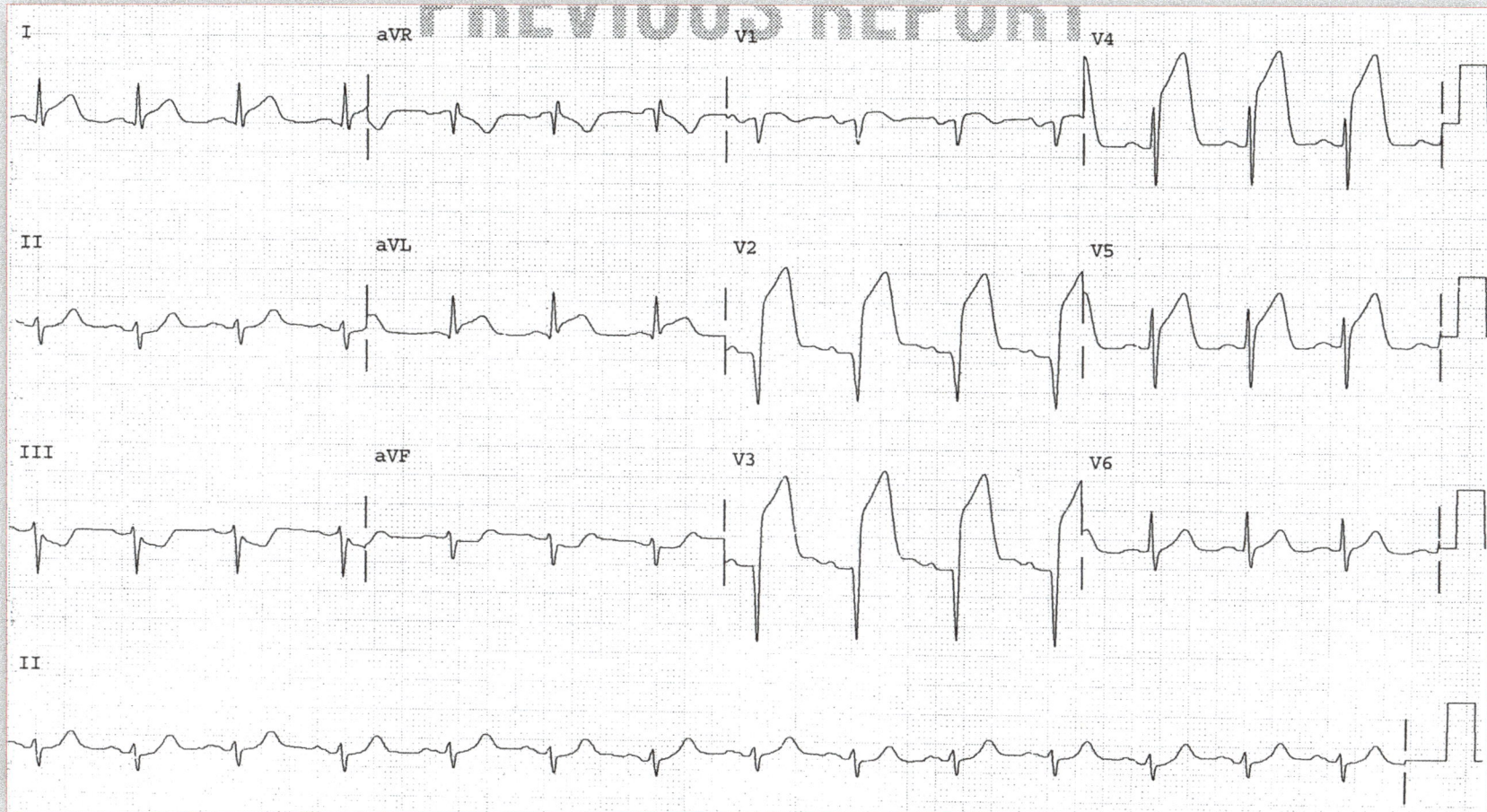

ECG 10 Analysis: Normal sinus rhythm, ST-segment elevation due to acute anterior wall myocardial infarction (MI), left anterior fascicular block (LAFB)

The ECG shows a regular rhythm at a rate of 90 bpm. There is a P wave (+) before each QRS complex, with a stable PR interval (0.20 sec). The P wave is positive in leads I, II, aVF, and V4-V6. Hence this is a normal sinus rhythm.

The QRS complex duration is normal (0.08 sec). The axis is extremely leftward, between −30° and −90° (positive QRS complex in lead I but a negative QRS complex in leads II and aVF with an rS morphology). An extremely leftward axis (in the absence of other etiologies for a left axis, specifically an inferior wall myocardial infarction [MI]) is termed left anterior fascicular block (LAFB). The criteria for LAFB include left axis deviation with an rS pattern in leads II and aVF. In contrast, a Qr complex in leads II and aVF is a pattern associated with a chronic inferior wall MI, not a conduction abnormality or fascicular block. Indeed, LAFB cannot be diagnosed in the presence of an inferior wall MI. The QT/QTc intervals are normal (320/390 msec).

The major abnormality is significant J-point (→) and ST-segment (↓) elevation (when compared with the TP segment, which is baseline) in leads V2-V5 and less marked ST-segment elevation in leads I and aVL (▲). The ST segments are no longer concave but are now convex in morphology and merged with the T waves. In addition there is loss of the R wave in leads V2-V3 (▼). These ECG changes are diagnostic for an acute MI involving the apex and anteroapical regions of the left ventricle. There is also involvement of the lateral wall, indicated by the ST-segment elevation in leads I and aVL as well as ST-segment depression (^) in leads III and aVF. In the setting of an acute MI, these ST-segment depressions do not represent ischemia in the inferior wall, but rather they are reciprocal changes due to the fact that these leads are seeing the infarcted region from an opposite direction. When an ST-segment elevation MI (STEMI) is present, immediate revascularization is indicated with either cardiac catheterization and percutaneous coronary intervention or thrombolytic therapy.

In the setting of an acute STEMI, the ECG demonstrates a typical progression of changes. During the first several minutes after the onset of chest discomfort, the earliest ECG changes indicating an acute MI are hyperacute (tall, peaked, and symmetric) T waves. This T-wave abnormality is the result of local hyperkalemia, which occurs early after the infarction as a result of loss of membrane integrity from the ischemia with a leaking of potassium; the potassium stays in the infarcted tissue as there is no blood flow into or out of the infarction zone. This initial ECG finding is often not seen because it is present soon after the onset of symptoms, while patients usually present several hours after symptoms begin. The T-wave changes are followed by ST-segment elevation. The ST segments initially maintain their normal concave morphology, but they become convex as the MI evolves, merging with the T waves. Over the ensuing hours to days, the ST-segment elevation persists, the R wave loses amplitude, and Q waves begin to

continues

develop. As the infarct evolves, the ST-segment elevation decreases, the Q waves become deeper, and T-wave inversions develop. In the absence of revascularization, the ST-segment elevations normalize over several days. The Q waves and T-wave inversions persist, and this is the pattern of a chronic MI.

Therefore, an acute MI is identified by the presence of localized ST-segment elevation; hyperacute T waves, which are tall, peaked, and symmetric; and reciprocal ST-segment depressions, which are the same ST-segment changes viewed from another direction. The leads that demonstrate these changes identify the location of the acute MI:

- Inferior wall MI: ST-segment elevation in leads II, III, and aVF (or any two of these three leads). An inferior wall MI may be associated with involvement of the posterior left ventricular wall or the free wall of the right ventricle. The presence of ST-segment elevation in lead V1 and ST-segment depression in lead aVR (which is actually elevation) suggests involvement of the right ventricle, which can be confirmed by obtaining right-sided precordial leads. The presence of ST-segment elevation in RV3-RV4 (right-sided leads V3-V4) confirms involvement of the free wall of the RV.

- Anterior wall MI: ST-segment elevation in any two contiguous precordial leads (V1-V6):
  - Anteroseptal MI: ST-segment elevation in leads V1-V2
  - Anteroapical MI: ST-segment elevation leads V3-V4
  - Anterolateral MI: ST-segment elevation leads V5-V6

- Lateral wall MI: ST-segment elevation leads I and aVL

- Posterior wall MI: ST-segment depression in leads V1-V2, particularly when there is an inferior wall MI, suggests posterior wall involvement, which is often associated with inferior wall MI. Leads placed on the back (V7-V8), below the left scapula and over the posterior wall, may show ST-segment elevation, confirming a posterior wall infarction. ◼

A 67-year-old man presents with chest pain, and the following ECG is obtained.

What is the underlying mechanism for the findings noted in leads V4-V6, I, and aVL?

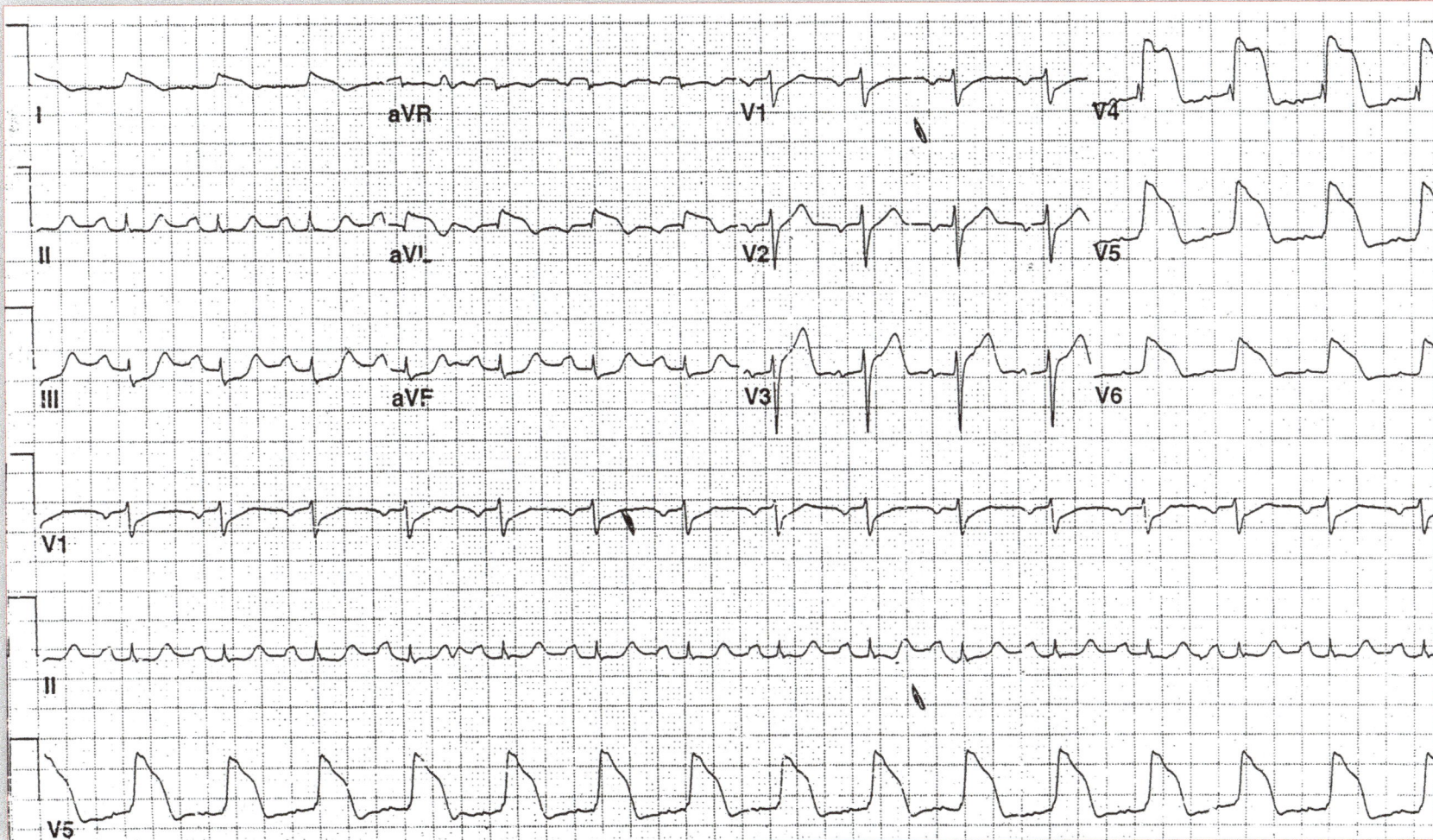

ECG 11 Analysis: Normal sinus rhythm, ST-segment elevation due to acute anterolateral and lateral myocardial infarction, left atrial hypertrophy, low voltage

The ECG shows a regular rhythm at a rate of 96 bpm. There is a P wave (+) before each QRS complex, with a stable PR interval (0.20 sec). The P wave is positive in leads I, II, aVF, and V4-V6. Hence this is a normal sinus rhythm. The QRS complex duration is normal (0.08 sec), and the axis is normal, between 0° and +90° (positive QRS complex in leads I and aVF). The QT/QTc intervals are normal (320/400 msec).

The major finding is localized ST-segment elevation (↓) in leads V4-V6, I, and aVL, diagnostic for an acute lateral and anterolateral myocardial infarction. The ST segments have become convex and are merged with the T waves, resulting in a QRS complex that looks like a monophasic action potential or a current of injury; this has also been referred to as "tombstoning." Reciprocal ST-segment depressions (▲) are seen in leads III and aVF. In addition, there is low voltage in the limb leads (QRS complexes of < 5 mm in each lead) and the precordial leads (QRS complexes of < 10 mm in each lead). Lastly, the deep and broad negative P waves in leads V1-V2 (^) are indicative of left atrial hypertrophy.

According to the diastolic current theory, injured myocardial cells release ions that result in partial depolarization of the territory at baseline. Thus, the original baseline voltage (TP segment) in the affected leads on the ECG is actually shifted downward. During electrical activation of the myocardium, the baseline is reset to true zero as there is no electrical activity in the infarcted tissue; thus on the ECG recording, the ST segments appear to be elevated from the original baseline. ■

Notes

A 47-year-old man with hypertension and dyslipidemia presents with acute-onset crushing substernal chest pressure. Initial vital signs are within the normal range, with a blood pressure of 135/85 and a pulse rate in the 90s. After an aspirin is administered, the patient receives sublingual nitroglycerin. He subsequently becomes pre-syncopal, with a blood pressure of 70/palp and a pulse rate in the 100s. He must be intubated for airway protection in the setting of altered mental status.

What is the diagnosis?

What is a likely explanation for the patient's hypotension?

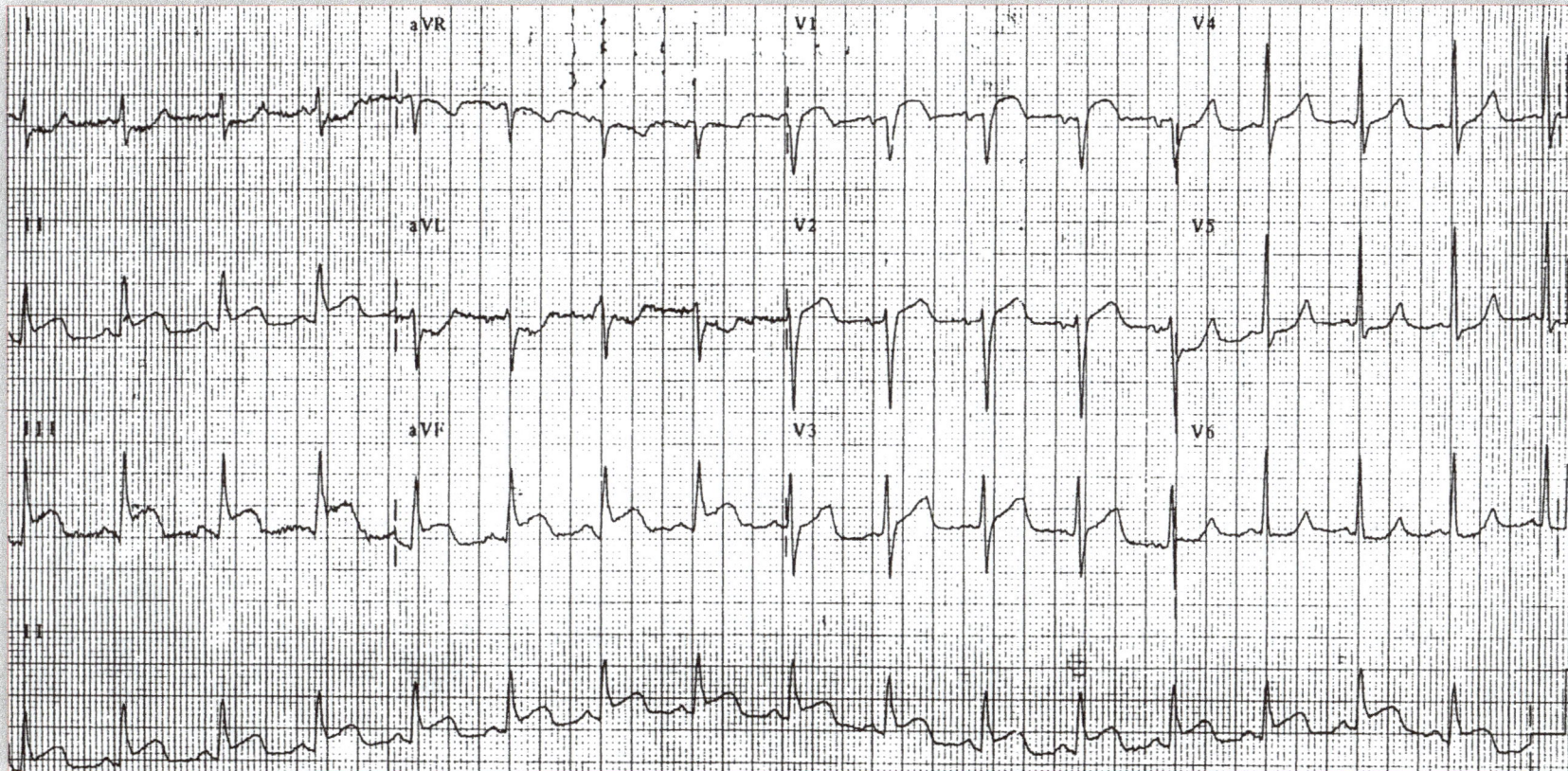

ECG 12 Analysis: Normal sinus rhythm, elevation due to acute interior wall myocardial infarction (MI), acute right ventricular infarction

The ECG shows a regular rhythm at a rate of 96 bpm. There is a P wave (+) before each QRS complex, with a stable PR interval (0.14 sec). The P wave is positive in leads I, II, aVF, and V4-V6. Hence this is a normal sinus rhythm. The QRS complex duration is normal (0.08 sec), and the axis is normal, between 0° and +90° (positive QRS complex in leads I and aVF). The QT/QTc intervals are normal (320/400 msec).

There is significant ST-segment elevation (↓) in leads II, III, and aVF, which is diagnostic for an acute inferior wall myocardial infarction (MI). The ST-segment elevation seen in lead V1 (▼) is strongly suggestive of right ventricular free wall infarction, which should be confirmed using right-sided chest leads (ie, the six chest leads placed on the right side of the chest in the same positions as used on the left side of the chest); the presence of ST-segment elevation in RV3-RV5 (right-sided leads V3-V5) would establish a right ventricular free wall infarction. Also noted are ST-segment depressions in leads I and aVL (▲), which represent reciprocal changes (ie, the same changes of the acute inferior infarction seen from another direction).

Hypotension in the setting of an acute coronary syndrome can be a manifestation of multiple etiologies. First, significant left ventricular dysfunction can lead to poor stroke volume and a resultant drop in blood pressure. Second, vagal reflexes (eg, the Bezold-Jarisch response), which often occur in the setting of inferior MI, can predominate, and the patient becomes bradycardic and hypotensive. However, this patient did not become bradycardic. Third, right ventricular infarction can result in a reduction in both right ventricular stroke volume and left ventricular filling and hence stroke volume. Therefore, patients with a right ventricular infarction are preload dependent, requiring adequate volume to maintaining cardiac output. Given the ST-segment elevation in lead V1, this patient likely has right ventricular involvement. In patients with right ventricular involvement, care should be taken in giving agents that reduce preload, such as nitrates, diuretics, and morphine. Indeed, these patients often require intravenous fluid to maintain blood pressure.

Because the acute right ventricular marginal branches of the right coronary artery supply the right ventricle, inferior infarctions are the type of MI most commonly associated with right ventricular infarcts. Anterior MIs can also result in right ventricular infarcts due to blood supply from septal branches. ■

A 74-year-old woman presents with progressive symptoms of dyspnea, orthopnea, and paroxysmal nocturnal dyspnea. She has noted a 15-lb weight gain over the past 2 months. She denies any current or past chest pain. On physical examination, jugular venous pressure is 12 cm, crackles are audible, and there is bilateral lower extremity edema. An ECG is obtained.

What is the most likely etiology for the patient's symptoms?

What is the initial step in management?

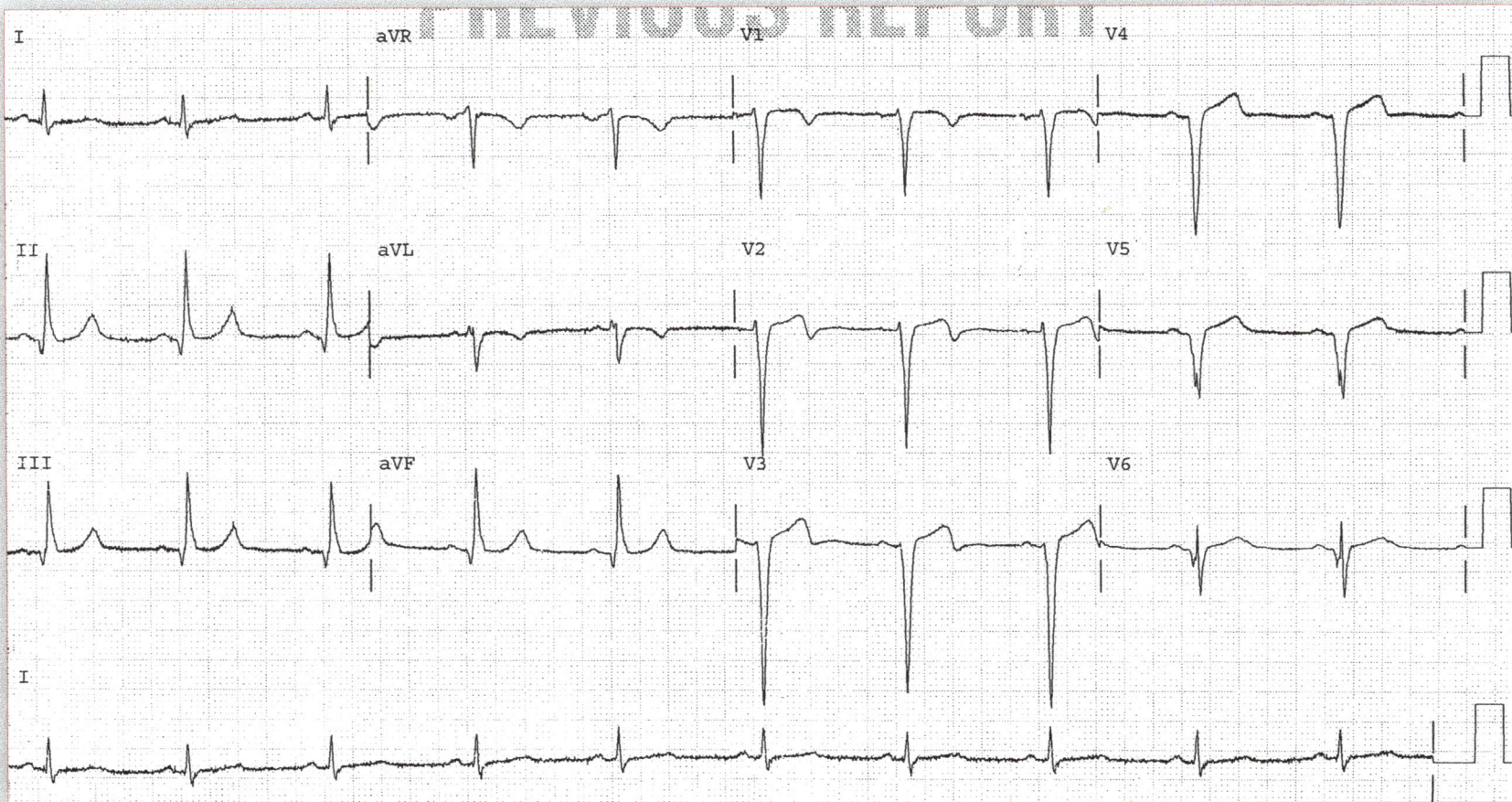

ECG 13 Analysis: Normal sinus rhythm, intraventricular conduction delay, chronic (old) anterior wall myocardial infarction (MI)

The ECG shows a regular rhythm at a rate of 60 bpm. There is a P wave (+) before each QRS complex, with a stable PR interval (0.16 sec). The P wave is positive in leads I, II, aVF, and V4-V6. Hence this is a normal sinus rhythm.

The QRS complex duration is prolonged (0.12 sec), and there is an intraventricular conduction delay. The QRS axis is normal, between 0° and +90° (positive QRS complex in leads I and aVF). The QT/QTc intervals are normal (400/400 msec). The major abnormality is the absence of R waves in leads V3-V5, resulting in complexes that have a QS pattern (↓) and also a pathologic Q wave (defined as being > 0.04 sec in duration) in lead V6 (^). The presence of significant Q waves indicates that the initial electrical forces are going away from the lead involved, which means that the tissue under the lead is electrically silent or infarcted. Hence, the QS complexes and Q wave on this ECG are indicative of an old or chronic myocardial infarction (MI) involving the anteroapical and anterolateral walls of the left ventricle. The T waves are biphasic in leads V2-V3 (*), although often they are inverted in the leads that demonstrate an infarction pattern. There are also small Q waves (↑) in leads II, III, and aVF; however, they are narrow and represent normal septal depolarization.

The patient is exhibiting symptoms of biventricular heart failure, likely resulting from an anterior MI she suffered sometime in the past. Since the patient denies any previous symptoms of chest discomfort, the infarction is determined to have been silent. The age of the Q wave or transmural infarction cannot be ascertained from the ECG. Initial steps in management include diuresis for fluid management and hydrazaline and nitrates or an angiotensin-converting enzyme (ACE) inhibitor for preload and afterload reduction. β-blockers have also been shown to have a significant mortality benefit in patients with heart failure with reduced ejection fraction. Revascularization of the coronary artery stenosis that resulted in the Q-wave MI (likely a lesion of the left anterior descending artery) has not been shown to be associated with a mortality benefit once the infarct is more than 3 days old (ie, a chronically occluded coronary artery). However, an ischemic evaluation with stress testing would be reasonable once the patient has been effectively treated for the heart failure to assess the level of any residual ischemic burden as well as establish functional capacity and status. ■

A 68-year-old man presents to his physician because of the recent onset of a productive cough associated with slight fever and shortness of breath. He has a history of a previous myocardial infarction (MI) but denies any recent cardiac symptoms. Physical examination demonstrates bilateral rhonchous sounds. An ECG is obtained and a chest X-ray is negative. The patient is diagnosed with bronchitis, and antibiotics are prescribed.

Does this patient have a posterior wall MI?

What is this patient's axis of ventricular depolarization in both the anterior (limb leads) and horizontal (precordial leads) planes?

What are the causes for these abnormal findings?

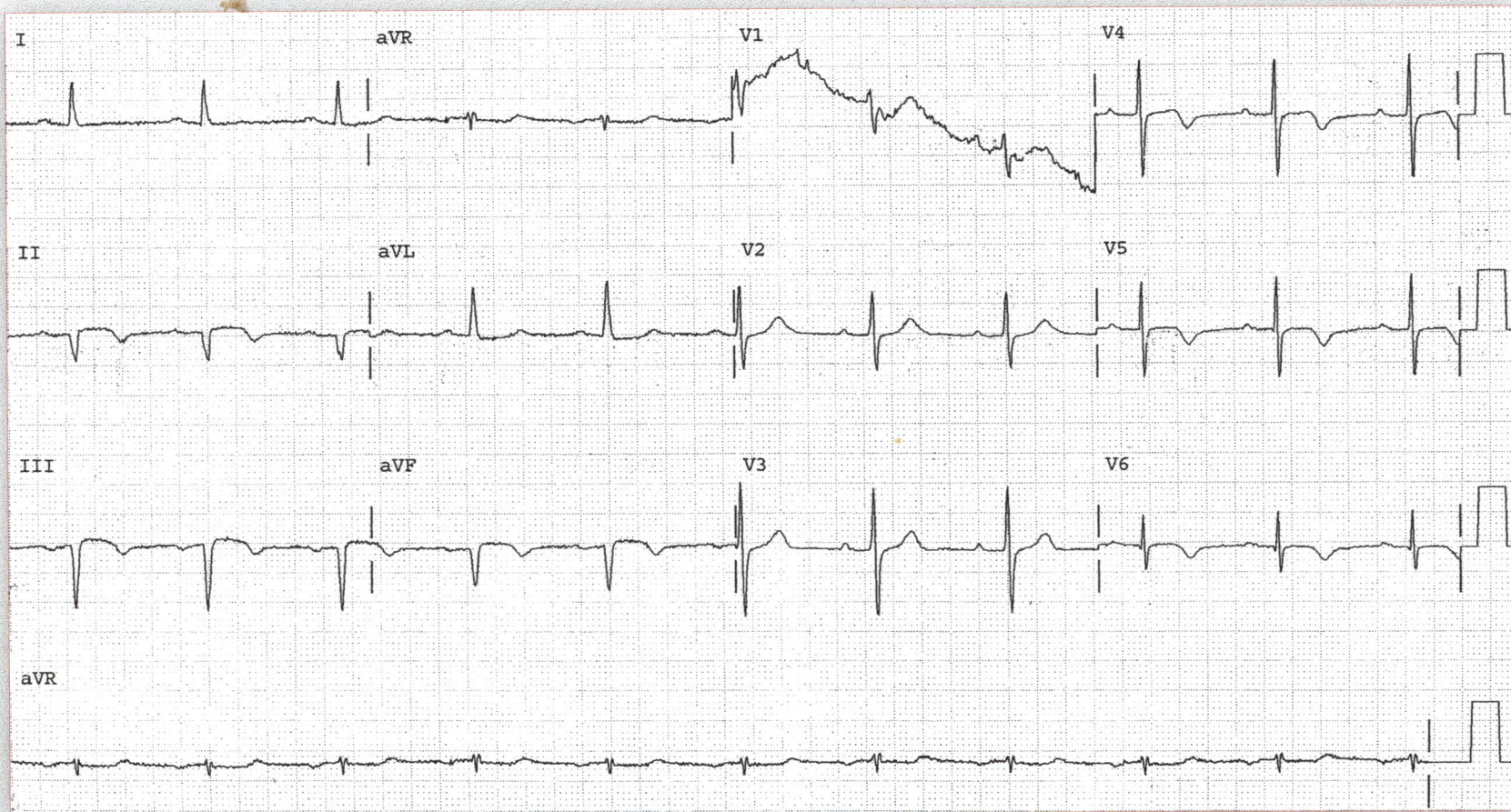

ECG 14 Analysis: Normal sinus rhythm, first-degree AV block, chronic (old) inferior wall MI, counterclockwise rotation

The ECG shows a regular rhythm at a rate of 64 bpm. There is a P wave (+) before each QRS complex, with a stable PR interval (0.22 sec). The P wave is positive in leads I, II, aVF, and V4-V6. Hence this is a sinus rhythm with a first-degree AV block.

The QRS complex duration is normal (0.08 sec), and the axis is extremely leftward, between −30° and −90° (positive QRS complex in lead I and negative QRS complex in leads II and aVF). However, the QRS complex in leads II, III, and aVF has a QS pattern (↓), indicating that the initial electrical forces are going away from the inferior wall. In addition, the T waves are inverted (↑) in these leads. This pattern represents an old or chronic inferior wall myocardial infarction (MI). The QT/QTc intervals are normal (360/370 msec).

Although the QRS complex is positive in lead I and negative in leads II and aVF, this does not represent a conduction abnormality (*ie*, left anterior fascicular block [LAFB], in which the QRS morphology in leads II and aVF would have an rS configuration). In this case the QRS complex has a QS pattern representing an inferior wall MI, which accounts for the left axis in the frontal plane. The diagnosis of an LAFB cannot made in the presence of an inferior wall MI.

Although there is a tall R wave in lead V2 (←), the R wave in lead V1 is not increased in amplitude. Hence this is not indicative of posterior wall involvement. Rather, the tall R wave in lead V2 (R/S > 1) is a result of counterclockwise rotation of the electrical axis in the horizontal plane. This is also called early transition. The axis in the horizontal plane can be determined by imagining the heart as viewed from under the diaphragm. The right ventricle is in front, while the left ventricle is to the left side. When there is counterclockwise rotation, the left ventricular forces are shifted anteriorly and are seen earlier in the precordial leads (*eg*, in lead V2), presenting with a tall R wave in this lead.

Also noted are T-wave inversions in leads V4-V6 (^). T-wave inversions are nonspecific, although in the setting of known coronary artery disease (*ie*, prior inferior wall MI) T-wave inversions are often interpreted as representing ischemia. However, T-wave inversions must be interpreted in association with the clinical situation. ■

A patient comes to your clinic for the first time and reports a history of prior myocardial infarction (MI). You obtain an ECG.

Is an infarction present?

If so, which myocardial territory or territories have been infarcted?

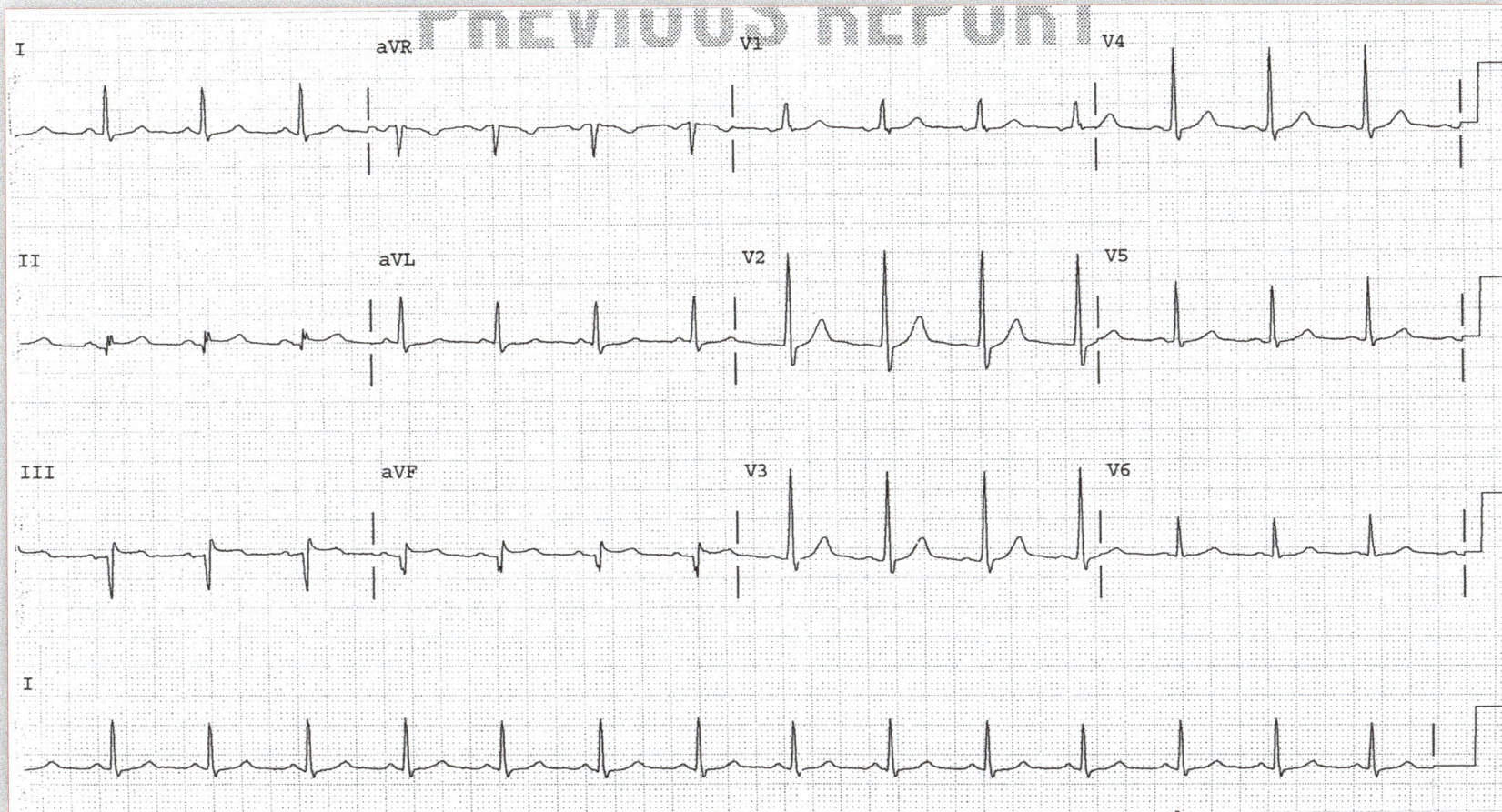

ECG 15 Analysis: Normal sinus rhythm, chronic (old) inferior wall MI, chronic (old) posterior wall MI, counterclockwise rotation

The ECG shows a regular rhythm at a rate of 90 bpm. There is a P wave (+) before each QRS complex, with a stable PR interval (0.16 sec). The P wave is positive in leads I, II, aVF, and V4-V6, indicating a normal sinus rhythm.

The QRS complex duration is normal (0.08 sec), and there is a leftward axis. However, the left axis is the result of significant Q waves (↑) (width of Q waves > 0.04 sec) in leads II, III, and aVF (Qr pattern) that indicate an old inferior wall myocardial infarction (MI). If this leftward axis were the result of a conduction abnormality, the QRS morphology in leads II, III, and aVF would have an rS pattern. In addition, there is a prominent R wave (←) in lead V1 (R/S > 1). When associated with an inferior wall MI, this represents posterior wall involvement. Although the R wave in lead V2 is also tall (→), this is in part the result of counterclockwise electrical rotation in the horizontal plane or early transition, which represents left ventricular forces occurring earlier in the precordial leads. Therefore, the patient has had an inferoposterior MI. The QT/QTc intervals are normal (320/390 msec). ■

A 72-year-old woman presents with worsening dyspnea over the past 2 days. She reports having an episode of nausea, vomiting, shortness of breath, and diaphoresis 2 weeks ago that lasted for 12 hours and then gradually resolved on its own. She also recalls feeling a strange sensation in her chest, described as mild substernal discomfort. Her past medical history is significant for diabetes, and she has no documented heart murmurs. However, on physical examination, she now has a blowing systolic murmur that is loudest at the lower sternal border. An ECG is obtained.

What is the diagnosis on ECG?

What is the likely cause for her dyspnea, and how would you confirm the diagnosis?

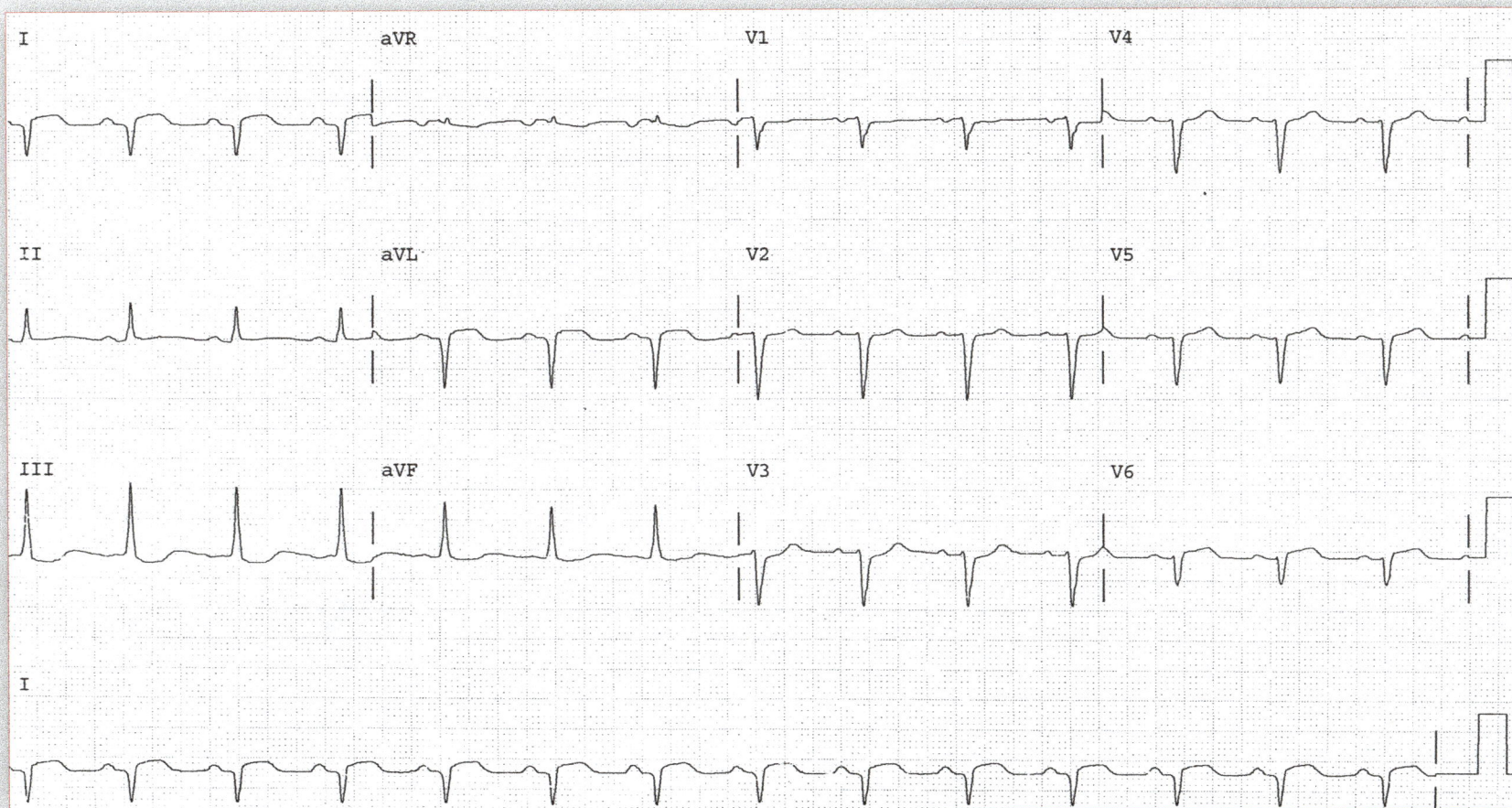

ECG 16 Analysis: Normal sinus rhythm, chronic (old) lateral wall myocardial infarction (MI), chronic (old) anterior wall MI

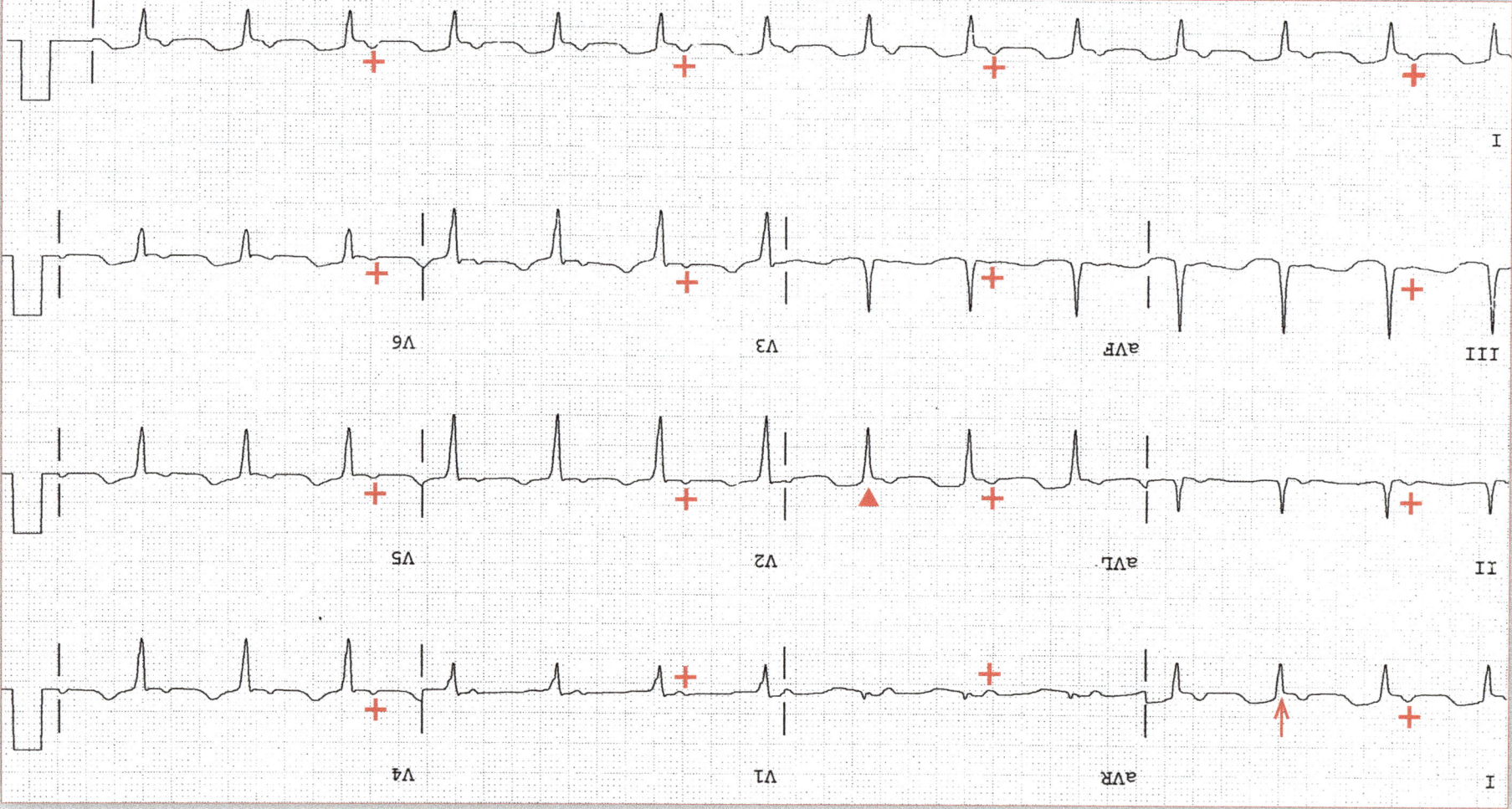

The ECG shows a regular rhythm at a rate of 82 bpm. There is a P wave (+) before each QRS complex, with a stable PR interval (0.18 sec). The P wave is positive in leads I, II, aVF, and V4-V6, indicating a normal sinus rhythm.

The QRS complex duration is normal (0.10 sec), and the axis is rightward, between +90° and +180° (QRS complex is negative in lead I and positive in lead aVF). A number of conditions and situations can cause a rightward axis, including right ventricular hypertrophy (RVH) (associated with a tall R wave in lead V1 and P pulmonale), a lateral wall myocardial infarction (MI) (with Q waves [ie, a QS or Qr morphology] in leads I and aVL), Wolff-Parkinson-White pattern (with a short PR interval and widened QRS complex resulting from a delta wave), right-to-left arm lead switch (associated with a negative P wave in leads I and aVL and a positive P wave and QRS complex in lead aVR), dextrocardia (which resembles right-to-left arm lead switch and is also associated with reverse R-wave progression across the precordium [ie, a tall R wave in lead V1 that becomes progressively shorter going to lead V6]), or a left posterior fascicular block (LPFB) (a diagnosis of exclusion that is established when other causes for a rightward axis have been ruled out).

In this case, there is a negative QRS complex in lead I that is the result of a QS morphology (↓) and not an rS morphology; this is diagnostic for an old or chronic lateral wall MI and not a rightward axis due to a conduction abnormality (eg, LPFB). There is also a QS complex in lead aVL (▼) that further confirms the lateral MI. In addition, the lack of significant R waves in leads V1-V6 is suggestive of an old or chronic anterior wall MI. The QT/QTc intervals are normal (340/400 msec).

The patient has had a large lateral and anterior wall MI, likely 2 weeks ago based on the timing of her described symptoms. Patients with diabetes can often have masking of anginal chest discomfort, and hence have "silent" (without pain or discomfort) ischemia. However, they will still often experience the other symptoms associated with angina, including nausea, vomiting, shortness of shortness of breath, and diaphoresis. Therefore, this is best termed discomfortless (or painless) ischemia.

Mechanical complications of an MI most commonly occur in the 5 to 10 days after infarction when granulation tissue develops. These complications include papillary muscle rupture of the mitral valve leading to severe mitral regurgitation, free wall rupture of the ventricular wall, and ventricular septal defects (VSDs). This patient's murmur is most consistent with a VSD. The diagnosis can be confirmed either with an echocardiogram (using Doppler color flow) or right heart catheterization and measurement of oxygen saturation within the cardiac chambers. A VSD with left-to-right shunting will have an oxygen step-up between the right atrial and right ventricular chambers. Most patients with acute VSD require surgical closure. ■

A patient with shortness of breath describes an episode of chest discomfort 1 week earlier that resolved after 12 hours. Since then, he has had progressive dyspnea on exertion and weight gain. Physical examination demonstrates a loud holosystolic murmur at the lower left sternal border. An ECG is obtained. Cardiac catheterization confirms single-vessel coronary disease.

What is the abnormality on the ECG?

What is the most likely mechanical complication associated with what the patient has experienced?

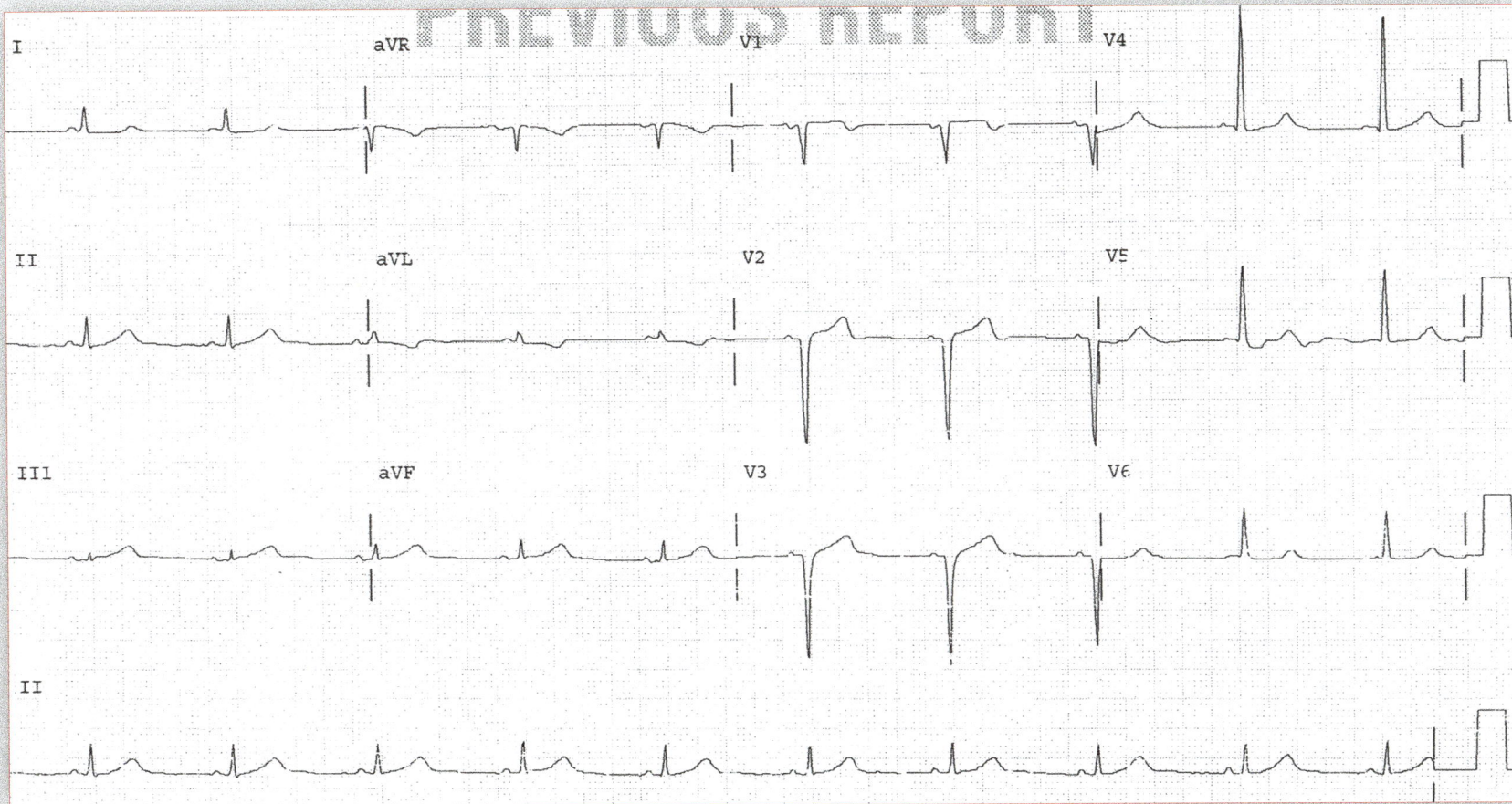

ECG 17 Analysis: Normal sinus rhythm, chronic (old) anteroseptal myocardial infarction

The ECG shows a regular rhythm at a rate of 60 bpm. There is a P wave (+) before each QRS complex, with a stable PR interval (0.14 sec). The P wave is positive in leads I, II, aVF, and V4-V6. The QRS complex duration is normal (0.08 sec), and the axis is normal, between 0° and +90° (the QRS complex is positive in leads I and aVF). The QT/QTc intervals are normal (440/440 msec).

The major finding is the presence of QS complexes in leads V1-V3 (↓), which are diagnostic for a myocardial infarction of the anteroseptal wall of the left ventricle. The QS complex indicates that all of the ventricular forces are directed away from leads V1-V3, meaning that the myocardium beneath these leads is electrically silent (*ie*, infarcted). This is consistent with an infarction in the territory of the left anterior descending artery. The most likely diagnosis is a mechanical complication (*ie*, a ventricular septal defect [VSD] of the apical septum). Other mechanical complications include rupture of the posteromedial papillary muscle, which is supplied by the posterior descending artery. This is usually associated with an inferior wall infarction. Rupture of the anterolateral papillary muscle is less common as this structure typically receives dual supply from the left anterior descending and circumflex arteries. It is, therefore, less likely to rupture in the setting of single-vessel disease. Conversely, VSDs are more likely to occur in patients with one-vessel disease since they have not developed an extensive degree of collateral circulation. Other risk factors for post–myocardial infarction VSD include large infarct sizes and ventricular aneurysm formation. An infarct in the territory of the left anterior descending artery will cause a VSD in the apical septum. Inferior infarcts will result in a VSD of the basal septum. ■

Notes

A 42-year-old man with no cardiac risk factors is brought to the emergency department by his wife, who states that he had acute-onset substernal chest pressure. She says that over the past 2 weeks he has had a viral syndrome with upper respiratory symptoms, fever, and myalgia.

On physical examination, his blood pressure is noted to be 70/palp, his neck veins are distended, and he is confused and disoriented. An arterial line is placed showing a systolic blood pressure ranging from 65 to 85 mm Hg, which varies with respiration. An ECG is obtained.

What is the most likely diagnosis?

Does the patient need to go to the cardiac catheterization lab?

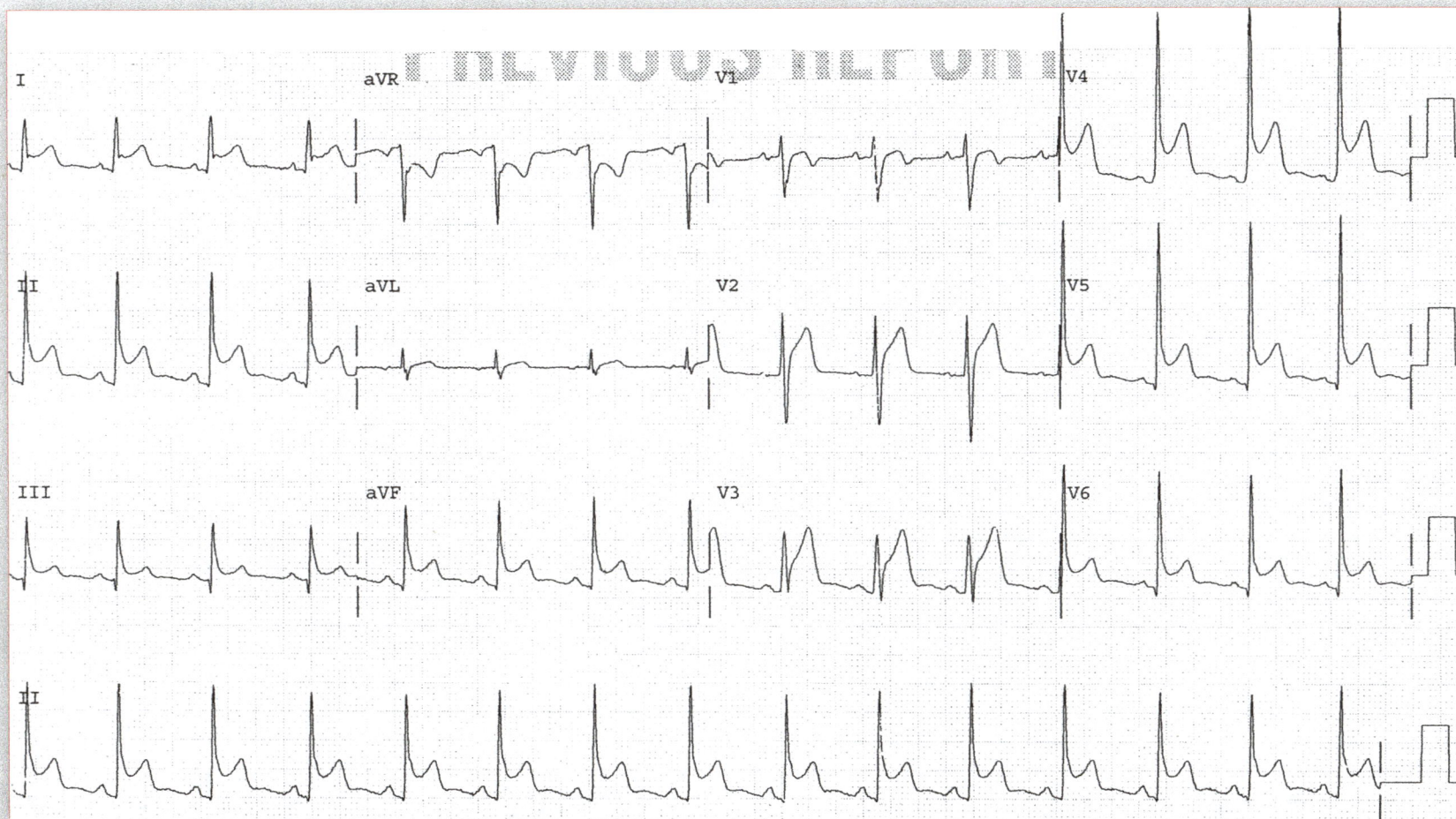

ECG 18 Analysis: Normal sinus rhythm, ST-segment elevation due to acute pericarditis

The ECG shows a regular rhythm at a rate of 88 bpm. There is P wave before each QRS complex (+), and the PR interval (0.16 sec) is stable. The P wave is positive in leads I, II, aVF, and V4-V6.

The QRS complex duration is normal (0.08 sec), and the axis is normal, between 0° and +90° (positive QRS complex in leads I and aVF). The QT/QTc intervals are normal (280/340 msec). There is widespread J-point (↑) and ST-segment elevation (▼) involving all leads except aVL; the ST-segment depression in lead aVR (▲) is actually ST-segment elevation. There are no reciprocal ST-segment depressions. The J point is elevated, up to 6 mm in lead V4, and the ST segment maintains its normal concave morphology. Also noted is the fact that the T waves retain their normal asymmetric pattern (*ie*, slower in upstroke and more rapid in downstroke). This ECG pattern is diagnostic for pericarditis, which also involves the epicardial pericardium and the surface of the myocardium (*ie*, there is an associated myocarditis). Although not always seen in pericarditis, there is evidence of PR-segment depression in leads II and aVF (^). There is also evidence of left ventricular hypertrophy (LVH), with an R wave in lead V5 that is 28 mm in height ([ ).

The ECG findings associated with pericarditis include:

- Diffuse ST-segment elevation. The ST segments maintain a normal concave morphology regardless of the height of ST-segment elevation or the duration of symptoms. There is no reciprocal ST-segment depression.
- The T waves are normal (*ie*, asymmetric).

- PR interval depression may be seen.
- T-wave inversion may occur after ST segments return to isoelectric baseline.

The changes with pericarditis should be distinguished from those seen with an acute myocardial infarction, in which the ST-segment elevation is localized; the ST-segment morphology becomes concave, merging with the T wave; T waves early on are often symmetric in configuration; and reciprocal ST-segment depressions are usually seen in other leads.

There is no indication for a coronary angiogram in the setting of acute pericarditis. However, hemodynamic instability and hypotension may occur, often due to a large pericardial effusion resulting in tamponade. Physical examination findings of tamponade include jugular venous distention, muffled heart sounds, and hypotension (Beck's triad) as well as pulsus paradoxus, which is a drop in systolic blood pressure of more than 10 mm Hg during inspiration. This patient does have pulsus paradoxus and most likely has tamponade. This could be confirmed on echocardiography, which would show a large pericardial effusion, right atrial and right ventricular diastolic collapse, and right and left ventricular interdependence. With inspiration, the right ventricular dimensions increase and there is increased flow across the tricuspid valve while the left ventricular dimensions decrease and there is decreased flow across the mitral valve. With expiration, the findings are reversed. If a large effusion and tamponade are confirmed, the patient will need to go to the cardiac catheterization lab urgently for drainage of his pericardial effusion. ■

A 40-year-old man presents to the emergency department with left-sided chest and shoulder pain. He reports that he was lifting heavy furniture over the past few days and may have "overdone it." His only medical history is hypertension, for which he takes a thiazide diuretic. Physical examination is normal except for a blood pressure of 170/90 mm Hg. An ECG is obtained.

What is the most likely diagnosis?

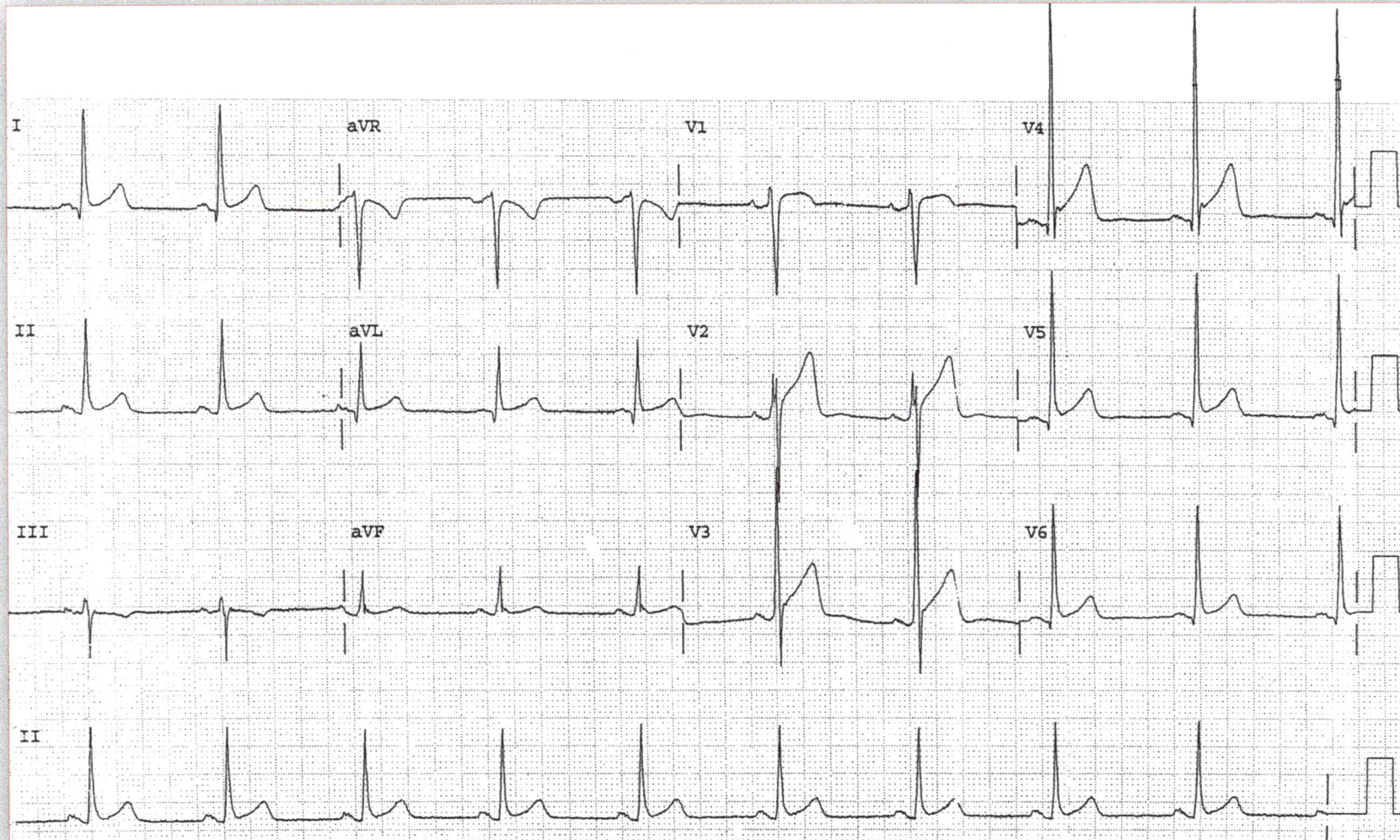

ECG 19 Analysis: Sinus bradycardia, left ventricular hypertrophy (LVH), early repolarization

The ECG shows regular rhythm at a rate of 54 bpm. There is a P wave (+) before each QRS complex, and the PR interval is stable (0.16 sec). The P wave is positive in leads I, II, aVF, and V4-V6. Therefore, this is a sinus bradycardia.

The QRS complex duration is normal (0.08 sec), and the axis is normal, between 0° and +90° (positive QRS complex in leads I and aVF). The QT/QTc intervals are normal (400/380 msec). There is markedly increased R-wave voltage seen in leads V3-V5 ( ]) (up to 40 mm in lead V4), which is characteristic of left ventricular hypertrophy (LVH). However, body habitus needs to be considered, and this might be a normal QRS amplitude in a young subject who is thin and has no lung disease. Also noted is J-point and ST-segment elevation (↑), particularly in leads V2-V5. In association with the prominent QRS complex amplitude, this pattern is termed early repolarization. It is often seen in the precordial leads in the presence of LVH, although it may also be present in younger patients who do not have LVH. It is a normal variant, although has occasionally been diagnosed as an early acute myocardial infarction when the ST-segment changes are very marked and the patient presents with chest pain. However, the presence of asymmetric T waves and the absence of reciprocal ST-segment depressions make the diagnosis of an acute myocardial infarction unlikely. ■

A routine ECG is obtained in an asymptomatic 30-year-old woman.

Is the ECG characteristic of ischemia?

What is the QT interval?

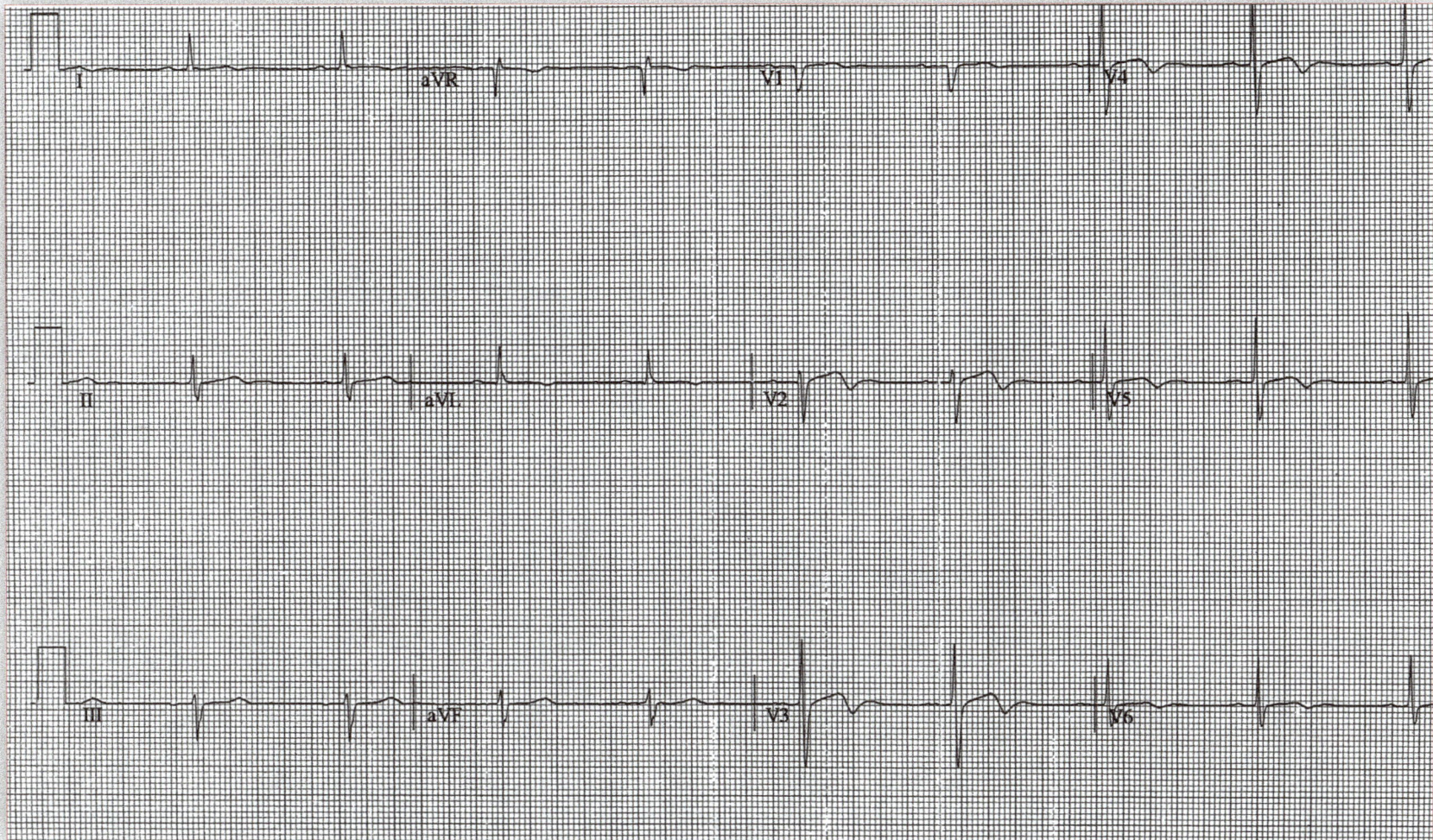

ECG 20 Analysis: Sinus bradycardia, left axis, nonspecific T-wave abnormalities

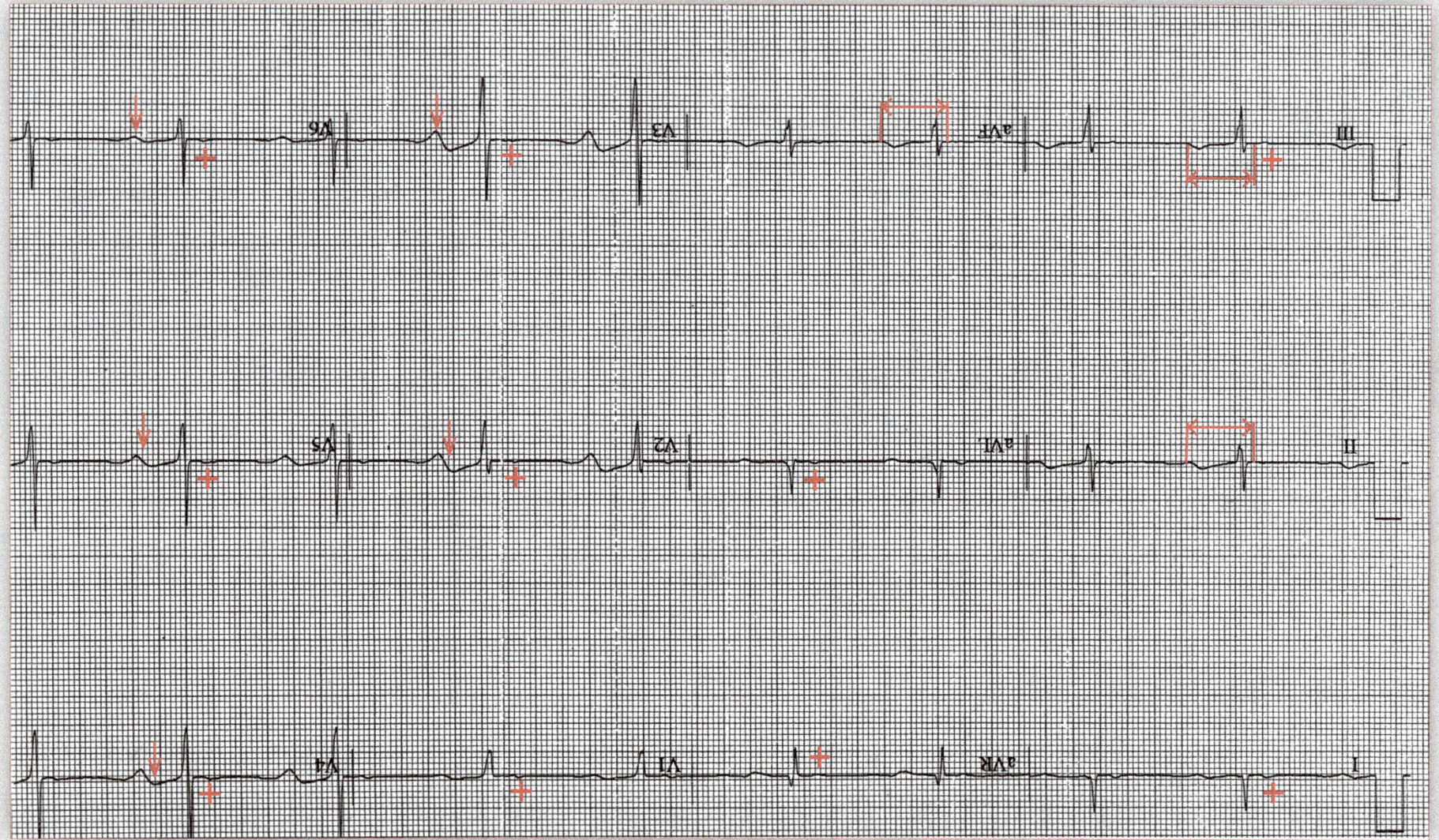

The ECG shows a regular rhythm at a rate of 54 bpm. There are P waves (+) before each QRS complex, with a stable PR interval (0.16 sec). The P waves are positive in leads I, II, aVF, and V4-V6. Therefore, this is a sinus bradycardia.

The QRS axis is between 0° and −30° (positive QRS complex in leads I and II, negative QRS complex in lead aVF), which represents a physiologic left axis. Although the QRS voltage in the limb leads is low, the criterion for low voltage is not met (ie, QRS complex < 5 mm in amplitude in each lead). Biphasic T waves (↑) are noted in leads V2-V6 (positive-negative); these are nonspecific T-wave abnormalities. Although of no particular importance, such abnormalities do affect the ability to accurately establish the QT interval, which should be measured in the lead in which a normal-looking T wave is seen and a distinct end of the T wave can be identified. In this case the best lead to use would be II, III, or aVF. The QT interval (↔) is 440 msec, or 420 msec when corrected for heart rate. Of note, in asymptomatic individuals, T-wave inversions or biphasic T waves can often represent normal variants. However, one must also consider pathologic etiologies, including coronary artery disease, hypertrophic cardiomyopathy, evolving pericarditis, and electrolyte abnormalities. T-wave abnormalities should be interpreted in association with the clinical picture of the patient. In the absence of a clinical story to suggest ischemia, the T-wave changes are "nonspecific." ◼

Notes

A 52-year-old woman comes for a clinic visit complaining of occasional palpitations. An ECG is obtained.

What is the most likely etiology for her symptoms?

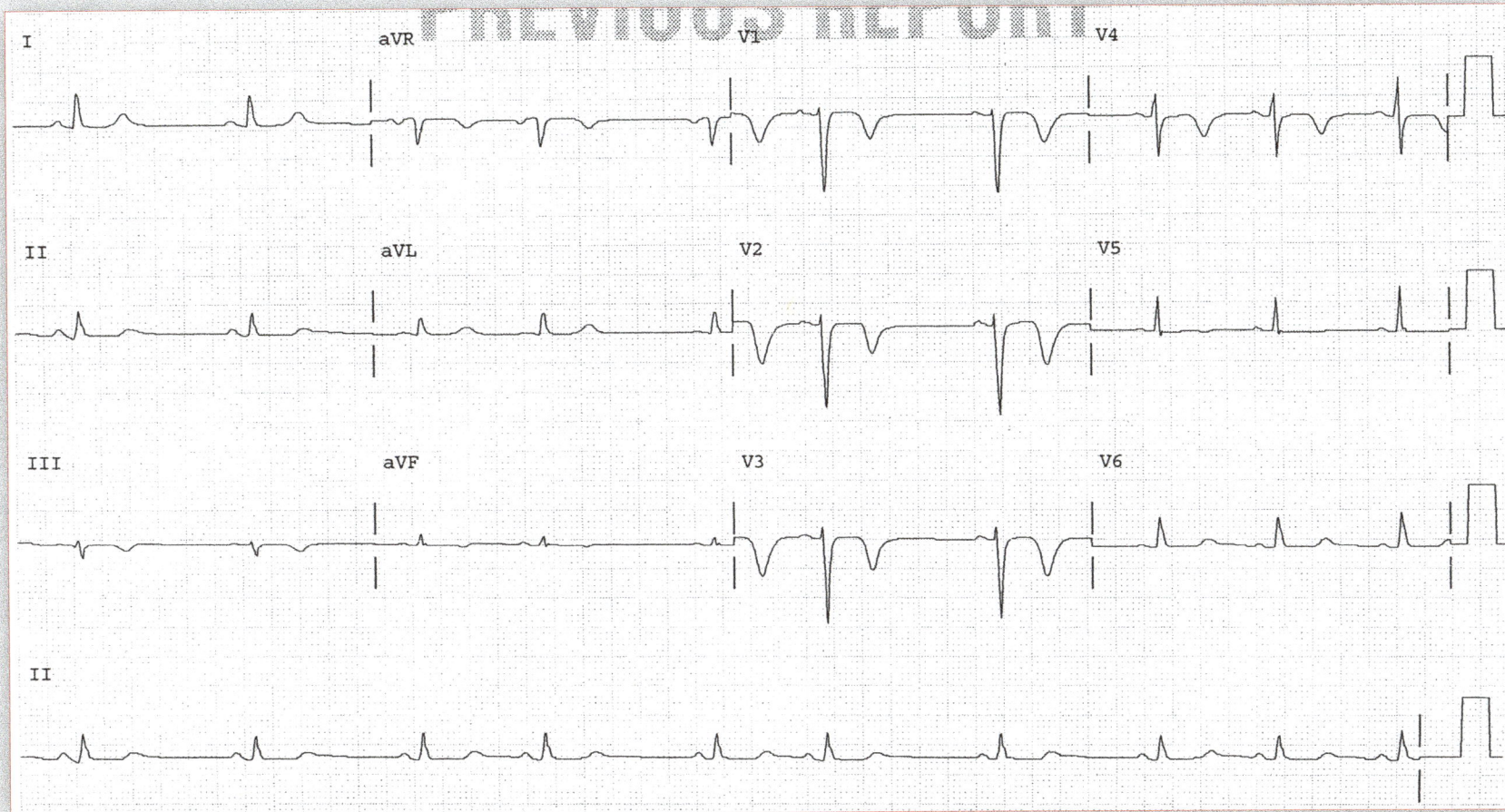

I aVR V1 V4

II aVL V2 V5

III aVF V3 V6

II

ECG 21 Analysis: Sinus bradycardia, premature atrial complexes, nonspecific T-wave changes, clockwise rotation

The ECG shows a regularly irregular rhythm at a rate of 50 bpm. The irregularity results from several early or premature QRS complexes (fourth, sixth, ninth, and 10th). The QRS complex duration is normal (0.08 sec), and the axis as normal, between 0° and +90°. The QT/QTc intervals are normal (480/440 msec). There is low voltage in the limb leads (< 5 mm in each lead). There are P waves (+) before each QRS complex, with a stable PR interval (0.16 sec). The P wave is positive in leads I, II, aVF, and V4-V6. Hence this is a sinus bradycardia.

However, as indicated, the rhythm is not regular as there are occasional early or premature P waves (*) and QRS complexes associated with a shorter RR interval (complexes 4, 6, 9, and 10). Although irregular, there is a pattern to the irregularity in that all of the shorter RR intervals are the same (⊔) and all of the longer intervals (⊓) are the same. Hence this is said to be regularly irregular. The early QRS complexes have a P wave (*) before them, and there are very subtle differences in the P-wave morphology when compared with the sinus P waves; this is seen best in leads aVF and V1-V6. Hence the early P waves and QRS complexes are called premature atrial complexes, and since the P-wave morphology is very similar to the sinus P waves they are originating very close to the sinus node.

Premature atrial premature complexes can often be symptomatic and cause the feeling of palpitations. The sensation of palpitations is not a result of the premature complex, however, but rather is due to the fact that after the premature complex there is a variable pause (longer RR interval) and a longer period of diastole during which there is continued left ventricular filling. Hence with the next sinus complex and ventricular contraction there is increased contractility and stroke volume (via the Starling effect) that accounts for the sensation of palpitations (post-extrasystolic potentiation). In this patient, it would be reasonable to obtain an event monitor in order to correlate her symptoms with any rhythm disturbance, such as frequent premature atrial complexes, or with other associated arrhythmias that may be initiated by these premature complexes, such as atrial tachycardia, atrial flutter, or atrial fibrillation.

In addition, asymmetric T-wave inversions can be seen in leads V1-V4 (^) along with flat T waves in leads aVF and V5 (▲). In the absence of any clinical history or other ECG changes, these T-wave inversions are nonspecific.

Lastly, there is poor R-wave progression from leads V1-V3 with late transition (R/S ratio becomes > 1) seen in lead V5. This is indicative of clockwise electrical rotation in the horizontal plane, determined by imagining the heart as viewed from under the diaphragm. With clockwise rotation the left ventricular forces are shifted posteriorly and are seen in the more lateral precordial leads. Poor R-wave progression may also be seen in women as a result of attenuation of forces, possibly as a result of breast tissue. ■

Which of the following is this patient most likely *not* to have?

A. Untreated hypertension
B. Critical aortic stenosis
C. Severe mitral regurgitation
D. Hypertrophic cardiomyopathy

ECG 22 Analysis: Normal sinus rhythm, left anterior fascicular block, counterclockwise rotation, ST-segment depression due to subendocardial ischemia

The ECG shows a regular rhythm at a rate of 68 bpm. There is a P wave (+) before each QRS complex, with a stable PR interval (0.16 sec). The P wave is positive in leads I, II, aVF, and V4-V6. Hence this is a normal sinus rhythm.

The QRS complex duration is normal (0.10 sec), and the axis is extremely leftward, between −30° and −90° (positive QRS complex in leads I and II and negative QRS complex in lead aVF). Because the complexes in leads II and aVF have an rS morphology, the leftward axis is not the result of an inferior wall myocardial infarction (in which there would be a QS or Qr morphology) but rather is the result of left anterior fascicular block, a conduction abnormality. In addition, there is a tall R wave in lead V2 (←), a result of early transition or counterclockwise rotation in the horizontal plane. This is established by imagining the heart as viewed from under the diaphragm. With counterclockwise rotation, the left ventricular forces are shifted anteriorly and are apparent earlier in the precordial leads (*ie*, the tall R wave in lead V2 [←]).

However, the amplitude of the QRS complex in lead V2 is increased (R wave = 30 mm), which likely represents left ventricular hypertrophy (LVH). The QT/QTc intervals (↔) are prolonged (520/550 msec).

The major finding, however, is the presence of diffuse, symmetric, deeply inverted T waves in leads II, III, aVF, and V3-V6 (^). The positive T wave in lead aVR (•) is actually T-wave inversion. In addition, there is J-point depression (▼) and downsloping ST-segment depression (↑). In this situation the symmetric T-wave inversions as well as the prolongation of the QT interval are reflective of diffuse subendocardial ischemia, which is likely the result of LVH. The presence of subendocardial ischemia may be the cause of the QT prolongation. The most common causes of LVH include uncontrolled hypertension, aortic stenosis, and hypertrophic cardiomyopathy. Mitral regurgitation results in a dilated left ventricle, which can often result in similar ST-segment and T-wave abnormalities but normally without the prominent voltages of LVH. ■

A 46-year-old man with polycystic kidney disease presents with new-onset left arm weakness and headache. The following ECG is obtained.

What is the most likely etiology of the abnormal findings?

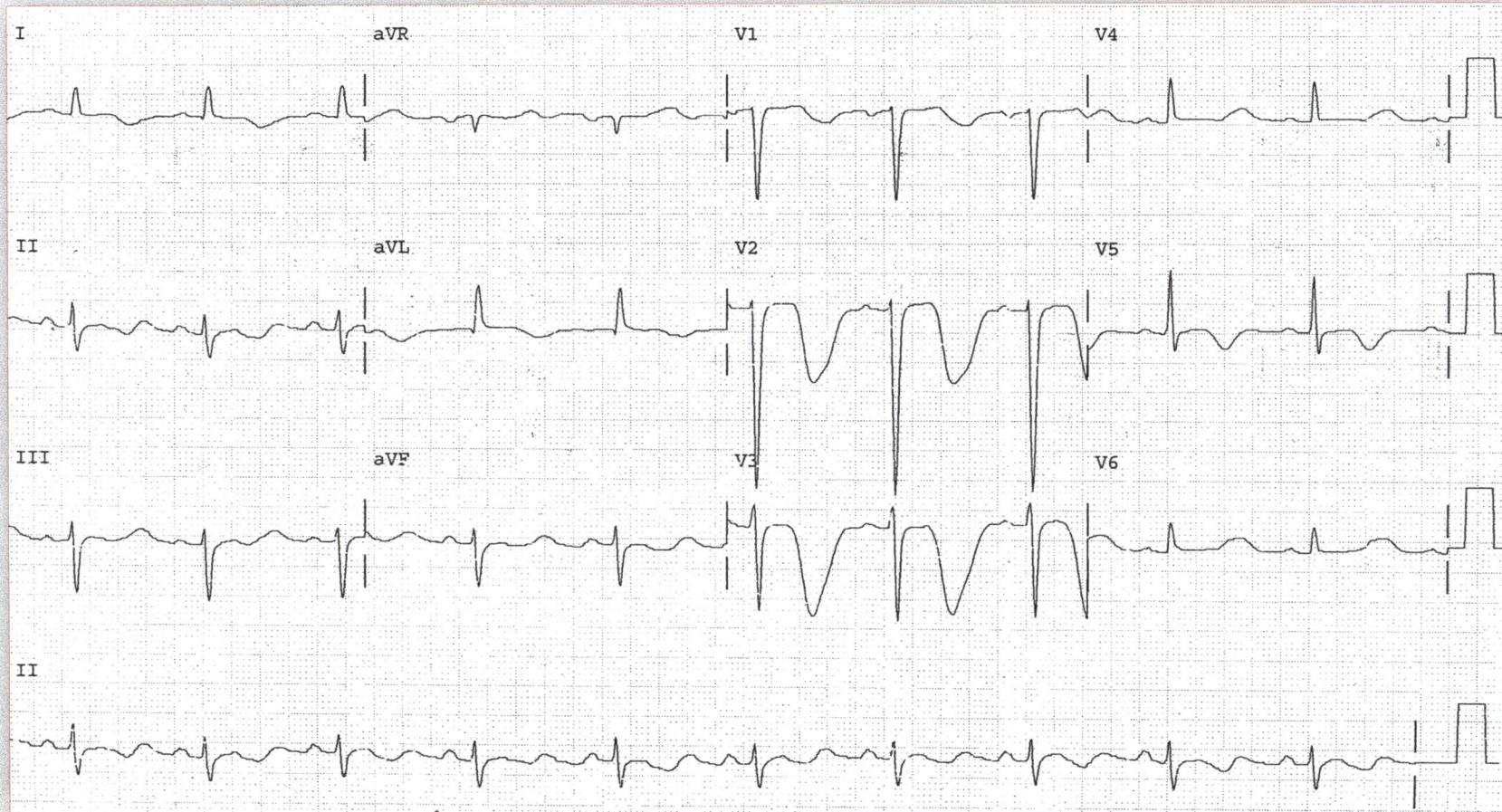

ECG 23 Analysis: Normal sinus rhythm, left axis, cerebral T waves, QT prolongation

The ECG shows a regular rhythm at a rate of 62 bpm. There is a P wave (+) before each QRS complex, with a stable PR interval (0.16 sec). The P wave is positive in leads I, II, aVF, and V4-V6. Hence this is a normal sinus rhythm. The axis is leftward and the QRS complex is positive in lead I, negative in lead aVF, and isoelectric in lead II, indicating that the axis is −30°. The major finding is prominent deep T-wave inversions in leads V1-V3 (↑). The T waves are asymmetric, with a more rapid upstroke and slower downstroke (the reverse of the normal T-wave morphology). Also present is significant prolongation of the QT/QTc intervals (↔) (620/630 msec). This is a pattern often seen with an intracerebral process, such as a subarachnoid or intracerebral hemorrhage, and the T waves are termed cerebral T waves. The QT interval prolongation is the result of autonomic imbalance. About 5% to 10% of patients with polycystic kidney disease have cerebral aneurysms. ■

A 57-year-old woman with a history of intermittent lightheadedness presents to the emergency department after having a syncopal episode. She denies any prodromal symptoms. An ECG is obtained while the patient is feeling dizzy.

What is the most likely diagnosis?

How should you treat this patient?

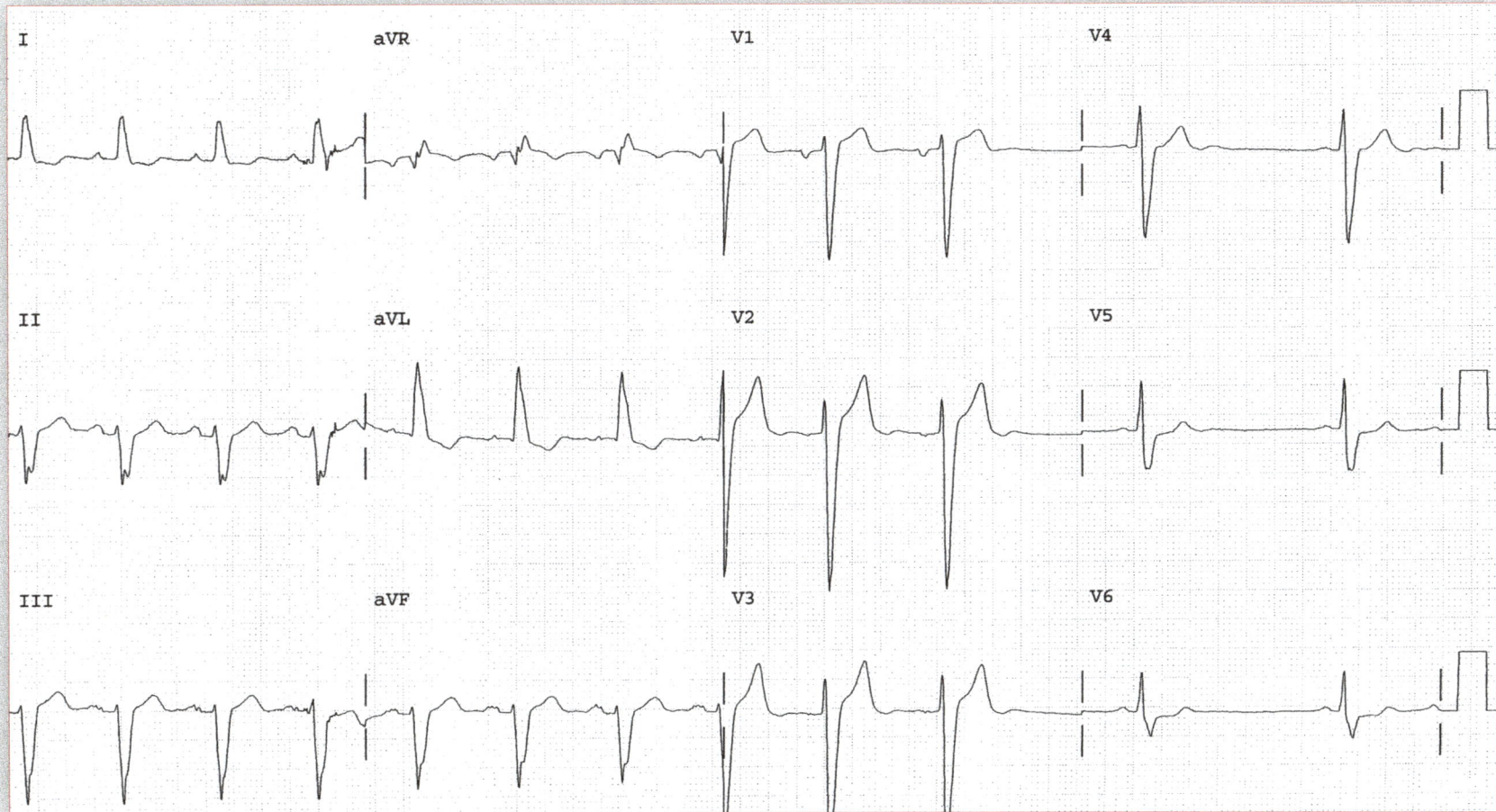

ECG 24 Analysis: Normal sinus rhythm, intraventricular conduction delay (IVCD), left anterior fascicular block, sinus node exit block

The ECG shows a regularly irregular rhythm at a rate of 84 bpm. There is a P wave (+) before each QRS complex, and the PR interval is stable (0.18 sec). The P wave is positive in leads I, II, aVF, and V4-V6. Hence this is a normal sinus rhythm. The QRS complex is widened (0.14 sec), but there is no specific pattern (there is a tall, broad R wave in lead I [→], suggesting left bundle branch block, but also terminal S waves in leads V5-V6 [←], suggesting right bundle branch block). Hence this is considered an intraventricular conduction delay (IVCD).

There is an important difference between a bundle branch block and an IVCD. With a bundle branch block, activation of the ventricle served by the affected bundle is no longer via the normal conduction system but rather by impulse conduction through an abnormal pathway and direct myocardial activation. Therefore, abnormalities affecting that ventricle cannot be interpreted. In contrast, an IVCD is diffuse slowing of conduction via the normal His-Purkinje system. As ventricular activation is still via the normal conduction pathway, abnormalities of the involved ventricle can be established. In this case, the axis is very leftward (between −30° and −90°), with a positive QRS complex in lead I and negative QRS complexes in leads II and aVF (rS morphology). This is a left anterior fascicular block, which can be diagnosed with an IVCD but could not be diagnosed if there was a true left bundle branch block. The QT/QTc intervals are prolonged (400/470 msec) but are normal after accounting for the prolonged QRS interval (340/400 msec).

The rhythm is regularly irregular as there are two long (and similar) RR intervals between the 10th, 11th, and 12th QRS complexes (⊓). The long RR intervals are the result of an abrupt slowing of the heart rate to 42 bpm. There is no evidence for a nonconducted P wave during the pause; this is termed a sinus pause. This type of sinus node abnormality can be a manifestation of either abnormal impulse formation (*ie*, sinus node arrest) or abnormal impulse propagation (*ie*, sinus node exit block). In this case, the PP interval around the pause is equal to two sinus intervals (⊔) and hence is termed sinus node exit block. The sinus node has discharged on time, but the impulse fails to propagate out of the sinus node area and does not activate the atrium, hence the absence of a P wave. Since the sinus node rate is unaffected, the next sinus impulse is on time and does activate the atrium, maintaining the regularity of the PP intervals.

continues

Another cause for a sinus node pause is termed a sinus node arrest. In this situation the sinus node fails to generate an impulse. Therefore, there is no relationship between the PP interval around the pause and the underlying sinus interval. The pause may be shorter than or longer than two sinus intervals. A pause that is longer than two sinus intervals may be indicative of underlying sinus node dysfunction, termed sick sinus syndrome.

A sinus node pause generally is transient, so there is usually no reason for any therapy. However, if there are continuous sinus node pauses, resulting in symptoms, therapy would involve atropine, isoproterenol, or a temporary pacemaker. In the absence of a reversible etiology, such as a medication effect, symptomatic sinus node disease that is persistently manifested (*ie*, a continuous symptomatic sinus bradycardia) is a class I indication for a permanent pacemaker. If this were an incidental finding in an asymptomatic patient, then no pacemaker would be indicated. However, sinus node dysfunction in an asymptomatic individual with a heart rate less than 40 bpm while awake is a class IIa indication for placement of a permanent pacemaker. ■

A 74-year-old man with known coronary artery disease is admitted to the hospital with atrial fibrillation and a rapid ventricular response. In addition to his known regimen of aspirin, β-blocker, and statin, he is prescribed verapamil for rate control. The next day, he begins to complain of intermittent dizziness. An ECG is obtained while the patient is symptomatic.

What is the most likely cause of the patient's dizziness?

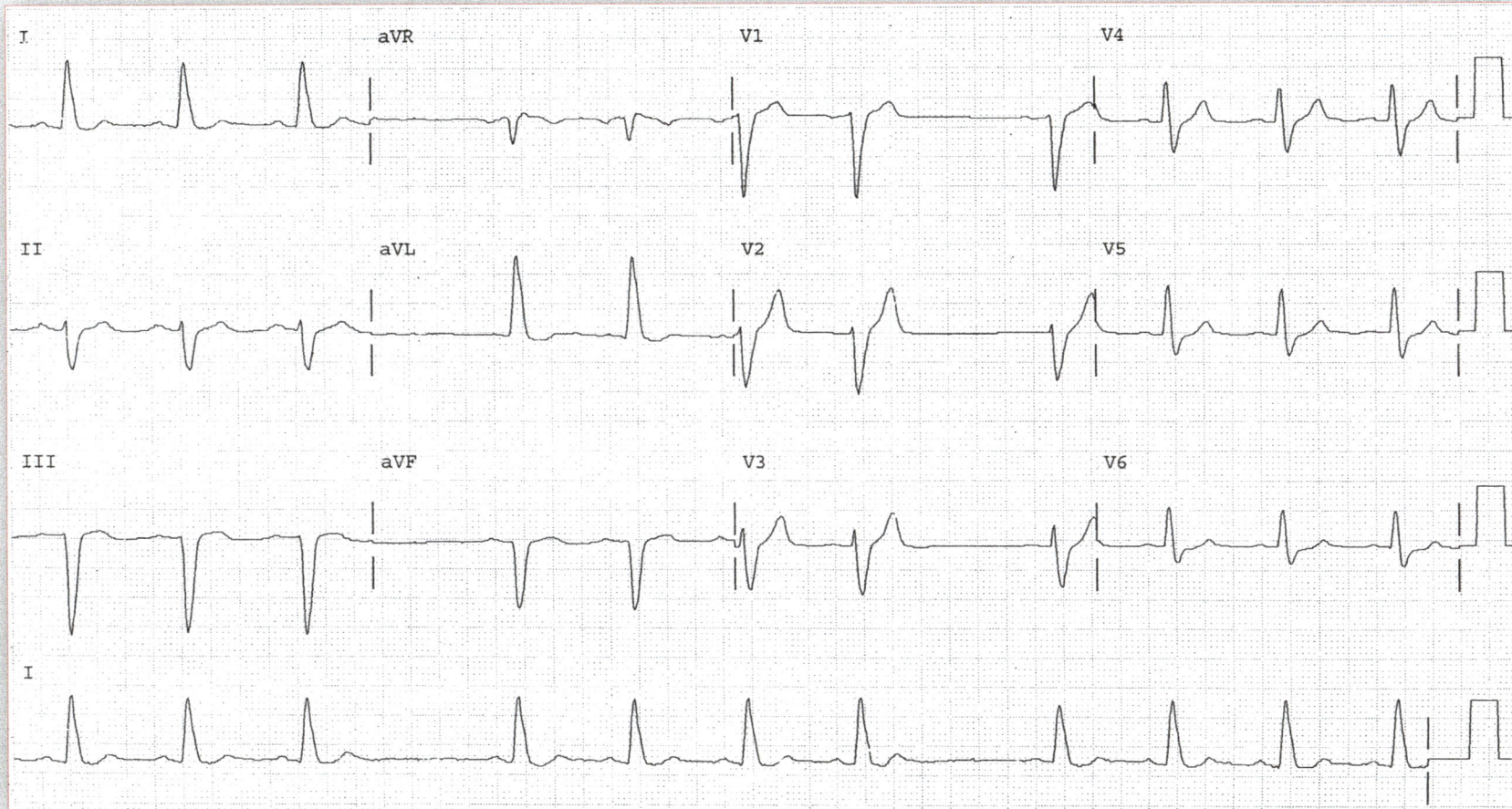

ECG 25 Analysis: Normal sinus rhythm, intraventricular conduction delay (IVCD), left anterior fascicular block (LAFB), sinus node arrest

The ECG shows an irregular rhythm at a rate of 76 bpm. There is a P wave (+) before each QRS complex, with a stable PR interval (0.20 sec). The P wave is positive in leads I, II, VF, and V4-V6. Hence this is a sinus rhythm.

The axis is extremely leftward (between −30° and −90°), and the QRS complex is positive in lead I but negative in leads II and aVF. The QRS complex is wide (0.16 sec), with a tall, broad R wave in leads I and V5-V6 (←), a wide QS complex in lead V1 (→), and no septal forces. This is characteristic of a left bundle branch block (LBBB). However, there are terminal S waves (left-to-right forces) in leads V5-V6 (↑), which suggests a right bundle branch block. Left-to-right forces are not seen in an LBBB. Hence this is an intraventricular conduction delay (IVCD). In this situation there is only diffuse slowing of conduction through the normal His-Purkinje system and no block in the left bundle. With an IVCD conduction is through the normal conducting system; it is just slower. Therefore, abnormalities of the left ventricle can be diagnosed. With an LBBB, left ventricular activation is not via the normal conduction system but directly through the myocardium, and hence left ventricular abnormalities cannot reliably be diagnosed. As an LBBB is not present, the extreme left axis is the result of a left anterior fascicular block (LAFB); if there were an LBBB, the diagnosis of LAFB would not be appropriate as both fascicles would be affected. The QT/QTc intervals are normal (360/410 sec).

The irregularity of the rhythm is due to two pauses (⊔) in the rhythm with absence of atrial activity or a P wave. These are termed sinus pauses. The PP interval of the pause is unrelated to the underlying sinus interval (⊓) (ie, it is shorter than two PP intervals). The PP intervals are otherwise fixed. This is termed sinus node arrest as the sinus node has failed to discharge but resumes its activity after a variable time. This may be an early manifestation of underlying sinus node dysfunction (ie, sick sinus syndrome).

The most likely cause of the patient's rhythm disturbance is polypharmacy. The combination of β-blocker and calcium-channel blocker can lead to significant bradyarrhythmias involving either the sinus or AV node. At this point, nodal agents should be withheld. However, if these agents are needed to control tachyarrhythmia, then this is a class I indication for a permanent pacemaker if the sinus node pauses are continuous and associated with symptoms or if the pauses become longer, indicating an underlying sick sinus syndrome.

It should be noted that ischemia is not the cause of sinus node abnormalities. The sinus and AV nodes generate an action potential that is based on calcium ion fluxes, which are energy independent and do not require an energy-dependent ATPase pump. Hence sinus and AV nodal activity is unaffected by ischemia. ■

A 62-year-old man with no cardiac history presents for a routine physical examination. An ECG is obtained as part of his evaluation.

Has this patient had an anterior myocardial infarction?

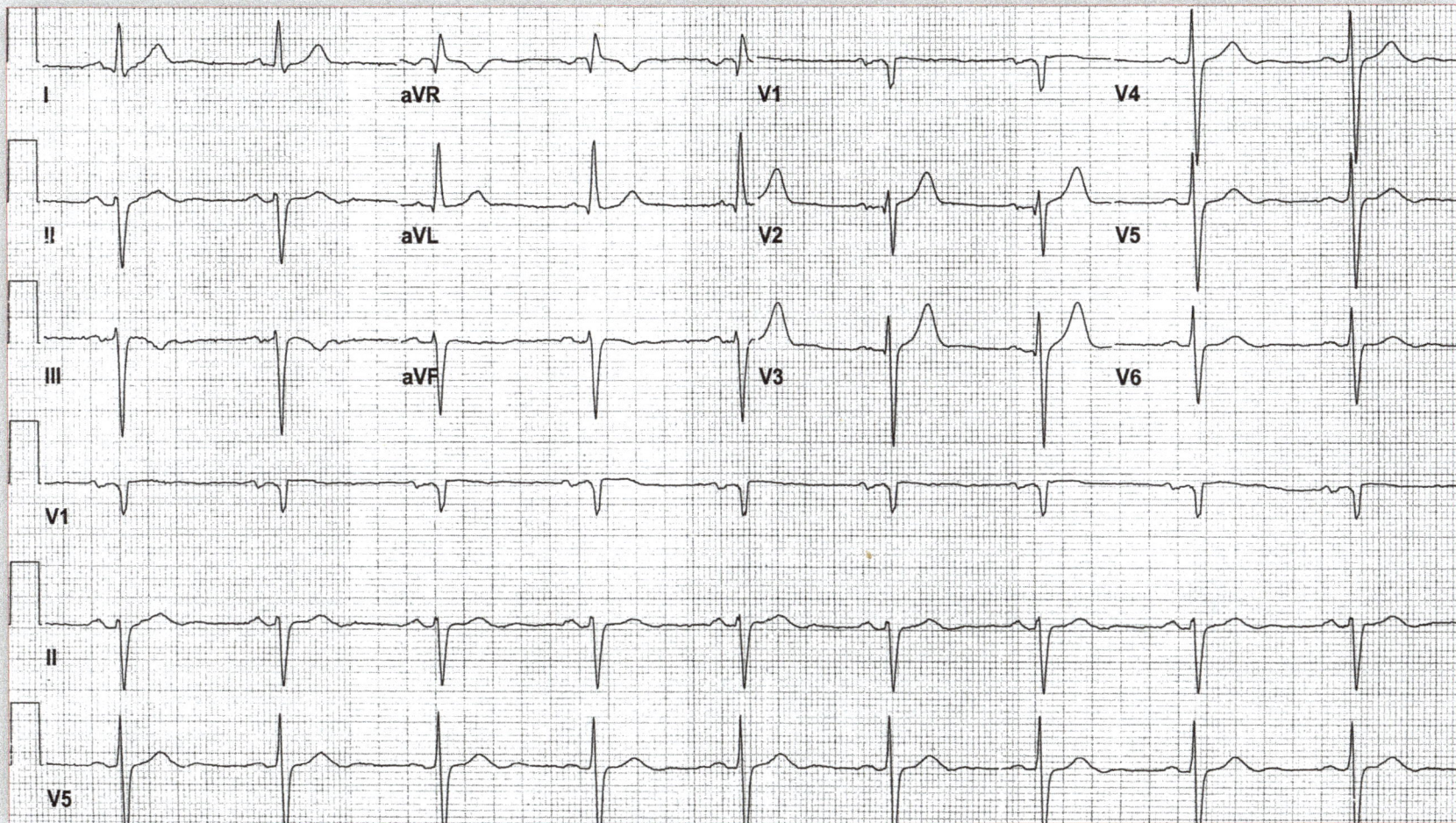

ECG 26 Analysis: Sinus bradycardia, intraventricular conduction delay (IVCD), left anterior fascicular block (LAFB)

The ECG shows a regular rhythm at a rate of 56 bpm. There is a P wave (+) before each QRS complex, and the PR interval is stable (0.18 sec). The P wave is positive in leads I, II, aVF, and V4-V6. Hence this is a sinus bradycardia.

The QRS complex duration is prolonged (0.12 sec). There is no pattern typical for a left or right bundle branch block; hence this is an intraventricular conduction delay (IVCD). The QT/QTc intervals are normal (400/350 msec). The axis is extremely leftward, between –30° and –90° (QRS complex is positive in lead I and negative in leads II and aVF with an rS morphology). This is called a left anterior fascicular block (LAFB), or hemiblock. The left bundle, which activates the left ventricle, divides into a minor fascicle (a median or septal branch that innervates the intraventricular septum) and two major fascicles, the left anterior and left posterior fascicle. The left anterior fascicle innervates the base of the left ventricle, while the left posterior fascicle travels along the inferior portion of the left ventricle. In the presence of an LAFB, activation of the left ventricle is via the left posterior fascicle and the direction of activation is upward and toward the left, producing the extreme leftward axis. There is no major delay in left ventricular activation and hence a fascicular block does not cause any IVCD (ie, the QRS duration is normal). When a wide QRS complex is present there is also an IVCD.

It is important to distinguish between an extreme left axis due to LAFB, in which the QRS complex has an rS morphology in leads II and aVF, and an inferior wall myocardial infarction, in which the QRS complex has a Qr morphology.

Small Q waves are noted in leads V2-V3 (↑). Although it has been suggested that any anterior Q waves represent a myocardial infarction, such small anterior Q waves may instead represent block of the septal branch of the left bundle. This may portend the development of a complete LBBB, which may be more likely in a patient who also has an LAFB.

Fascicular blocks are often due to idiopathic conduction system disease (called Lev's or Lenègre's disease), which results in fibrosis or a calcificofibrosis of the bundles. They may be due to ischemic heart disease with prior infarction and fibrosis of the conduction system, idiopathic cardiomyopathy with diffuse fibrosis of the myocardium, hypertension, or drugs that may alter conduction through the His-Purkinje system. Fascicular blocks may be permanent, intermittent, or rate related. ■

A 64-year-old asymptomatic patient is seen for a routine physical examination.

What is the most likely etiology for this patient's abnormal QRS axis?

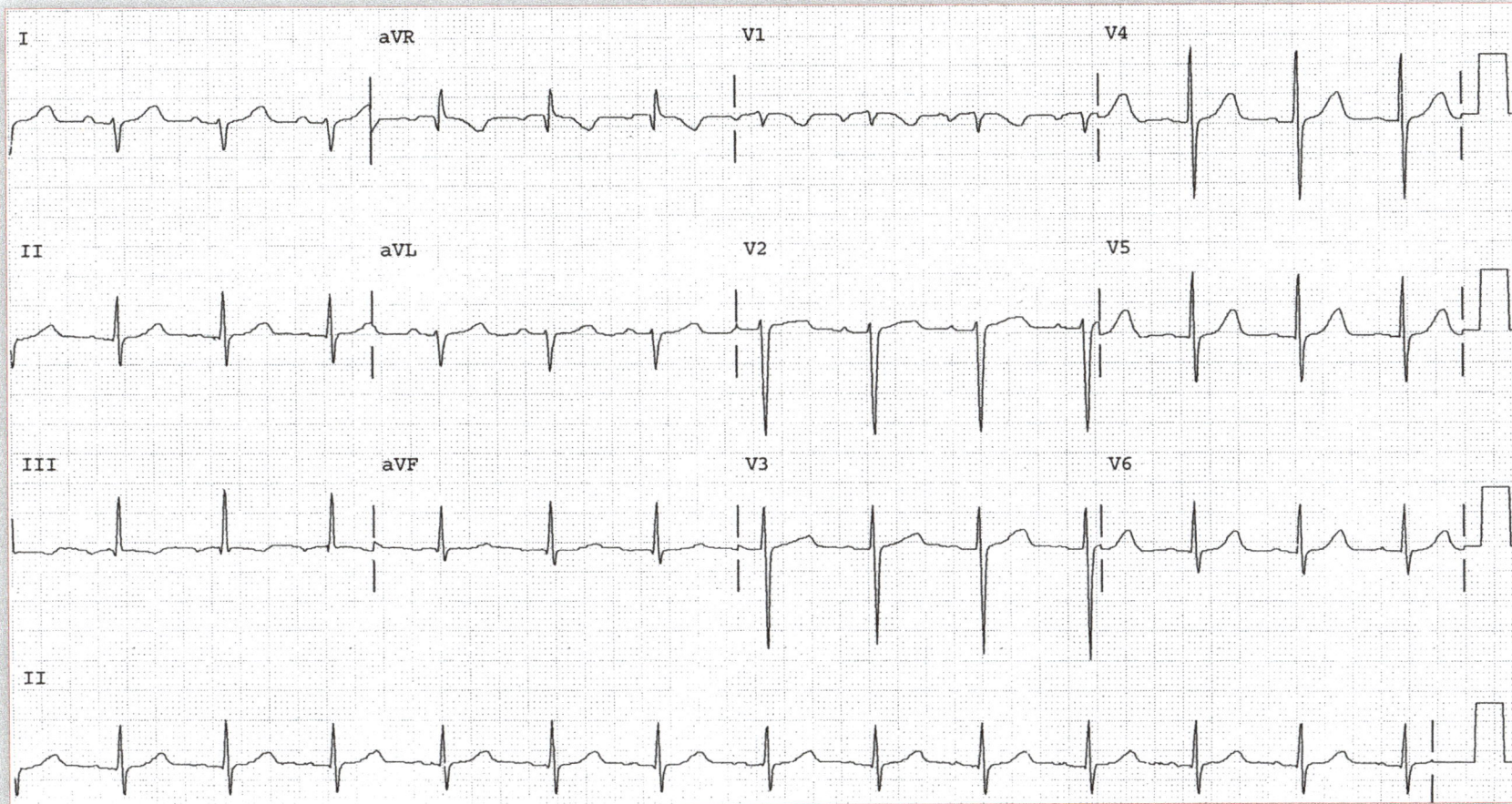

ECG 27 Analysis: Normal sinus rhythm, right axis due to a left posterior fascicular block (LPFB)

The ECG shows a regular rhythm at a rate of 82 bpm. There is a P wave (+) before each QRS complex, with a stable PR interval (0.20 sec). The P wave is positive in leads I, II, aVF, and V4-V6. Hence this is a normal sinus rhythm.

The QRS complex duration is normal (0.08 sec), as are the QT/QTc intervals (380/440 msec). The axis is rightward, between +90° and +180° (the QRS complex is negative in lead I and positive in lead aVF). The QRS complex in lead I has an rS morphology.

A rightward axis is always abnormal and may be due to:

- Right ventricular hypertrophy (RVH), in which case there is a tall R wave in lead V1 and often evidence of right atrial hypertrophy with P pulmonale, which is indicated by a tall, narrow, and peaked P wave.

- A lateral wall myocardial infarction, in which case the initial waveform of the QRS complex in leads I and aVL is a Q wave (a Qr complex).

- Right-to-left arm lead switch, in which case negative P waves are also seen in leads I and aVL.

- Dextrocardia, as evidenced by negative P waves in leads I and aVL as well as reverse R-wave progression across the precordium (ie, there is a tall R wave in lead V1 that becomes progressively shorter from leads V1 to V6).

- Wolff-Parkinson-White pattern, in which the PR interval is short and the QRS complex is wide as a result of a delta wave. The rightward axis results from an initial Q wave in leads I and aVL (QS complex) and not an rS complex. This is a pseudo lateral infarction pattern.

- Left posterior fascicular block (LPFB), in which the initial QRS waveform in lead I is an R wave (an rS complex). The diagnosis of an LPFB is established when the other causes of a rightward axis have been excluded.

The rightward axis in this ECG is a result of an LPFB (with an rS complex in leads I and aVL) as there are no features to suggest any other causes for a rightward axis (*ie*, evidence of RVH, dextrocardia, right-to-left arm lead switch, lateral wall myocardial infarction, or Wolff-Parkinson-White pattern). Although less common than a left anterior fascicular block (LAFB), the causes for an LPFB are the same as for an LAFB, including idiopathic conduction system disease (Lev's or Lenègre's disease), hypertension, ischemic heart disease, or a cardiomyopathy. ■

A healthy 26-year-old presents with an ankle fracture that resulted from a sports injury. A routine ECG is obtained, and an abnormality is noted.

Would further cardiac workup be necessary?

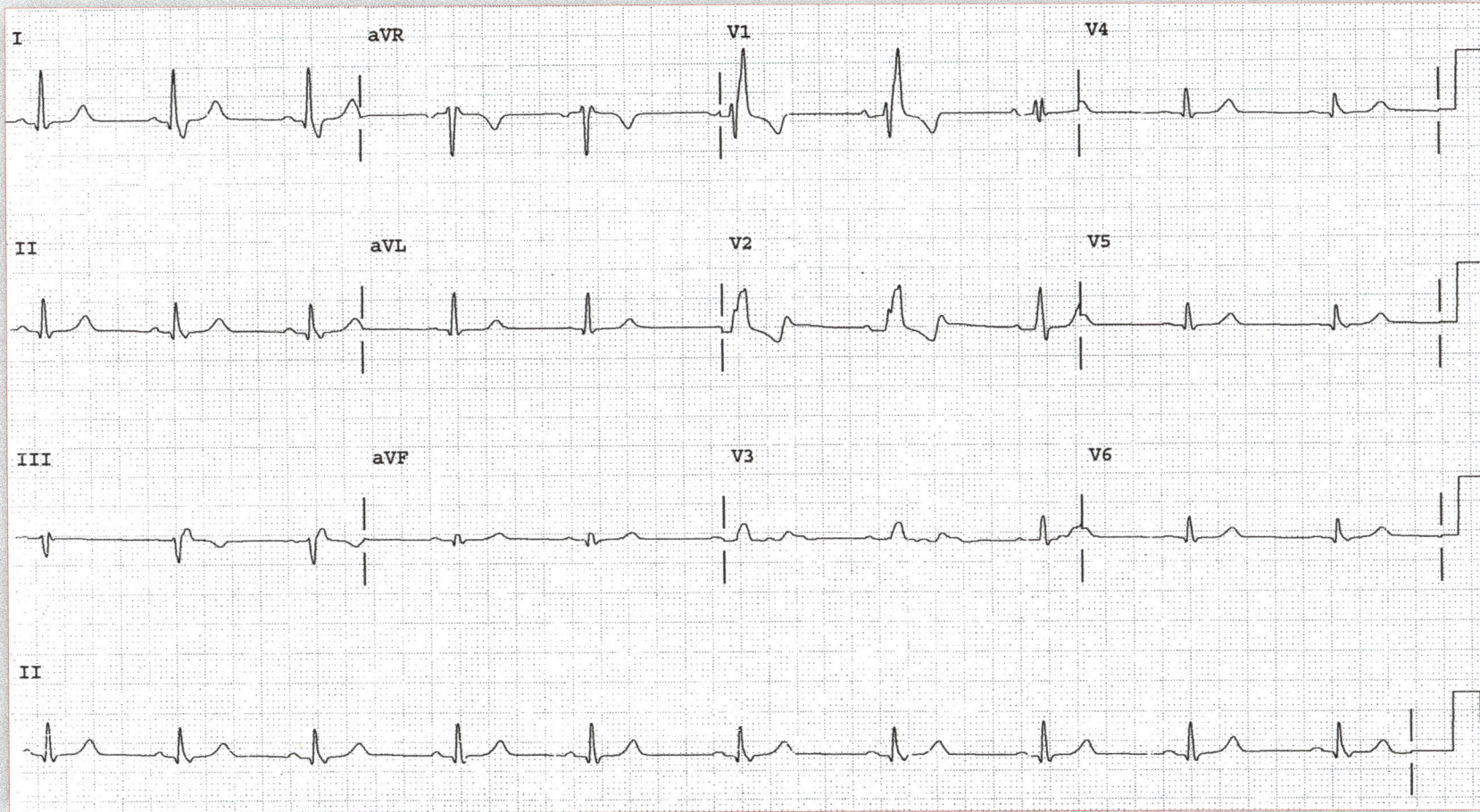

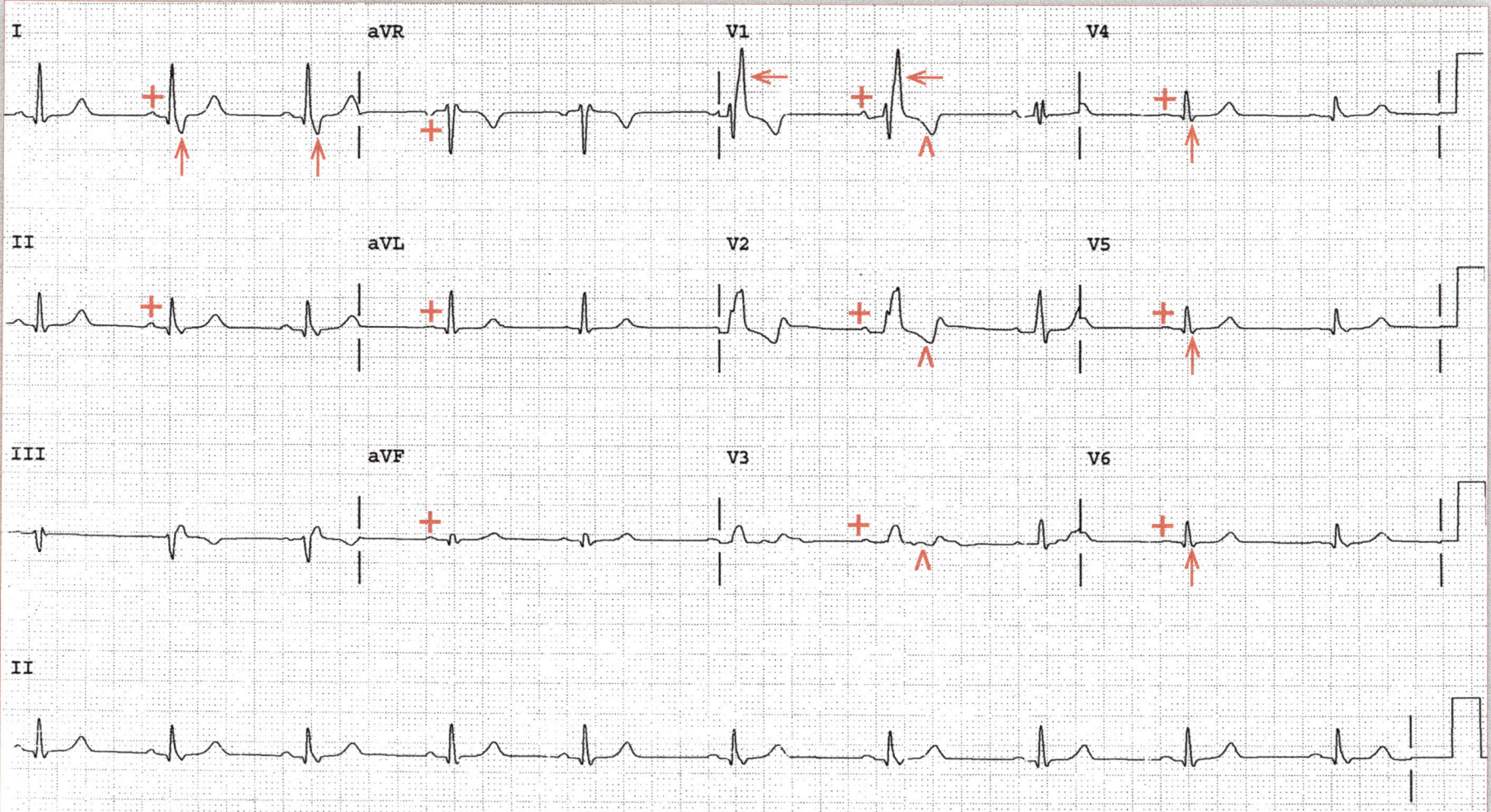

ECG 28 Analysis: Normal sinus rhythm, right bundle branch block (RBBB)

The ECG shows a regular rhythm at a rate of 60 bpm. There is a P wave (+) before each QRS complex, and the PR interval is stable (0.18 sec). The P wave is positive in leads I, II, aVF, and V4-V6. Hence this is a normal sinus rhythm.

The QRS complex duration is increased (0.14 sec). There is an RSR′ complex in lead V1, and the R′ (←) is broad and tall. A broad terminal S wave (↑) is seen in lead I; although not well seen on this ECG, there are usually broad S waves in leads V5-V6 (↑). This is a typical pattern of right bundle branch block (RBBB) in which there is delayed activation of the right ventricle. The ST-T wave abnormalities noted in leads V1-V3 (^) are associated with an RBBB. The QRS complex has a normal axis, between 0° and +90° (positive QRS complex in leads I and aVF). The QT/QTc intervals are normal when the prolonged QRS duration is considered (420/430 and 360/370 msec).

The diagnosis of an RBBB is based on the following:

- The QRS duration is ≥ 0.12 second due to delayed activation of the right ventricle.
- Right ventricular activation is from left bundle and left ventricle, directly through the myocardium. Therefore, the terminal forces of the QRS complex are directed from left to right.

- As a result of the terminal forces going from left to right, the QRS complex has a secondary R wave in lead V1 (*ie*, an RSR′ morphology) with a broad terminal R wave (R′) in leads V1-V2 and a broad terminal S wave in leads I and V5-V6. The broad terminal waveforms are due to prolonged time for right ventricular activation as the impulse is conducted directly through the ventricular myocardium and not the normal Purkinje system.
- Right ventricular repolarization is abnormal, and secondary ST-T wave changes can be seen in leads V1-V3.
- As right ventricular activation is abnormal, right ventricular hypertrophy cannot be reliably diagnosed.
- Left ventricular activation is normal. Therefore, the initial portion of the QRS complex is normal and abnormalities of the left ventricle (*eg*, left ventricular hypertrophy, infarction, ischemia, pericarditis) can be recognized.

RBBB can be seen in healthy individuals as well as in several pathologic conditions, including idiopathic conduction system disease (Lev's or Lenègre's), ischemic heart disease with previous myocardial infarction, myocarditis, hypertension, cardiomyopathy, acute elevation of right ventricular pressure (as with a pulmonary embolism), and chronically elevated right ventricular pressure (such as cor pulmonale) or a left-to-right shunt (such as with an atrial septal defect). ■

Notes

A 75-year-old patient is seen in the emergency department for an acute abdomen that is believed to be due to acute cholecystitis. Just before going to the operating room, an ECG is obtained and an abnormality is noted.

Is any further workup or therapy indicated prior to surgery?

ECG 29 Analysis: Normal sinus rhythm, right bundle branch block (RBBB), left anterior fascicular block (LAFB), bifascicular block

The ECG shows a regular rhythm at a rate of 74 bpm. There is a P wave (+) before each QRS complex, with a stable PR interval (0.16 sec). The P wave is positive in leads I, II, aVF, and V4-V6. Hence this is a normal sinus rhythm.

The QRS complex duration is increased (0.16 sec), and the morphology shows a typical right bundle branch block (RBBB) pattern, with an RSR′ in leads V1-V2 (←) and broad terminal S waves (↑) in leads I, aVL, and V5-V6. The T-wave abnormalities seen in leads V1-V3 (^) are associated with an RBBB. In addition, the axis is very leftward, between −30° and −90° (positive QRS complex in lead I and negative QRS complexes in leads II and aVF with an rS morphology). The extreme left axis is not the result of an inferior wall MI, in which the QRS complexes would have a QS or Qr morphology. Here the QRS complex has an rS morphology, indicating that the extreme leftward axis is the result of a left anterior fascicular block (LAFB). Therefore,

there is conduction block in two of the three major fascicles (right bundle and left anterior fascicle); this is termed bifascicular block. The QT/QTc intervals are normal when accounting for the prolonged QRS complex duration (400/440 msec).

The presence of bifascicular block has been a concern in patients who are to undergo surgery because of the potential development of complete heart block as a result of further conduction problems. However, there are no data to indicate that this will definitely occur, and the presence of bifascicular block is not an indication for temporary pacing prior to surgery or permanent pacing after surgery. Pacing would be indicated for a symptomatic patient who had evidence of disease also affecting the left posterior fascicle (*ie*, trifascicular disease), such as alternating left bundle branch block and RBBB, RBBB with alternating LAFB and left posterior fascicular block, evidence of Mobitz type II block, or intermittent complete heart block with a ventricular escape rhythm. ■

The following ECG was obtained from a patient who sustained a myocardial infarction (MI). The patient's baseline ECG 6 months earlier was completely normal.

What is the most likely territory of this patient's MI?

What is the patient's overall prognosis given the presence of new conduction system disease?

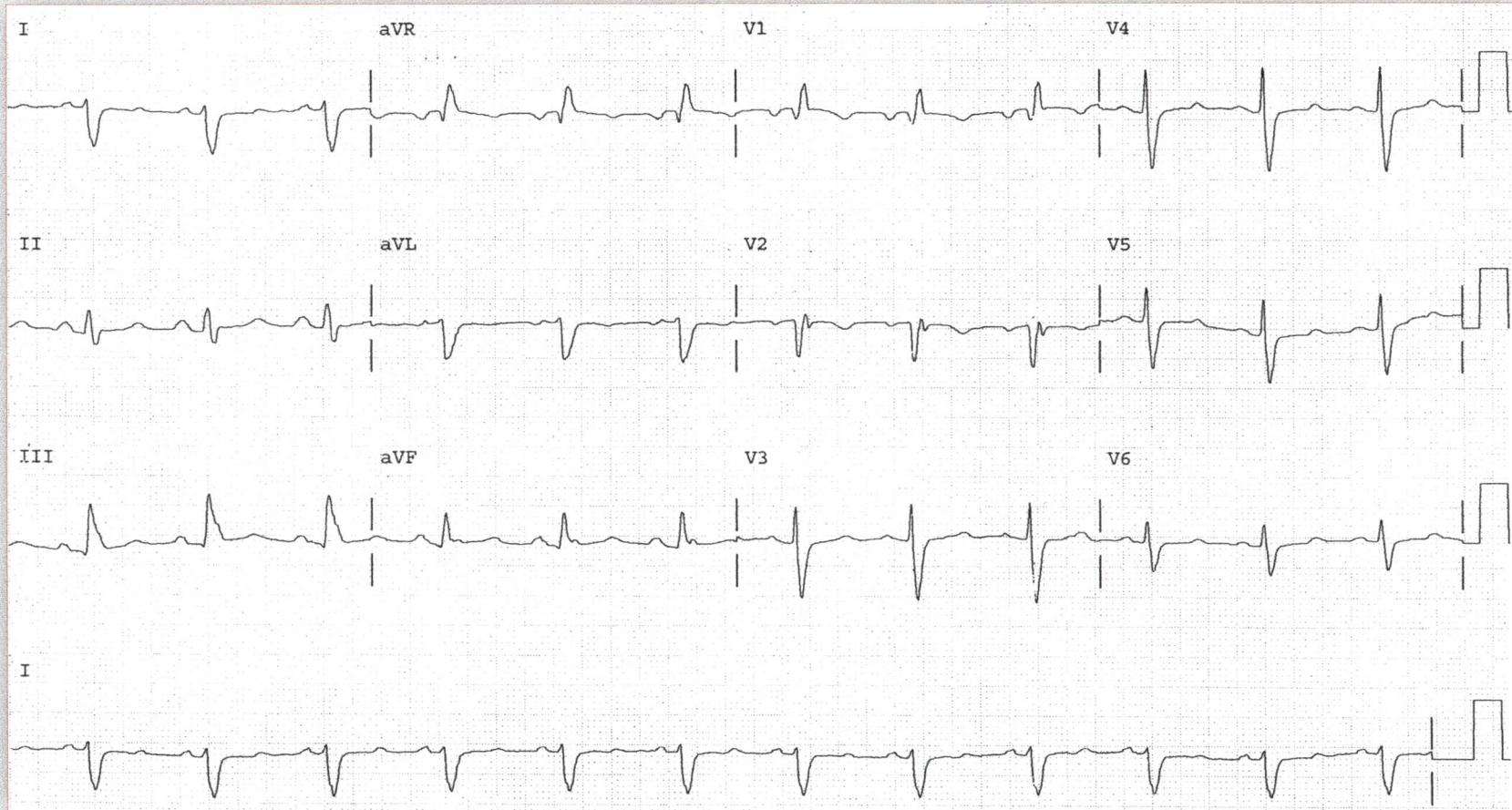

S wave

ECG 30 Analysis: Normal sinus rhythm, right bundle branch block (RBBB), right axis due to left posterior fascicular block (LPFB), bifascicular block, old anteroseptal myocardial infarction (MI)

The ECG shows a regular rhythm at a rate of 72 bpm. There is a P wave (+) before each QRS complex, with a stable PR interval (0.16 sec). The P wave is positive in leads I, II, aVF, and V4-V6. Hence this is a normal sinus rhythm.

The QRS complex duration is prolonged (0.16 sec) and has a right bundle branch block (RBBB) morphology, with a broad R wave or qR complex in lead V1 (←) and a broad S wave (→) in leads I, aVL, and V5-V6. The axis is rightward, between +90° and +180° (positive QRS complex in lead aVF and negative QRS complex in lead I). The broad terminal S wave in lead I is a result of the RBBB, so it is important that this waveform not be included in determination of the axis because this represents right ventricular depolarization. For axis determination, only the first 0.08 second of the QRS complex is considered. However, even ignoring the terminal S wave, the QRS complex in lead I is still negative and hence the axis is indeed rightward. In the absence of any other ECG features accounting for the rightward axis (*ie*, right ventricular hypertrophy, right-to-left arm lead switch, lateral infarction, dextrocardia, Wolff-Parkinson-White pattern), it is the result of a left posterior fascicular block (LPFB). The presence of an RBBB and

LPFB is termed bifascicular block, similar to what was discussed for Case 29. There are also Q waves in leads V1-V2 (▼), consistent with an old anteroseptal MI.

Isolated LPFB (or hemiblock) is uncommon and is the least common of the fascicular conduction diseases because of its anatomic location; the left posterior fascicle often spreads out within the posterior and infero-posterior walls and is less likely to be affected by disease processes. In addition, it has dual blood supply from the septal branches of the left anterior descending artery and the AV nodal branch from the posterior descending artery. It may have an idiopathic etiology (*ie*, Lev's or Lenègre's disease) or may occur in association with a cardiomyopathy, hypertension, myocarditis, or extensive coronary artery disease and myocardial infarction (MI). When isolated LPFB does occur in the setting of coronary artery disease and previous MI, it generally indicates more extensive disease. The presence of LPFB and RBBB is associated with a 21% to 75% increased risk for complete heart block compared with RBBB and left anterior fascicular block. Mortality is increased when an LPFB occurs in the setting of acute MI, primarily as a result of the presence of more extensive coronary disease. ◼

Notes

A 24-year-old man presents for a routine physical exam before entering graduate school. He has no known heart disease and no cardiac symptoms.

Is the QRS complex abnormal in this ECG?

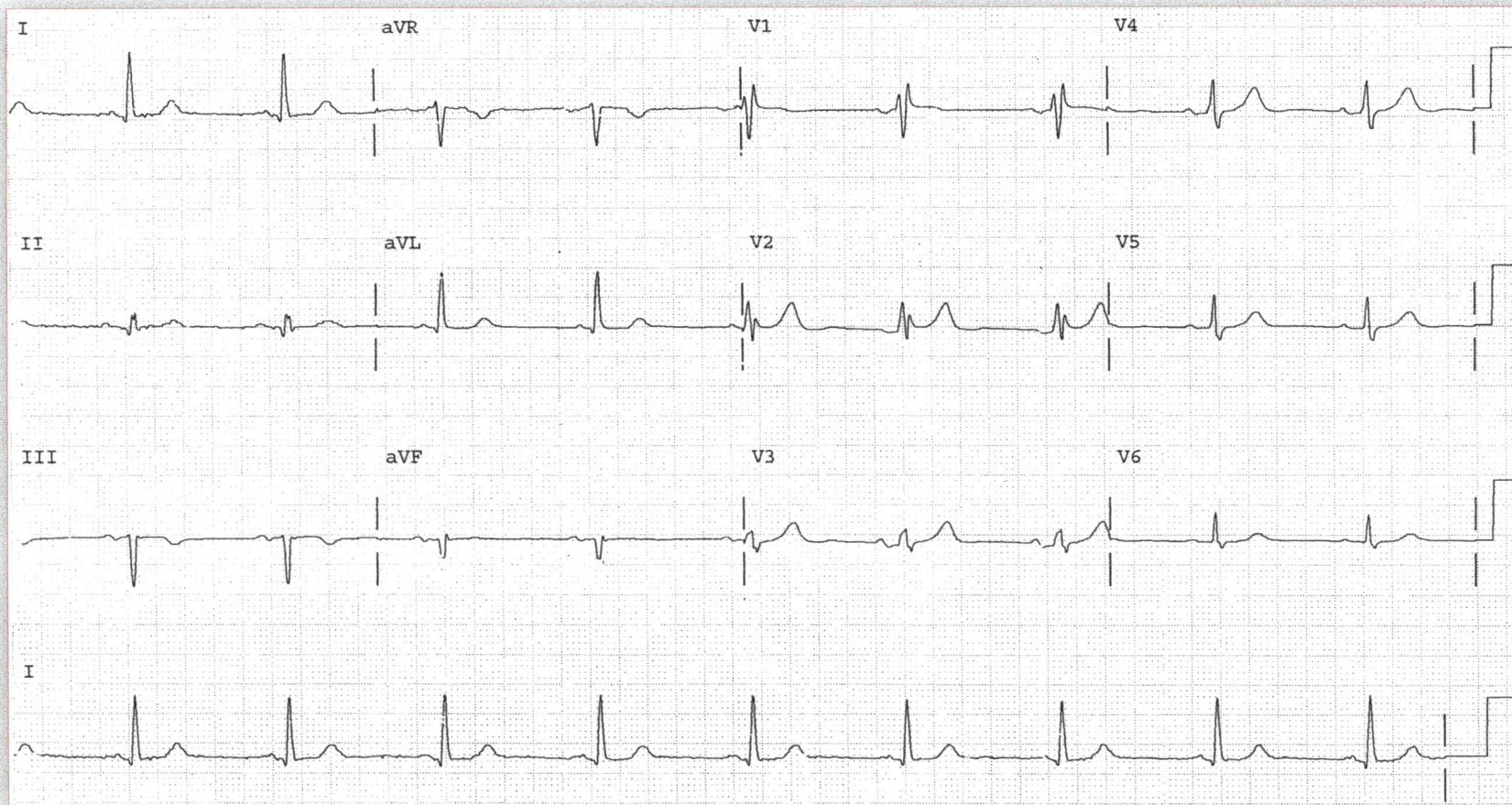

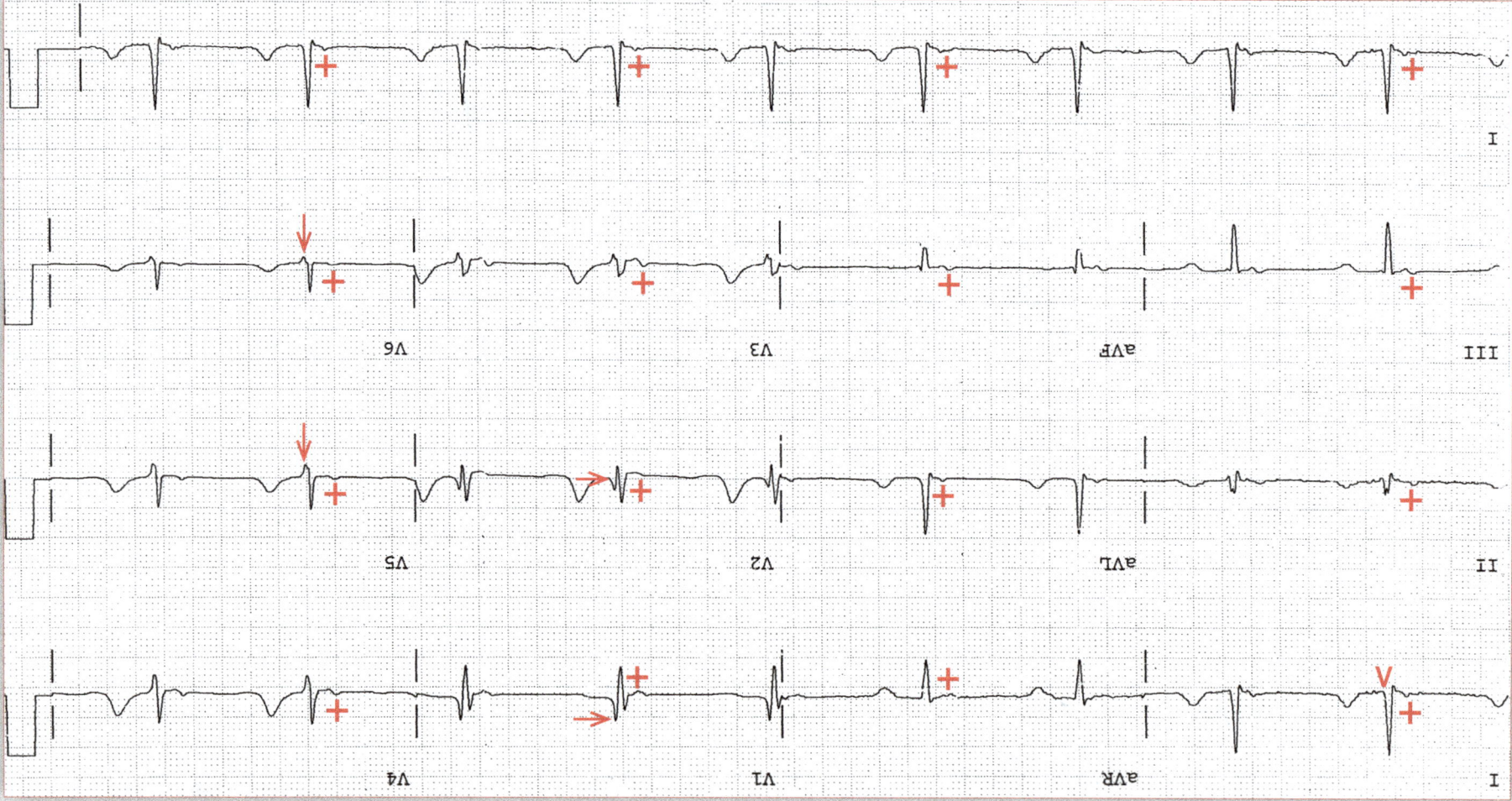

ECG 31 Analysis: Sinus bradycardia, left axis, intraventricular conduction delay (IVCD) to the right ventricle (incomplete RBBB)

The ECG shows a regular rhythm at a rate of 54 bpm. There is a P wave (+) before each QRS complex, with a stable PR interval (0.16 sec). The P wave is positive in leads I, II, aVF, and V4-V6.

The QRS complex duration is normal (0.10 sec), and there is a physiologic left axis, between 0° and –30° (negative QRS complex in lead aVF and positive QRS complex in leads I and II). The QT/QTc intervals are normal (400/380 msec). Although the QRS duration is normal, there is an RSR′ complex in leads V1-V2 (←). As a result, the QRS complex morphology resembles a right bundle branch block (RBBB). However, the QRS complex duration is not prolonged, there is no broad S wave in lead I (^), and the S wave in leads V5-V6 (↑) has a normal duration. When the QRS width is greater than 0.10 but less than 0.12 second, the pattern is often referred to as an incomplete RBBB, although it is best termed an intraventricular conduction delay (IVCD) to the right ventricle. As conduction through the bundles (*ie*, right bundle) is all or none, incomplete conduction is actually an IVCD. When the QRS width is normal (*ie*, ≤ 0.10 sec), the RSR′ pattern is a normal variant, representing a minor right ventricular conduction delay; this is referred to as a crista pattern, indicating a delay in the activation of the crista supraventricularis of the right ventricle. ■

The following ECG is obtained from a 66-year-old patient who came to your clinic for a routine physical. The patient is doing well and complains of no symptoms. However, blood pressure is found to be elevated at 170/100 mm Hg.

What further evaluation needs to be performed?

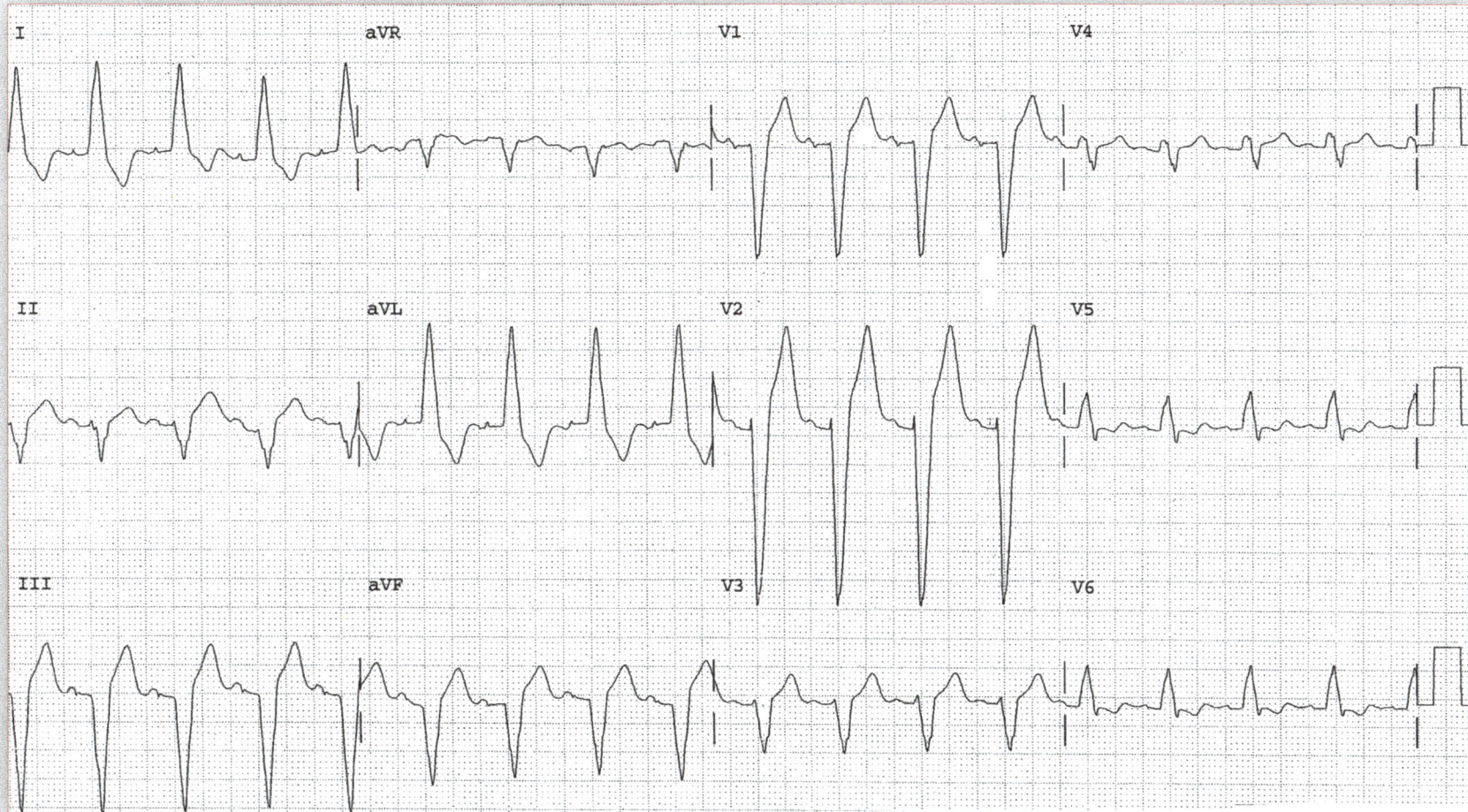

I	aVR	V1	V4
II	aVL	V2	V5
III	aVF	V3	V6

ECG 32 Analysis: Sinus tachycardia, left bundle branch block (LBBB)

The ECG shows a regular rhythm at a rate of 100 bpm. There is a P wave (+) before each QRS complex, with a stable PR interval (0.20 sec). The P wave is positive in leads I, II, aVF, and V4-V6. Hence this is a sinus tachycardia.

The QRS complex duration is prolonged at 0.16 second. The QT/QTc intervals are prolonged (400/520 msec) but normal when accounting for the prolonged QRS complex duration (320/410 msec). There is a broad R wave in leads I and V5-V6 (←), with a wide and deep QS complex in lead V1 (→). This is a typical pattern of left bundle branch block (LBBB). The axis is extremely leftward, between –30° and –90° (positive QRS complex in lead I and negative QRS complex in leads II and aVF). However, since LBBB involves both the left posterior and left anterior fascicles, it would not be appropriate for this extreme left axis to be called a left anterior fascicular block. There are ST-T wave changes in leads I, aVL, and V5-V6 (^) that are secondary to the left bundle branch block.

Characteristics of an LBBB include the following:

- The QRS duration is 0.12 second or longer due to delayed activation of the left ventricle.

- Left ventricular activation is from the right bundle and right ventricle and is directly through the myocardium. Therefore, all ventricular forces are directed from right to left and there is a

slow velocity of activation as the impulse is via the ventricular muscle and not the Purkinje system. This results in a broad, tall R wave in leads I, aVL, and V5-V6 and a wide and deep QS complex in leads V1-V2. Not uncommonly, a QS pattern may be seen across the entire precordium (*ie*, from leads V1-V6).

- Since the septum is innervated by a small septal branch from the left bundle, there are no septal forces seen and hence no Q waves in lead I, aVL, or V5-V6 and no R wave in lead V1.

- All forces are directed from right to left. No forces are directed from left to right, and hence terminal S waves in leads I and V6 are not present.

- Since depolarization is abnormal, there is also abnormal repolarization (*ie*, diffuse ST-T wave abnormalities).

- The axis may be normal or leftward. Since both the left posterior and left anterior fascicles are involved, axis shift is not related to fascicular block but to the abnormal activation sequence of the left ventricle that occurs directly through the left ventricular myocardium and not the Purkinje system. A rightward axis is not seen.

- Since left ventricular activation is abnormal and does not occur via the normal His-Purkinje system, left ventricular abnormalities (eg, left ventricular hypertrophy [LVH], infarction, ischemia, pericarditis, myocarditis) cannot be recognized.

continues

LBBB is an uncommon finding in young patients, but when present it is not associated with heart disease. It is more common in older patients, as it a frequent finding associated with heart disease. However, an LBBB does not suggest the presence of active ischemia but is seen with ischemic heart disease when there has been a previous infarction, primarily of the septum. However, ischemia (if present) cannot be reliably detected on the surface ECG in the setting of an LBBB as there are ST-T wave changes that are due to the LBBB. As indicated, an old infarction cannot be reliably diagnosed in the setting of an LBBB. An LBBB is often the result of idiopathic conduction system disease (Lev's or Lenègre's) and may also occur in the setting of LVH, left ventricular scar or fibrosis, cardiomyopathy, infiltrative processes of the myocardium, aortic valve endocarditis, rheumatic fever, and after cardiac surgery. Even though the patient is asymptomatic, obtaining an echocardiogram is indicated in light of the elevated blood pressure to assess for any structural heart disease, particularly LVH. ■

A 47-year-old man with a known history of an idiopathic dilated cardiomyopathy, severe mitral regurgitation, and low ejection fraction now presents with congestive heart failure.

How would the conduction abnormalities be classified in this ECG?

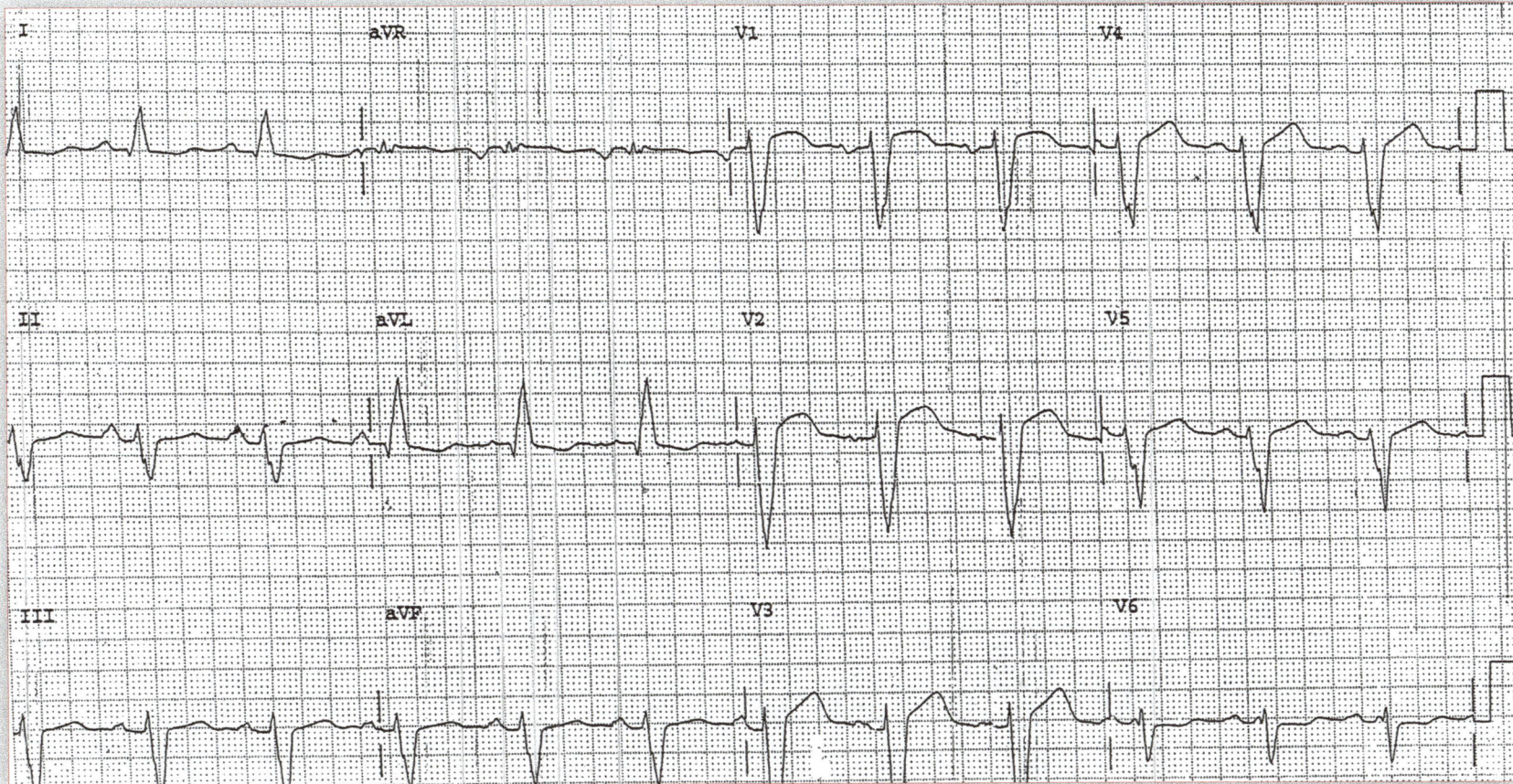

ECG 33 Analysis: Normal sinus rhythm, first-degree AV block,
left anterior fascicular block, intraventricular conduction delay (IVCD)

The ECG shows a regular rhythm at a rate of 68 bpm. There is a P wave (+) before each QRS complex, with a stable PR interval (0.24 sec). The P wave is positive in leads I, II, aVF, and V4-V6. Hence this is a normal sinus rhythm with a first-degree AV block. The P waves are broad, there is a prominent negative component in leads V1 and V2 (↑), and some notching is noted in leads V3-V4 (▼), features that are consistent with left atrial hypertrophy.

The QRS complex is widened (0.16 sec), and the axis is extremely leftward, between −30° and −90° (positive QRS complex in lead I and negative QRS complex in leads II and aVF). Although there is a broad R wave in lead I (→) and a deep S wave in lead V1 (←), a pattern that resembles left bundle branch block (LBBB), there are septal Q waves (^) seen in leads I and aVL as well as a prominent septal R wave (↓) in lead V1. As the septal branch activating the septum arises from the left bundle, septal forces cannot be present with an LBBB. In addition, there is a terminal S wave in lead V6 (▲), indicating terminal forces that are directed in a left-to-right direction. In an LBBB all forces are directed right to left and there should not be any left-to-right forces, which are indicative of a conduction delay to the right ventricle. Therefore, this is not an LBBB but rather an intraventricular conduction delay (IVCD).

This QRS pattern, with a very wide QRS complex duration resembling an LBBB, is commonly seen in patients with severe dilated cardiomyopathy. There is a correlation between QRS width and left ventricular ejection fraction: The wider the QRS complex, the lower the ejection fraction is. The QT/QTc intervals are prolonged (480/510 msec) but are normal after correcting for the prolonged QRS complex duration (400/430 msec).

With an LBBB, left ventricular activation is abnormal as impulse conduction does not travel through the normal His-Purkinje system but rather travels directly through the ventricular myocardium. Therefore, abnormalities of the left ventricle cannot be reliably diagnosed. Since the widened QRS complex is not the result of an LBBB, left ventricular activation is via the normal His-Purkinje system, but it is prolonged or slowed, usually as a result of diffuse and severe fibrosis affecting the terminal Purkinje system. Hence abnormalities of the left ventricular myocardium, such as infarction, ischemia, inflammation (as with pericarditis or myocarditis), and hypertrophy can be diagnosed. In addition, axis shifts resulting from block of the left anterior or posterior fascicle can be identified. On this ECG the axis is very leftward (more negative than −30°); hence there is a left anterior fascicular block present. ■

An 80-year-old woman presents with an acute fracture of her left hip. She denies any previous cardiac history. Prior to surgery, an ECG is obtained and a cardiology consult requested for further advice.

Has this patient suffered from a prior myocardial infarction (MI)?

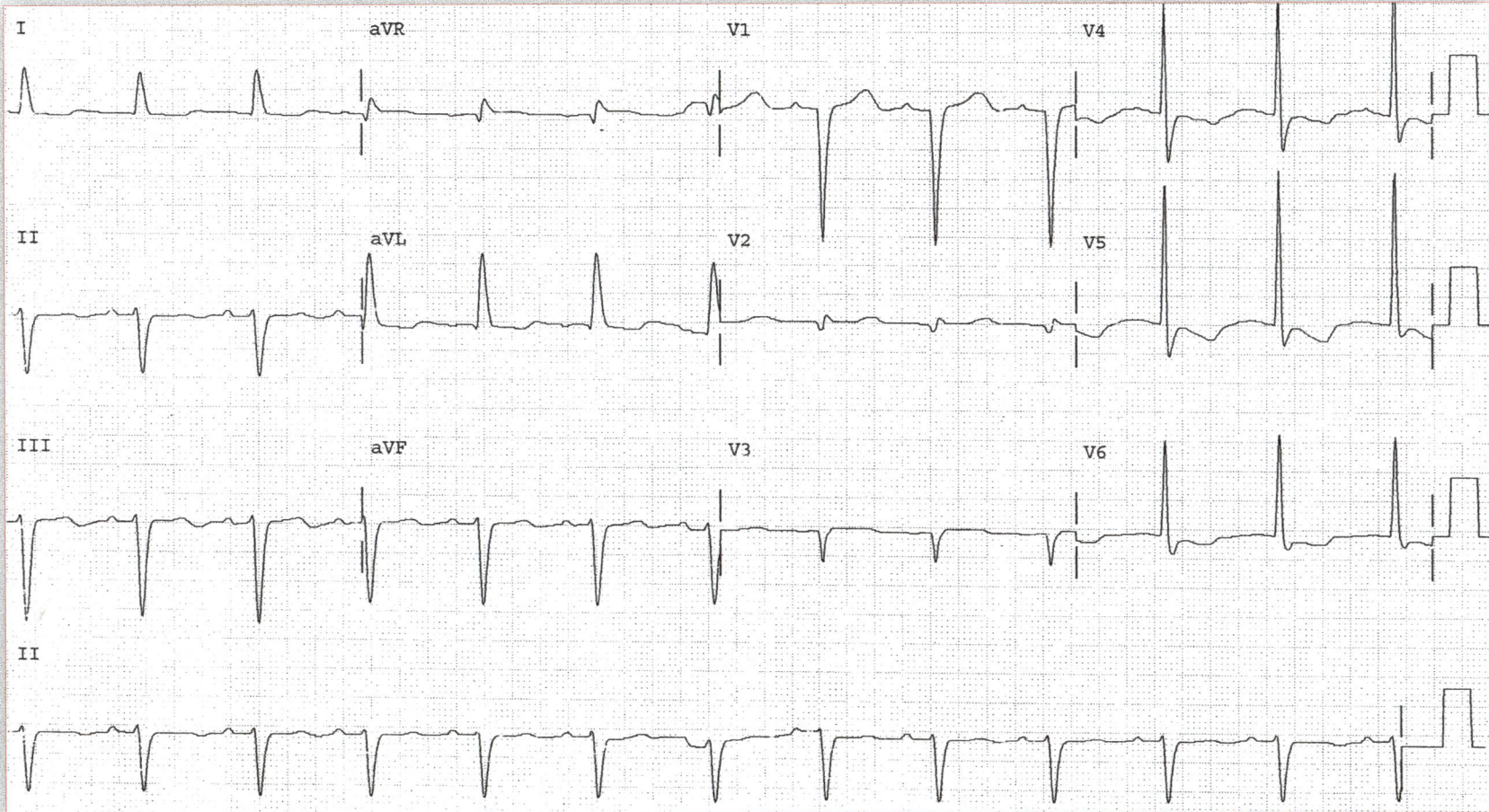

ECG 34 Analysis: Normal sinus rhythm, intraventricular conduction delay (IVCD), left anterior fascicular block, old anteroseptal MI, nonspecific ST-T wave changes

The ECG shows a regular rhythm at a rate of 74 bpm. There is a P wave (+) before each QRS complex, with a stable PR interval (0.20 sec). The P wave is positive in leads I, II, aVF, and V4-V6. Hence this is a normal sinus rhythm.

The QRS complex duration is slightly less than 0.12 second, and the axis is extremely leftward, between –30° and –90° (positive QRS complex in lead I and negative QRS complex in leads II and aVF with an rS morphology). The QT/QTc intervals are slightly prolonged (440/490 msec), even when adjusted for the prolonged QRS complex duration (410/450 msec). Although the QRS complex has a pattern that resembles a left bundle branch block (LBBB) (monophasic R wave in leads I and V5-V6 [←], deep S wave in lead V1 [→]), the QRS duration is not quite 0.12 second and hence is slightly less than that which defines an LBBB (ie, ≥ 0.12 sec). In addition, there is a small septal Q wave (▲) in lead aVL. This pattern has often been termed an incomplete LBBB. However, impulse conduction through the bundles is "all or none"; therefore, incomplete conduction is actually an intraventricular conduction delay (IVCD). This distinction is important because left ventricular abnormalities, such as infarction, ischemia, and hypertrophy, can be identified on the ECG in the setting of IVCD but not LBBB. An IVCD is due to diffuse slowing of conduction through the left ventricle as a result of diffuse involvement of the terminal Purkinje fibers. Therefore, impulse conduction is still along the normal His-Purkinje system, although it is slower. In an LBBB, left ventricular activation is not via the normal His-Purkinje system but rather is directly through the left ventricular myocardium (ie, an alternative pathway).

Since this is not an LBBB, the extreme leftward axis indicates that a left anterior fascicular block is present. In addition, the initial QRS force in leads V1-V3 is a Q wave (▼), which is diagnostic for an anteroseptal myocardial infarction (MI). Also present are nonspecific ST-T wave changes (↑) in leads V4-V6. As the patient is without any symptoms, no further cardiac evaluation is necessary prior to orthopedic surgery. However, an echocardiogram would be useful to confirm the old anteroseptal MI as well as to evaluate left ventricular function. ■

A 56-year-old man with bicuspid aortic valve undergoes surgical valve replacement for aortic stenosis. His postoperative course is unremarkable, and his ECG is shown below.

What is the principal abnormality?

How would you manage this?

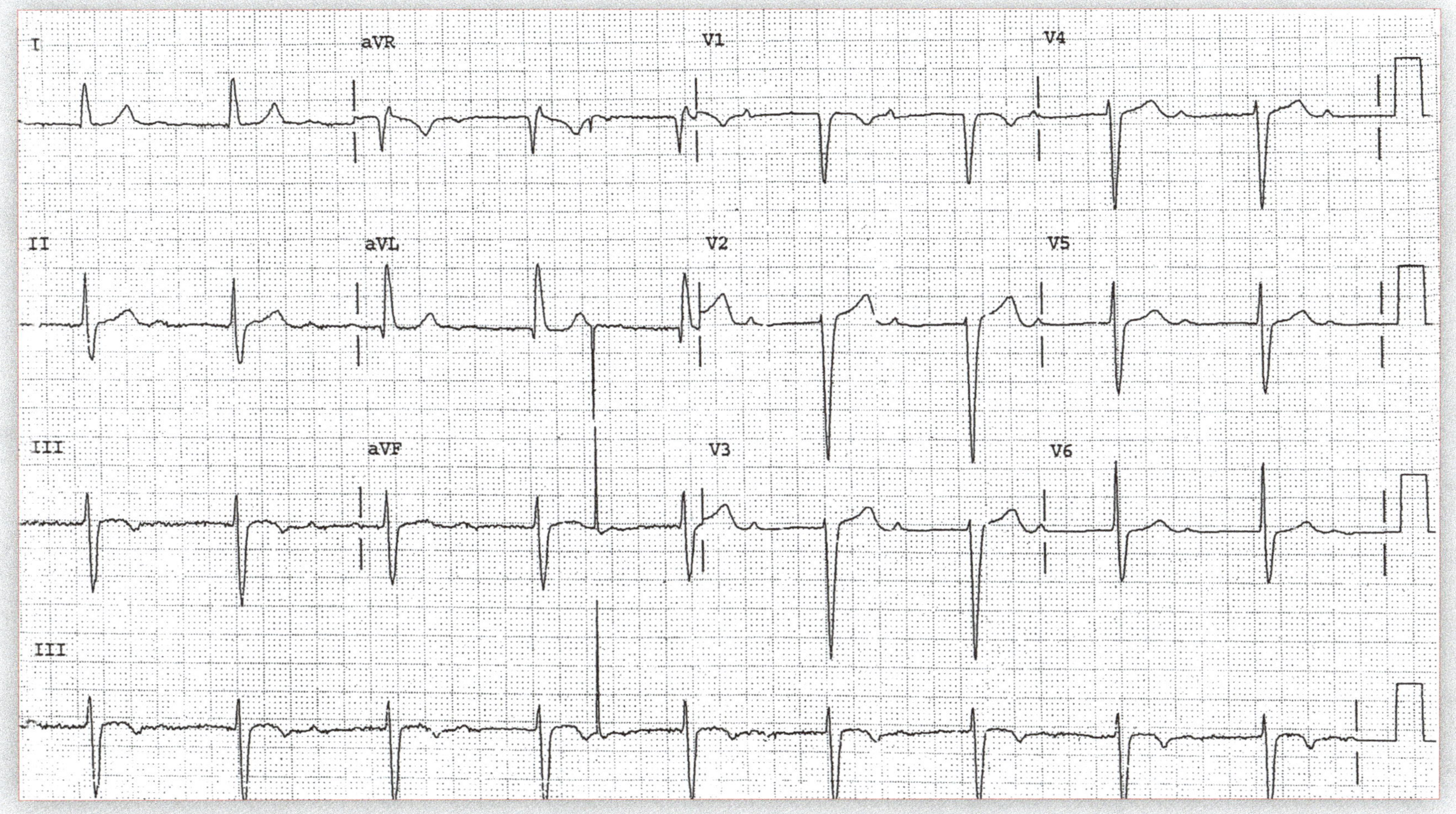

ECG 35 Analysis: Sinus bradycardia, first-degree AV block, intraventricular conduction delay, left axis, clockwise rotation

The ECG shows a regular rhythm at a rate of 56 bpm. There is a P wave (+) before each QRS complex, with a stable PR interval (0.58 sec) (↔). The P wave is positive in leads I, II, aVF, and V4-V6. Hence this is a sinus bradycardia with first-degree AV block, defined as a PR interval longer than 0.20 second.

The QRS complex duration is 0.12 second. However, there is no specific pattern suggesting either a right or left bundle branch block. While there is a QS complex in lead V1 (←) and a broad R wave in lead I (→), there is also a broad S wave in leads V5-V6 (^) and a septal Q wave (↑) in lead aVL. As the septal branch innervating the septum comes from the left bundle, septal forces are not present with a left bundle branch block. In addition, all forces are directed from right to left and there are no left-to-right forces; terminal S waves in leads V5-V6 are not present. Hence this is a nonspecific intraventricular conduction delay. The QT/QTc intervals are normal (400/390 msec and 360/350 msec when corrected for prolonged QRS complex duration). The axis is leftward, between 0° and −30° (the QRS complex is positive in leads I and II and negative in lead aVF). There is poor R-wave progression in leads V1-V3 and late transition (ie, R/S > 1 in lead V6), which are the result of clockwise rotation, as determined by imagining the heart as viewed from under the diaphragm. With counterclockwise rotation, the left ventricular forces are more posteriorly directed and seen in the more lateral (left-sided) precordial leads.

The major finding is a very long PR interval (primarily PR segment) that is 0.58 second and is termed a first-degree AV block. It may result from a slowing of conduction through the AV node or the His-Purkinje system. As there is no actual block of impulse conduction, a more appropriate term is prolonged AV conduction.

The PR interval includes the P wave (intraatrial conduction time) and the PR interval (conduction through the AV node and His-Purkinje system). Therefore, it represents the time for AV conduction between the atrium and ventricle. It is measured from the beginning of the P wave to the beginning of the QRS complex (Q or R wave). The normal PR interval is between 0.14 and 0.20 second. The PR interval changes with heart rate; that is, it lengthens with sinus bradycardia as a result of slower conduction through the AV node due to enhanced vagal tone or decreased sympathetic inputs, and it shortens with sinus tachycardia as a result of enhanced AV nodal conduction due to increased sympathetic tone. The PR interval, regardless of its length, is constant for each QRS complex.

A first-degree AV block is a common complication after aortic valve surgery as the aortic valve is close to the AV annulus and the AV node. No pacemaker is needed unless there is evidence of high-grade AV block, primarily complete heart block. Further PR interval prolongation or development of higher-grade AV block during follow-up may be a sign of aortic valve endocarditis in the appropriate clinical setting. ■

A 22-year-old college student comes to the emergency department with episodic lightheadedness and dizziness. A few days after returning from a hiking trip in Connecticut, she developed an erythematous, circular rash on her left leg with central clearing. Over the past several weeks the rash spread to other areas of her legs. She has had fatigue and myalgia but denies any fevers. An ECG is obtained while the patient is asymptomatic.

What is the major abnormality?

What is the overall clinical diagnosis?

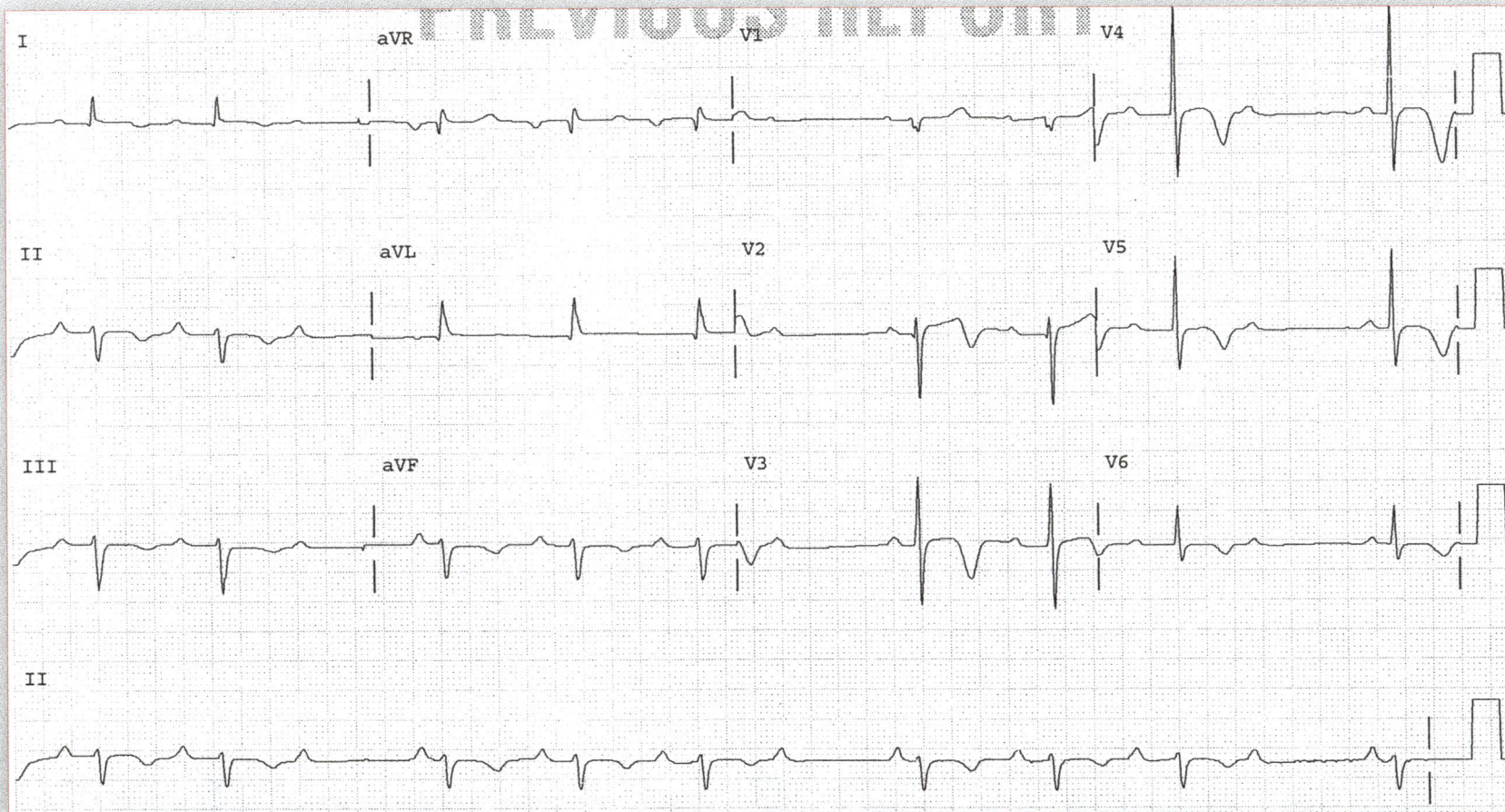

I aVR V1 V4

II aVL V2 V5

III aVF V3 V6

II

0.20 sec   0.28 sec   0.32 sec

ECG 36 Analysis: Normal sinus rhythm, second-degree AV block (Mobitz type I or Wenckebach), left anterior fascicular block, nonspecific T-wave abnormalities

The ECG shows a rhythm that is irregular, but there is a pattern of group beating with all the short RR intervals being the same and three longer RR intervals that are all the same. Hence the rhythm is regularly irregular. There is an underlying sinus rhythm of 70 bpm, established by finding sequential P waves (+). The PP intervals are regular throughout (⊔). The P waves are upright in leads I, II, aVF, and V4-6; hence they are originating from the sinus node. The PR interval is not constant. The baseline PR interval is established as the PR interval that is present after the pause in the RR interval. Hence the baseline PR interval (↔) is 0.20 second. The second PR interval is lengthened to 0.28 second, and the third is 0.32 second. The fourth P wave (^) is nonconducted (ie, it is not followed by a QRS complex). The pattern of PR interval lengthening then repeats itself. In addition, there is a slight shortening of the RR interval, from 0.92 to 0.84 second. This represents a second-degree AV block, Mobitz type I or Wenckebach pattern. There is a pattern of 4:3 Wenckebach.

A second-degree AV block is identified by a pause in the RR interval due to occasional nonconducted P waves. The sinus rate or PP intervals are constant. First-degree AV block may also be present.

A second-degree AV block as a result of Wenckebach is identified by a progressive prolongation of the PR interval prior to a single nonconducted P wave. After the nonconducted P wave (^), conduction resumes with a resetting of the PR interval back to its baseline. Thus there is always one more P wave than QRS complexes and Wenckebach is termed 3:2, 4:3, 5:4, etc. The pattern of block may be stable (ie, always 3:2, 4:3, etc) or may have variable pattern (ie, alternating periods of 4:3 with 3:2, etc). Often the increment of PR lengthening may progressively decrease with each complex, with the greatest degree of lengthening in the first interval and then a progressive decrease in the increment of lengthening, as is seen in this case (the PR interval increased from 0.20 to 0.28 and then to 0.32 sec). As a result there is a shortening of the RR interval, as can be seen between the first and second RR intervals (ie, 0.92 and 0.84 sec). However, shortening of the RR interval may not be observed and is not necessary to establish Wenckebach.

continues

Mobitz type I second-degree AV block results from a conduction abnormality involving the AV node. As the action potential generated by the AV node is mediated by calcium currents, the conduction velocity through this structure may not be constant (*ie*, it is not all or none) but can change depending on the presence of AV nodal disease, changes in autonomic tone, or drugs that affect the AV node such as digoxin, calcium-channel blockers (specifically verapamil or diltiazem), or β-blockers. Therefore, the AV node manifests decremental conduction (*ie*, conduction through it slows as the heart rate increases), which likely accounts for the Wenckebach pattern of progressive slowing of impulse conduction through the AV node.

Mobitz type I AV block is generally not serious. If the patient is asymptomatic, no further therapy is warranted. However, if there are symptoms from a bradycardia and the patient is not receiving AV nodal blocking agents, then a pacemaker would be indicated for symptomatic bradycardia. Should complete heart block develop, the escape rhythm will originate in the AV node (*ie*, a nodal or junctional rhythm), which is typically stable. Unless the escape rhythm is slow and/or associated with symptoms, there is no indication for the acute insertion of a temporary pacemaker.

Additional findings on this ECG include a normal QRS complex duration (0.08 sec) and the presence of an extreme leftward axis, between −30° and −90° (positive QRS complex in lead I and negative QRS complex in leads II and aVF with an rS morphology). An extreme leftward axis may be seen with an inferior wall myocardial infarction, which is associated with a deep initial Q wave in leads II and aVF. When the QRS complexes in leads II and aVF do not show evidence of an inferior wall myocardial infarction, but rather have an rS morphology, the cause of the left axis is a left anterior fascicular block. There are also diffuse T-wave inversions (↑), which are nonspecific. The QT/QTc intervals are slightly prolonged (420/450 msec).

The patient presents with fatigue, myalgias, and AV block after a camping trip in Connecticut. This, along with the rash she has developed, which is a typical pattern for erythema migrans, supports a diagnosis of Lyme disease. The fact that she has AV nodal Wenckebach that is asymptomatic is concerning for the occurrence of intermittent episodes of higher-grade AV block as an etiology of her dizziness. Observation with continuous monitoring would be useful to establish the presence of more advanced conduction problems, which, if present, are an indication for temporary pacing. The AV nodal conduction abnormalities associated with Lyme disease are transient and reversible, although the time course for recovery is variable. ■

A 92-year-old woman with chronic hypertension treated with atenolol presents with significant pre-syncopal symptoms of dizziness over the past day. She reports significant watery diarrhea over the past 3 days with nausea, resulting in poor oral intake. She denies fevers, sweats, or blood in her stools. Her physical exam reveals a blood pressure of 90/45 mm Hg, jugular venous pressure of 5 cm, dry mucous membranes, a regularly irregular heartbeat, and a soft abdomen with prominent bowel sounds. An ECG is obtained.

What is the primary ECG abnormality?

What is the most likely cause of her dizziness?

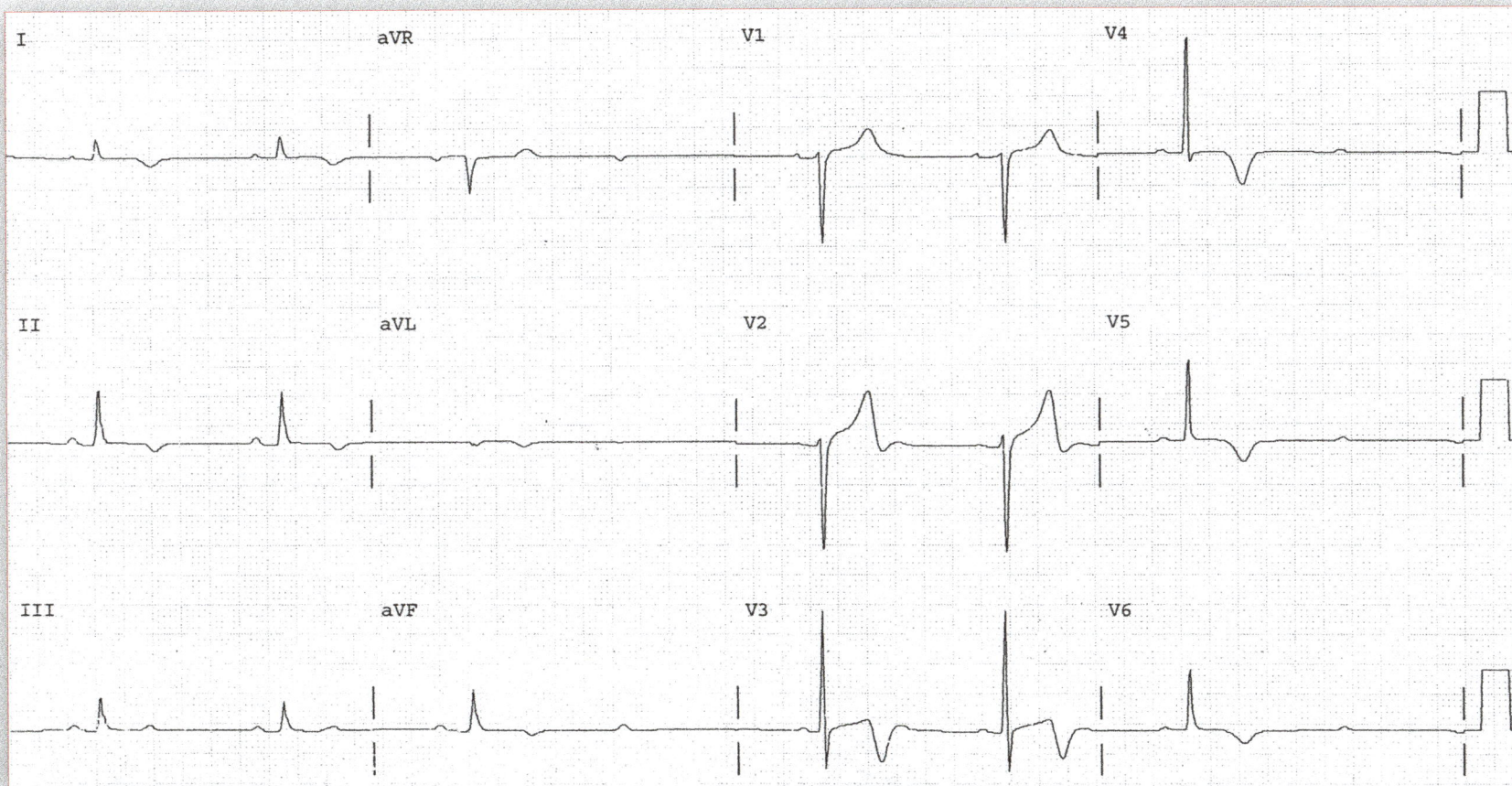

ECG 37 Analysis: Sinus bradycardia, second-degree AV block (Mobitz type II), left ventricular hypertrophy, nonspecific ST-T wave changes

The ECG shows P waves (+) occurring at regular intervals (⊔) and a heart rate of 48 bpm. The P waves are upright in leads I, II, aVF, and V4-V6. Hence this is a sinus bradycardia. However, the ventricular rate is not regular as a result of an occasional long RR interval (⊓) that occurs because of a single nonconducted P wave (▼). Hence the rhythm is regularly irregular. There is a stable PR interval at 0.20 second (↔). Every fourth P wave (▼) lacks a conducted QRS. Hence this represents a second-degree AV block (*ie*, a pause in the RR interval due to an occasional nonconducted P wave). The fact that the PR intervals of each of the conducted complexes is constant defines this as Mobitz type II AV block. The QRS complex duration is normal (0.08 sec), and the axis is normal, between 0° and +90° (positive QRS complex in leads I and aVF). The QT/QTc intervals are normal (460/410 msec).

Mobitz type II second-degree AV block results from conduction failure within the His-Purkinje system. The His-Purkinje system generates a fast action potential that is mediated by sodium currents. It is all or none (*ie*, it either conducts the impulse or does not conduct the impulse). It does not manifest decremental conduction. With a Mobitz II block, therefore, the His-Purkinje system intermittently fails to conduct an impulse, but when an impulse is conducted the rate of conduction is stable, accounting for the constant PR interval.

Mobitz type II second-degree AV block is a more serious condition than Mobitz type I, which involves the AV node. This is because, should complete heart block develop, the escape rhythm will be ventricular and possibly unstable and unpredictable. In contrast, complete heart block with Mobitz type I is associated with an escape junctional rhythm that is stable. Hence a Mobitz type II second-degree AV block is an indication for a pacemaker if there are symptoms suggesting bradycardia or if there is transient complete heart block.

continues

The ECG also shows a borderline criterion for left ventricular hypertrophy (S-wave depth in lead V2 [[ ] + R-wave amplitude in lead V4 [ ]] = 36 mm), and there are diffuse T-wave abnormalities (↑).

The patient's clinical history and physical examination are significant for profound dehydration, likely resulting in a pre-renal state of acute renal insufficiency. Although blood urea nitrogen and creatinine are not reported, low blood pressure in a normally hypertensive patient generates concern for the potential of renal insufficiency due to reduced renal perfusion. One would expect a reflex tachycardia in the setting of hypotension. However, the patient has been taking atenolol, which can blunt this effect. Since atenolol is primarily cleared renally, it is likely that the patient's bradycardia is a result of high atenolol levels in the setting of a pre-renal state.

However, the β-blocker will not affect conduction through the His-Purkinje system. Therefore, another etiology for Mobitz II should be sought. It may be the result of other metabolic abnormalities associated with renal insufficiency that will alter His-Purkinje conduction. Another possible cause is underlying disease of the His-Purkinje system that was exposed by the metabolic abnormalities. Although the symptoms of pre-syncope and dizziness can be explained by dehydration and hypotension, Mobitz II with subsequent complete heart block could also account for the symptoms. Complete heart block in this situation would be associated with a ventricular escape rhythm. Therefore, continued monitoring after correction of dehydration, metabolic abnormalities, and renal insufficiency would be indicated to evaluate for the presence of continued conduction abnormalities. ■

A 49-year-old man with diabetes and hypertension presents acutely to the emergency department following 6 hours of substernal chest pressure. When an ECG on presentation shows inferior ST-segment elevations, the patient is taken urgently for cardiac catheterization; a stent is placed in the distal right coronary artery. His ST segments normalize and his chest pain resolves. The next morning, the patient continues to be asymptomatic. A routine ECG is obtained.

How would you classify the rhythm disturbance?

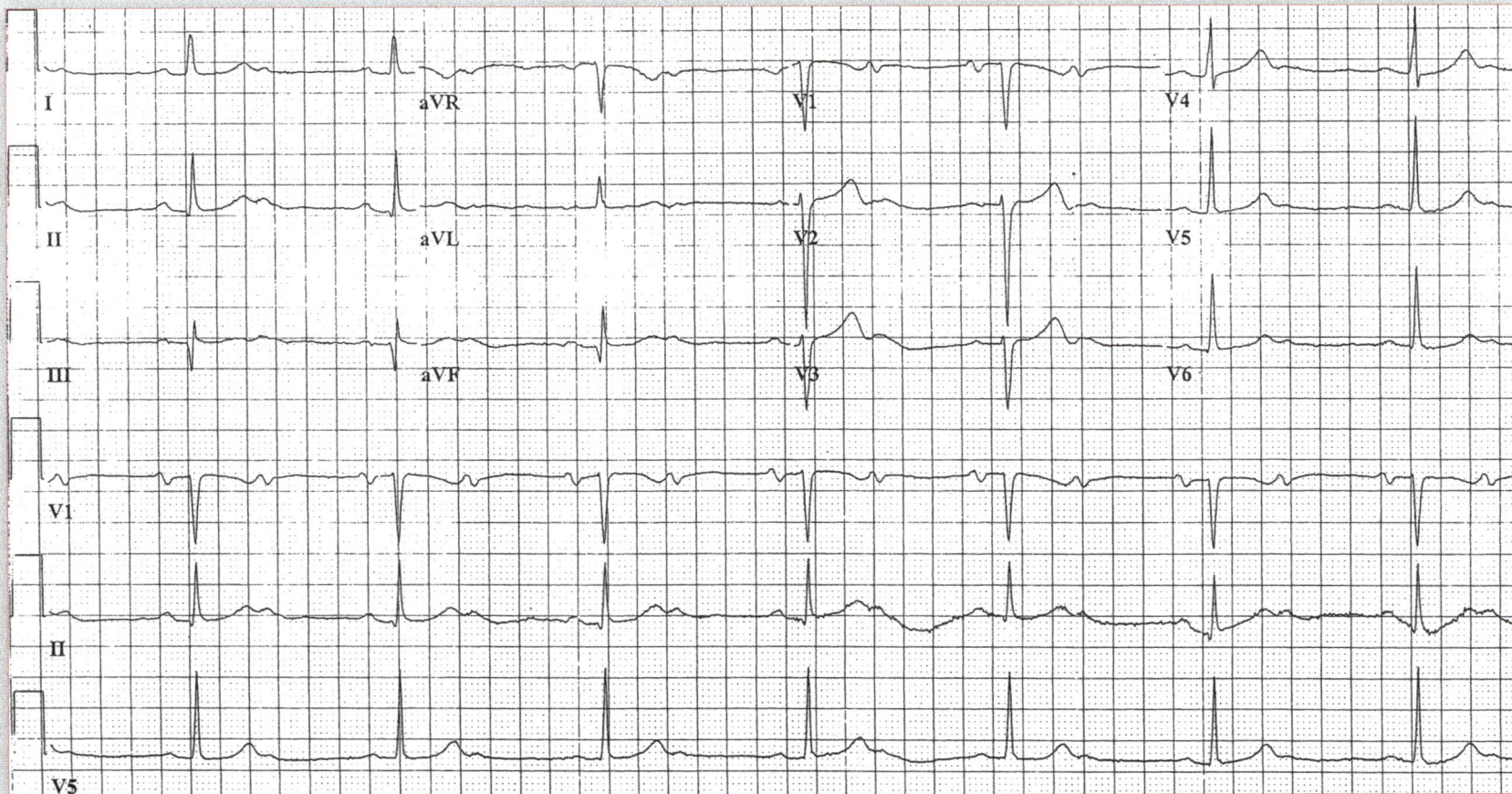

ECG 38 Analysis: Normal sinus rhythm, second-degree AV block (2:1 AV conduction or block), clockwise rotation, old inferior wall myocardial infarction (MI)

The ECG shows an underlying regular ventricular rate of 45 bpm. There is a P wave (+) before each QRS complex. The P waves are positive in leads I, II, aVF, and V4-V6. Hence there is a sinus rhythm. A second on-time but nonconducted P wave (^) can be seen between each QRS complex. Therefore, there is a stable normal sinus rhythm (⊔) at a rate of 90 bpm. The P waves that are conducted have a stable PR interval of 0.20 second (↔).

The QRS complex duration is normal (0.08 sec), and the axis is normal, between 0° and +90° (positive QRS complex in leads I and aVF). The QT/QTc intervals are normal (420/360 msec). Noted is poor R-wave progression, which is the result of clockwise rotation of the electrical axis in the horizontal plane, established by imagining the heart as viewed from under the diaphragm. With clockwise rotation, left ventricular forces occur later (more leftward) in the precordial leads. Also noted are Q waves (↑) in leads III and aVF, which are characteristic of an inferior wall myocardial infarction (MI). There are also U waves (▲) in leads V2-V4; these are normal.

Therefore, this ECG demonstrates second-degree AV block with 2:1 AV conduction, although it cannot be established if this is a Mobitz I with 2:1 AV conduction or AV block or Mobitz II with 2:1 conduction.

In the acute setting of an MI, the indications for temporary pacing include Mobitz type II AV block, given the high risk for progressing to complete heart block with an escape ventricular rhythm that could be unstable. Therefore, making the distinction between Mobitz type I and II is clinically important. Since this patient had an inferior wall MI, which is often associated with transient AV nodal conduction abnormalities resulting from either increased vagal tone or inflammation and/or edema around the AV junction, it may be assumed that this is a Mobitz type I and will resolve. In the presence of an anterior wall MI, there is often permanent damage to the septum and His-Purkinje system, which would be associated with a Mobitz type II block and, given the permanently damaged conduction system, with a risk for complete heart block and an escape ventricular rhythm.

However, the only way to establish the etiology with certainty is to see another pattern develop during monitoring. Therefore, if a pattern typical for Mobitz type I or complete heart block with an escape junctional rhythm developed, then the 2:1 AV block would be due to Mobitz type I. A subsequent pattern of Mobitz II or the development of complete heart block with a ventricular escape rhythm would confirm that the 2:1 AV block was the result of Mobitz II. ■

An 18-year-old Olympic track and field competitor needs a complete medical evaluation prior to running in her upcoming competitions. She has no medical complaints, her medical history reveals no major problems, and her physical examination is completely normal. An ECG is obtained.

How would you classify the rhythm disturbance?

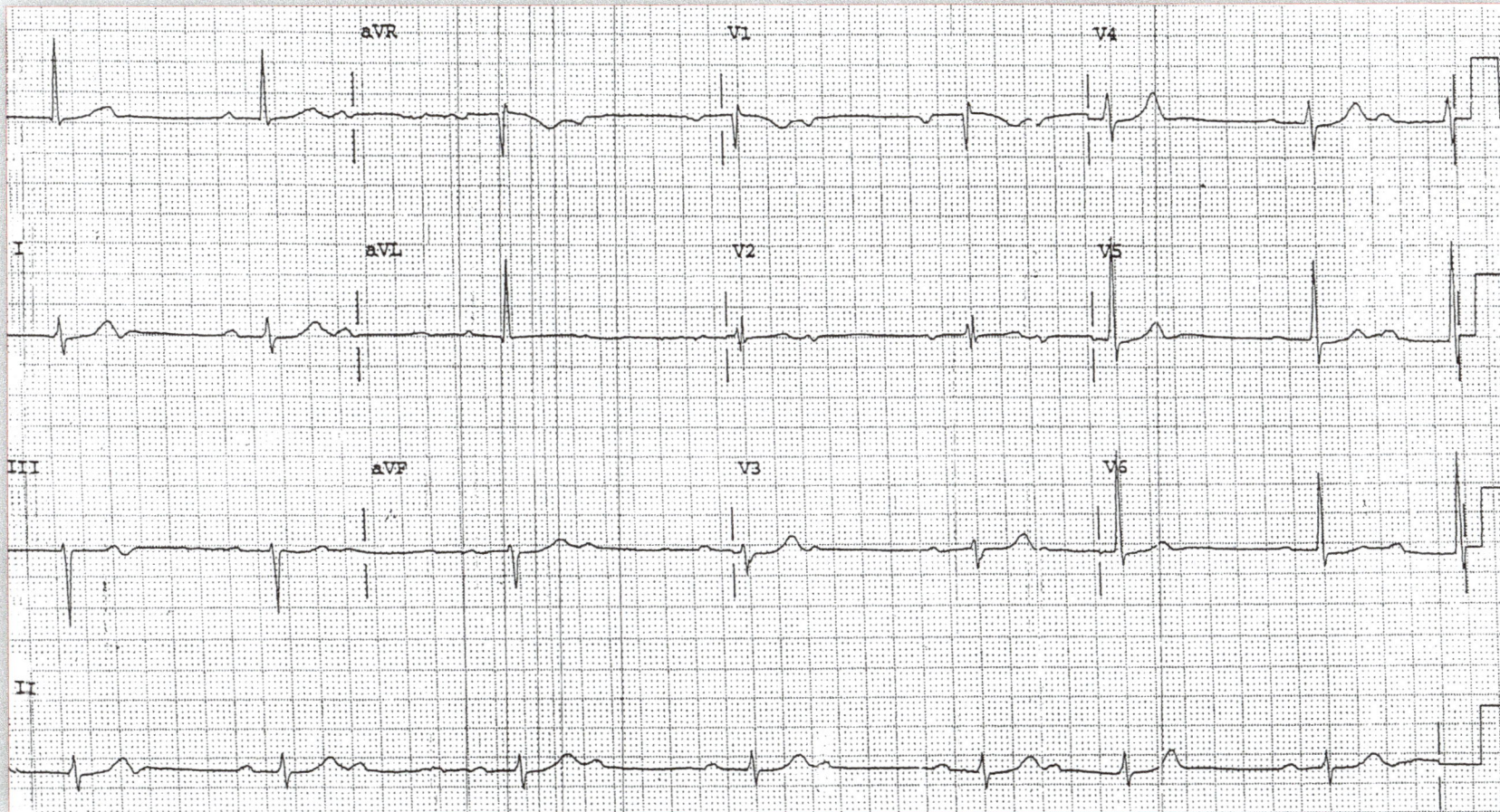

ECG 39 Analysis: Normal sinus rhythm, left axis, first-degree AV block, second-degree AV block (Mobitz type I)

The heart rate (36 bpm) is stable initially, with a consistent RR interval. There are P waves (+) before each QRS complex, with a stable PR interval (↔) (0.28 sec). A second on-time but nonconducted P wave is seen after each QRS complex (^). The PP intervals are constant (⊔), at a rate of 72 bpm. The P waves are upright in leads I, II, aVF, and V4-V6. Hence there is an underlying sinus rhythm. The QRS complex duration is normal (0.08 sec), and the axis is leftward, between 0° and −30° (positive QRS complex in leads I and II and negative QRS complex in lead aVF). The QT/QTc intervals are normal (400/310 msec).

Therefore, the initial portion of the ECG has a pattern of second-degree AV block with 2:1 AV conduction or 2:1 AV block (*ie*, every other P wave is nonconducted [^]). The baseline PR interval is stable but prolonged at 0.28 second, indicating that a first-degree AV block (prolonged AV conduction) is also present. At the end of the ECG recording (fifth and sixth QRS complexes), there is a change in the QRS pattern. The fifth QRS complex (*) is conducted with a PR interval of 0.28 second, which is the baseline PR interval. However, the sixth QRS complex (↓), which is preceded by an on-time P wave (●), is early and

the PR interval preceding it is longer (0.52 sec). After the sixth QRS complex there is a nonconducted P wave (▼), which can be timed out by marching out the PP intervals; this occurs on top of the T wave of the sixth QRS complex (▼), altering its morphology. Hence there is a brief period of a second-degree heart block with a pattern of a Mobitz type I and 3:2 conduction. Therefore, the 2:1 AV block in this situation represents a Wenckebach pattern (Mobitz type I) and not Mobitz type II.

The presence of Mobitz type I, an AV nodal conduction problem, in a young athlete is the result of high vagal tone, which can reduce the rate of conduction through the AV node and result in decremental conduction at a slower rate, and hence the Mobitz type I. High vagal tone also occurs at night, while sleeping, so Mobitz type I is not uncommon at this time. Other causes for Mobitz type I could be AV nodal blocking agents or intrinsic AV nodal disease. This conduction abnormality does not require any additional therapy and often resolves when there is an increase in sympathetic tone and a reduction in vagal tone, as with exercise. ■

A 17-year-old male high school senior comes to your clinic with worsening exercise tolerance. He has noticed that over the past 6 months he has been unable to keep up during his track and field practices. He remembers being told that he was born with a slow heart rate, but no treatment was needed at the time. The following ECG is obtained. An echocardiogram confirms that there is no structural heart disease.

What is the rhythm disturbance?

What is the most likely underlying etiology for this ECG finding?

What is the next step in management?

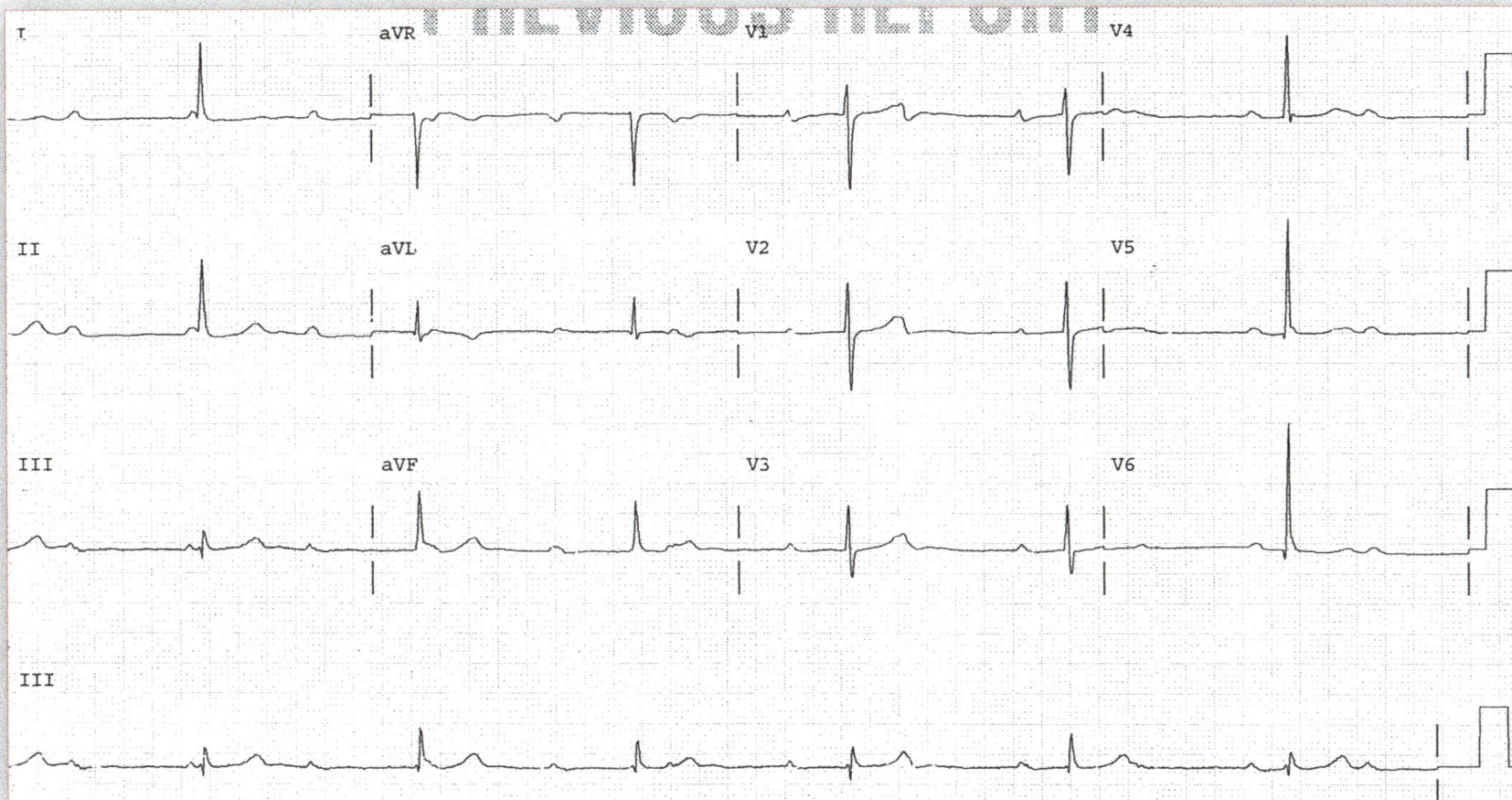

ECG 40 Analysis: Normal sinus rhythm, complete heart block (third-degree AV block), escape junctional rhythm

The ECG shows an underlying regular atrial rate (⊔) (regular PP interval) of 72 bpm. The P waves (+) are positive in leads I, II, aVF, and V4-V6. Some of the P waves are not obvious as they are at the end of the QRS complex (*), in the ST segment (^), or on T waves (▼). Hence there is a normal sinus rhythm. The QRS complex duration is normal (0.08 sec), and there is a normal morphology and axis, between 0° and +90° (positive QRS complex in leads I and aVF).

However, the ventricular rate is 40 bpm and the RR intervals are constant (⊓). The QT/QTc intervals are normal (460/380 msec). Additionally, the PR intervals (↔) are variable without any notable pattern (*ie*, there is no association between the P waves and the QRS complexes). This is termed AV dissociation as the atrial rate is independent of the ventricular rate. The atrial rate is faster than the ventricular rate, which is characteristic of third-degree or complete AV block. The QRS complexes are narrow and normal in morphology; therefore, the escape rhythm is nodal or junctional, meaning that the location of the conduction block is the AV node. The location of the escape rhythm is based not on its rate but rather on the morphology of the QRS complexes, which is normal in this case. Junctional escape rhythms tend to be predictable, better tolerated, and more stable than ventricular escape rhythms.

In view of the history of a slow heart rate since birth and the finding of complete heart block at a young age, the most likely etiology for the patient's complete heart block is neonatal lupus, an immunologic process involving transplacental migration of maternal antibodies (anti-Ro and anti-La antibodies) that bind to fetal cardiac tissue and destroy the AV node. Neonatal lupus is responsible for the majority of cases of congenital complete heart block. The diagnosis is often missed due to a lack of symptoms. Because some affected individuals do not develop complete heart block until later in life, they often present for the first time in childhood. The major indications for pacemaker placement in this setting include symptomatic bradycardia, significant exercise intolerance, heart failure related to bradycardia, left ventricular systolic dysfunction, or a wide QRS escape rhythm. ■

A 56-year-old man with known coronary artery disease and ischemic cardiomyopathy with an ejection fraction of 25% presents to the emergency department with syncope. He is currently experiencing symptoms of lightheadedness. You perform a physical examination and are able to diagnose a rhythm disturbance. An ECG confirms your suspicions.

What is the rhythm abnormality?

What findings on the physical exam support this diagnosis?

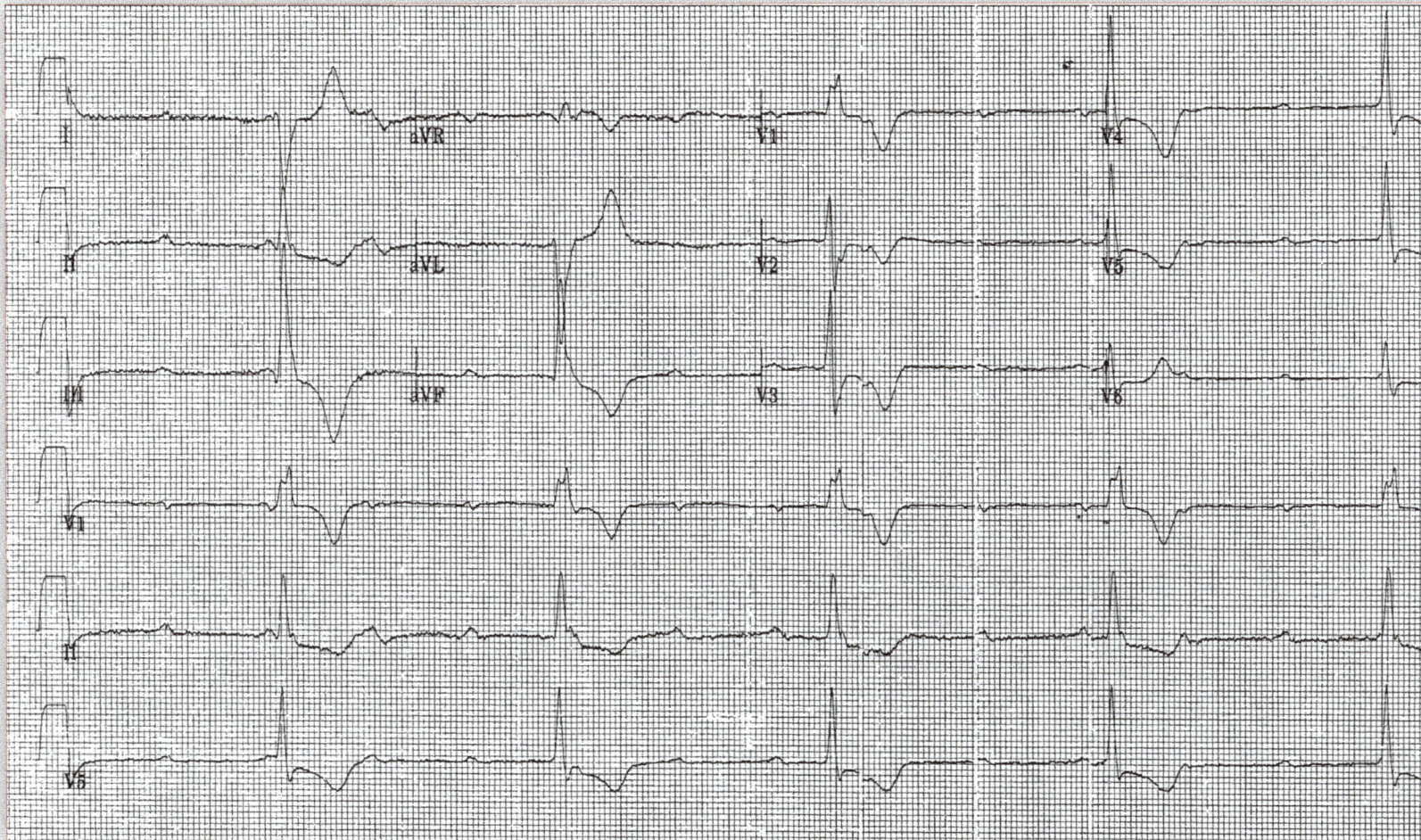

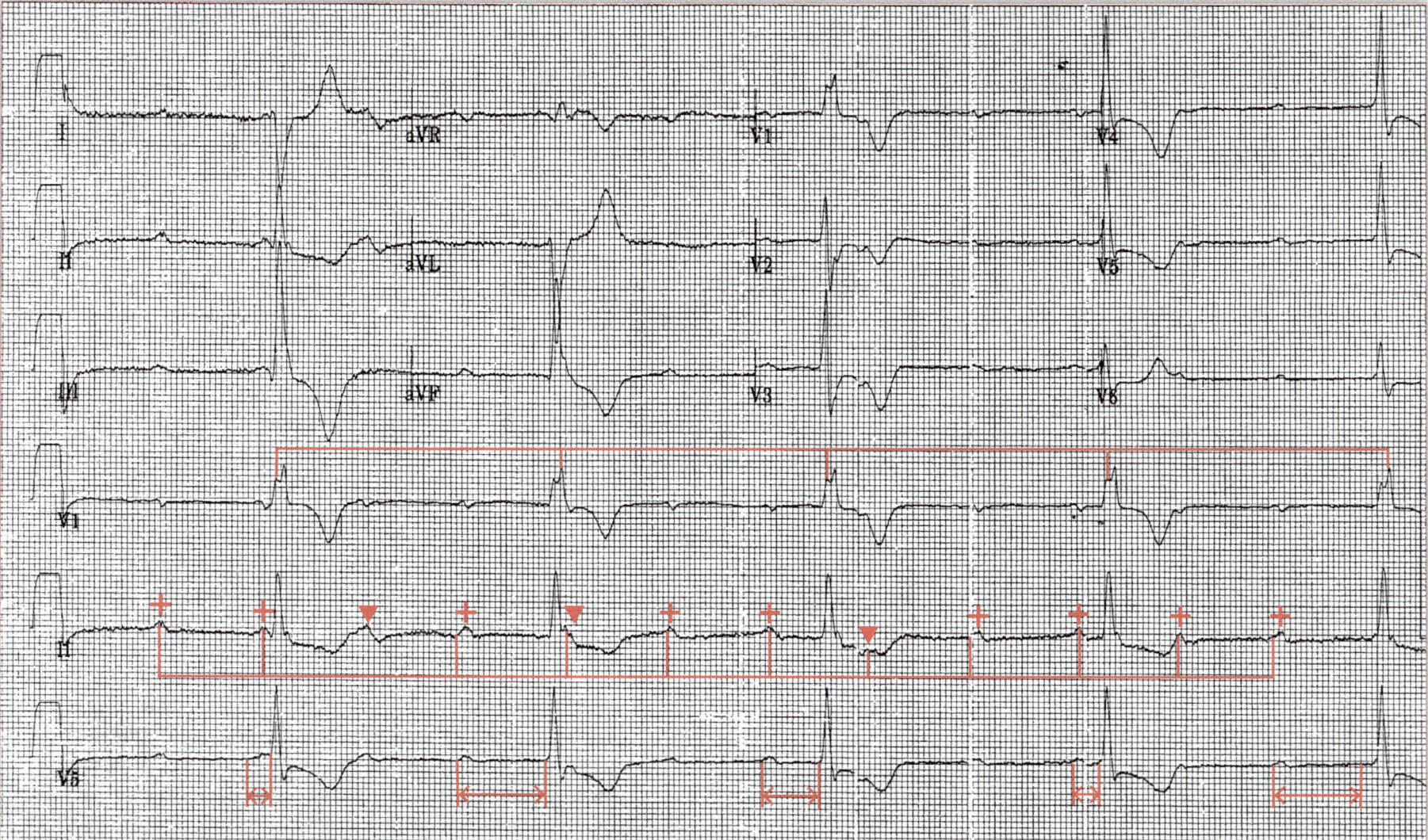

ECG 41 Analysis: Normal sinus rhythm, complete heart block
(third-degree AV block), escape ventricular rhythm

The ECG shows P waves (+) at a rate of 80 bpm. Some of the P waves are within the ST segments or T waves (▼) and not obvious. The PP intervals are constant (⊔). The P waves are positive in leads I, II, aVF, and V4-V6. Hence there is a normal sinus rhythm. The ventricular rate (RR intervals) is also regular (⊓), but at a rate of 30 bpm. There is no stable relationship between the P waves and the QRS complexes (PR intervals are variable [↔]), and hence there is AV dissociation. The atrial rate is faster than the ventricular rate; therefore, this is third-degree or complete AV block.

The QRS complexes are wide (0.16 sec) and abnormal in morphology, without a typical pattern for a right or left bundle branch block. Therefore, the escape rhythm is ventricular in origin and the location of the AV block is within the His-Purkinje system. The QRS complexes are ventricular, so abnormalities of the ventricular myocardium cannot be diagnosed because neither left nor right ventricular activation occurs via the normal His-Purkinje system. Among the most common etiologies for this rhythm is ischemic heart disease (especially with a previous myocardial infarction), severe cardiomyopathy, or idiopathic conduction system disease (Lev's or Lenègre's disease).

The major physical exam findings of complete heart block besides bradycardia include cannon A waves in the neck, a variable S1, and fluctuations in blood pressure reflecting the independent contraction of the atria and ventricles. Cannon A waves, which are irregular A waves with increased volume and amplitude, are visible in the jugular venous pulsation when the right atrium intermittently contracts against a closed tricuspid valve. This occurs when a P wave (atrial activation) occurs simultaneously with a QRS complex (ventricular activation). In complete heart block, the P waves are more frequent than the QRS waves, so the cannon A waves are interspersed with A waves that have a normal amplitude. The intensity of S1 is determined by the extent to which the AV valve leaflets (mitral and tricuspid) are open just before they close with ventricular contraction. When the AV valve leaflets are farther apart (ie, with a short PR interval), S1 intensity is increased. When the AV valve leaflets are closer together (ie, with a long PR interval in which the leaflets float back together), the S1 intensity is reduced. In complete heart block, since the P waves are at variable times in relation to the QRS complexes, the mitral and tricuspid valve leaflets are open to varying degrees before each ventricular contraction. This results in a variable S1 sound. The variability of the blood pressure results from changes in beat-to-beat stroke volume caused by variability in ventricular filling from left atrial contraction. ■

A 75-year-old woman presents with intermittent lightheadedness and dyspnea. An ECG is obtained. She is otherwise healthy and is taking no medications. An echocardiogram reveals significant calcification of the mitral annulus and ventricular septum.

What is the rhythm disturbance?

What is the anatomic location of the abnormality?

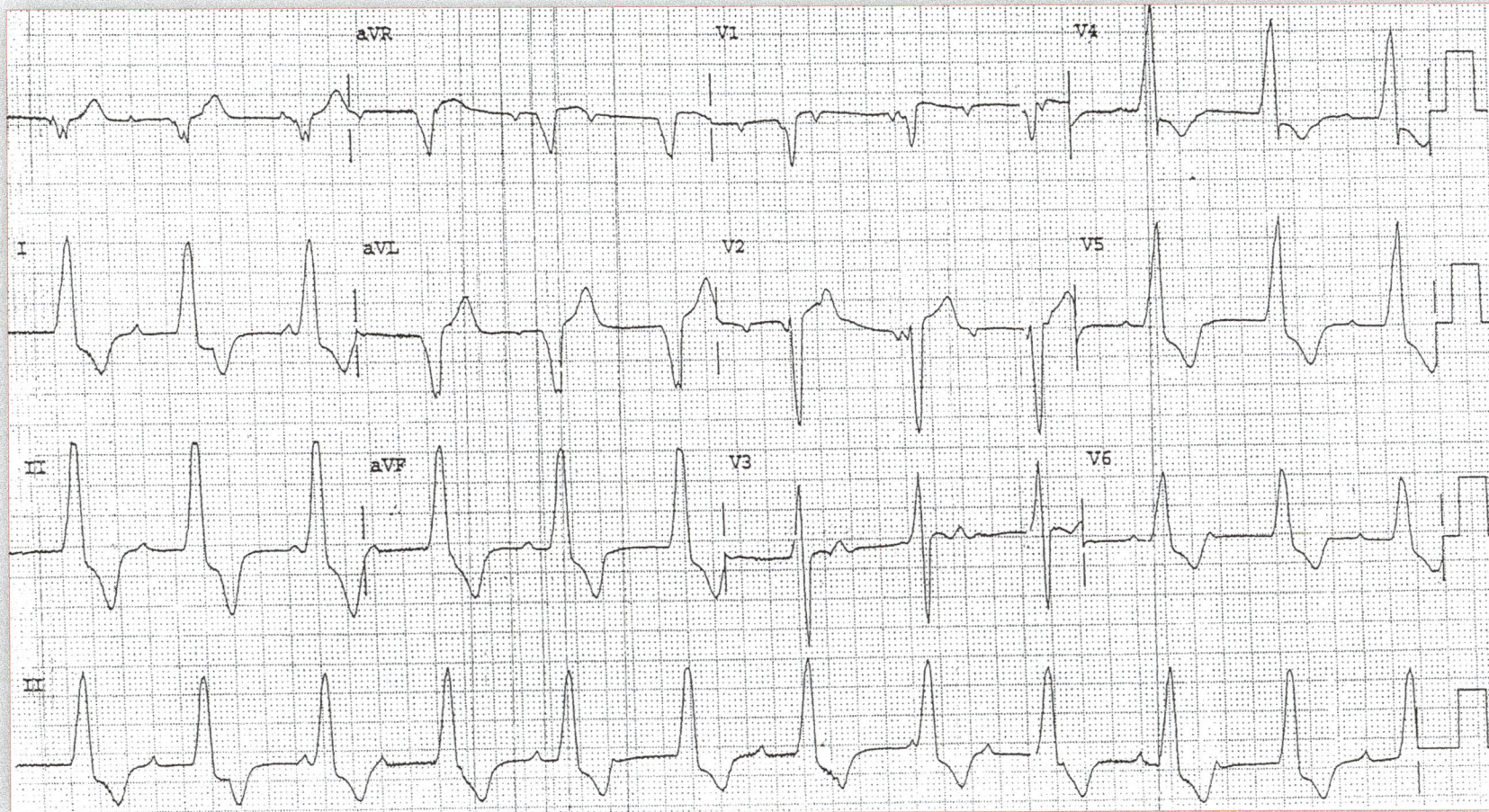

ECG 42 Analysis: Sinus tachycardia, complete heart block (third-degree AV block), ventricular escape rhythm

The ECG shows regular P waves (+) with a stable PP interval (⊔) at a rate of 120 bpm. It is important to determine the sinus rate by identifying two sequential P waves and then making certain that the P waves, when seen, are on time (ie, they "march out," or occur at a regular interval). They should be at a regular interval even if they are not apparent everywhere (^); that is, they may occur simultaneously with the QRS complex and hence not be obvious. This is best seen in the lead II rhythm strip. The P waves are positive in leads I, II, aVF, and V4-V6. Hence this is a sinus tachycardia. The ventricular rate is stable at 75 bpm (constant RR intervals [⊓]). There is no relationship between the P waves and QRS complexes as the PR intervals are variable (↔); hence there is AV dissociation. As the atrial rate is faster than the ventricular rate, this represents third-degree or complete heart block.

The QRS complexes are wide (0.14 sec) and abnormal in morphology, resembling neither a right or left bundle branch block. This represents a ventricular escape rhythm, even though the ventricular rate is 75 bpm, faster than what is expected from a ventricular escape focus. The etiology of the escape rhythm in complete heart block is based on the QRS morphology and not the ventricular rate. The ventricular rate is faster than expected in this case because of enhanced sympathetic stimulation, indicated by the fact that the sinus rate is 120 bpm. As the escape rhythm originates in the ventricle, the site of the AV conduction block is within the His-Purkinje system. This patient has no history of underlying heart disease and hence the most likely etiology is Lev's or Lenègre's disease, conditions involving fibrosis and calcification of left-sided cardiac structures, including the mitral annulus and ventricular septum, that often result in AV conduction system disease. ■

Notes

The following ECG is from a 72-year-old man who is in the recovery room after undergoing an elective cholecystectomy. His vital signs are normal.

What is the diagnosis?

How would you manage this patient?

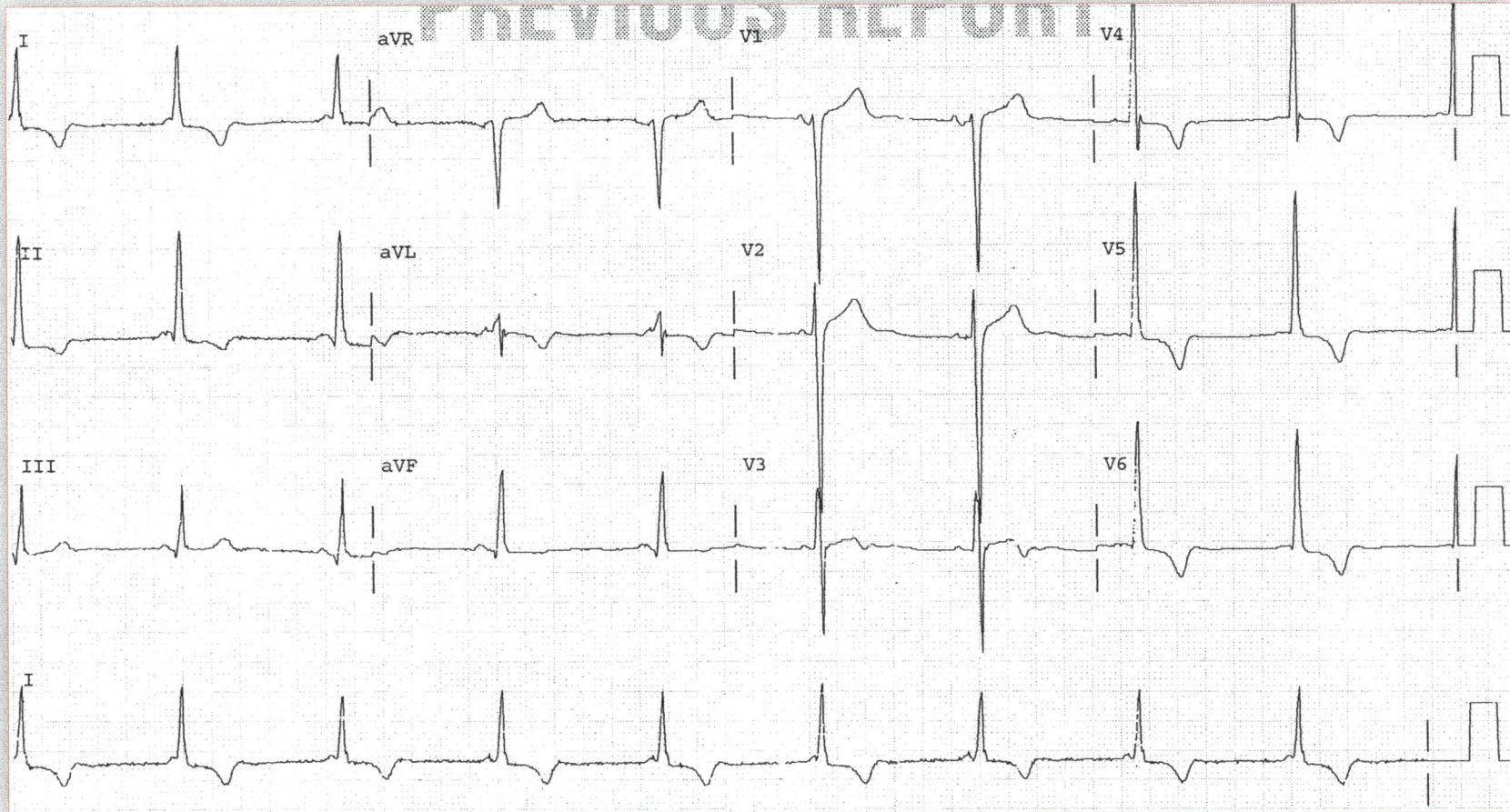

ECG 43 Analysis: Normal sinus rhythm, isorhythmic dissociation, junctional rhythm, left ventricular hypertrophy (LVH), ST-T wave abnormalities

The ECG shows a stable ventricular rate of 54 bpm. The QRS complex duration is normal (0.09 sec), and the axis is normal, between 0° and +90° (positive QRS complex in leads I and aVF). The QT/QTc intervals are normal (400/380 msec). P waves (+) can be seen in front of each QRS complex at a rate of 54 bpm. The P waves are upright in leads I, II, aVF, and V4-V6; hence they are sinus in origin. However, the PR intervals are short and not stable. Therefore, AV dissociation is present. Nevertheless, the atrial (PP intervals [⊔]) and ventricular (RR intervals [⊓]) rates are identical. When the atrial rate is faster than the ventricular rate, third-degree or complete heart block is present. In contrast, when AV dissociation is present but the ventricular rate is faster than the atrial rate, the etiology is an accelerated lower ectopic focus (either junctional or ventricular). However, when the atrial and ventricular rates are identical, the etiology for the AV dissociation cannot be established and this is termed isorhythmic dissociation.

If this were an accelerated junctional rhythm, any maneuver to increase the sinus rate (*eg*, administration of atropine) would result in restoration of normal conduction as the increased sinus rate would overdrive the lower focus and result in sinus captures and a sinus rhythm with a stable PR interval. In contrast, with complete heart block, an increase in the sinus rate would not result in capture and AV dissociation would persist, with now an atrial rate that is faster than the ventricular rate. Isorhythmic dissociation can be seen in the post-anesthesia setting and often resolves on its own. As long as the patient is stable, there is no specific treatment other than avoidance of any nodal blocking agents.

Also noted on this ECG is a deep S wave in lead V2 ([ ) and a tall R wave in lead V5 ( ]). Together they have an amplitude of 55 mm, which meets one of the criteria for left ventricular hypertrophy (LVH) (*ie*, S-wave depth in leads V1-V2 + R-wave amplitude in leads V5-V6 ≥ 35 mm). Also, ST-T wave (↑) abnormalities are noted in leads I, II, aVL, and V4-V6; these are associated with LVH and probably represent chronic subendocardial ischemia. ■

Case 44

A 21-year-old college student is seen at his student health service for intermittent palpitations. He otherwise has no complaints, and his physical examination is normal. An ECG is obtained.

What is the abnormality seen on this ECG?

What is the most likely etiology for the patient's palpitations?

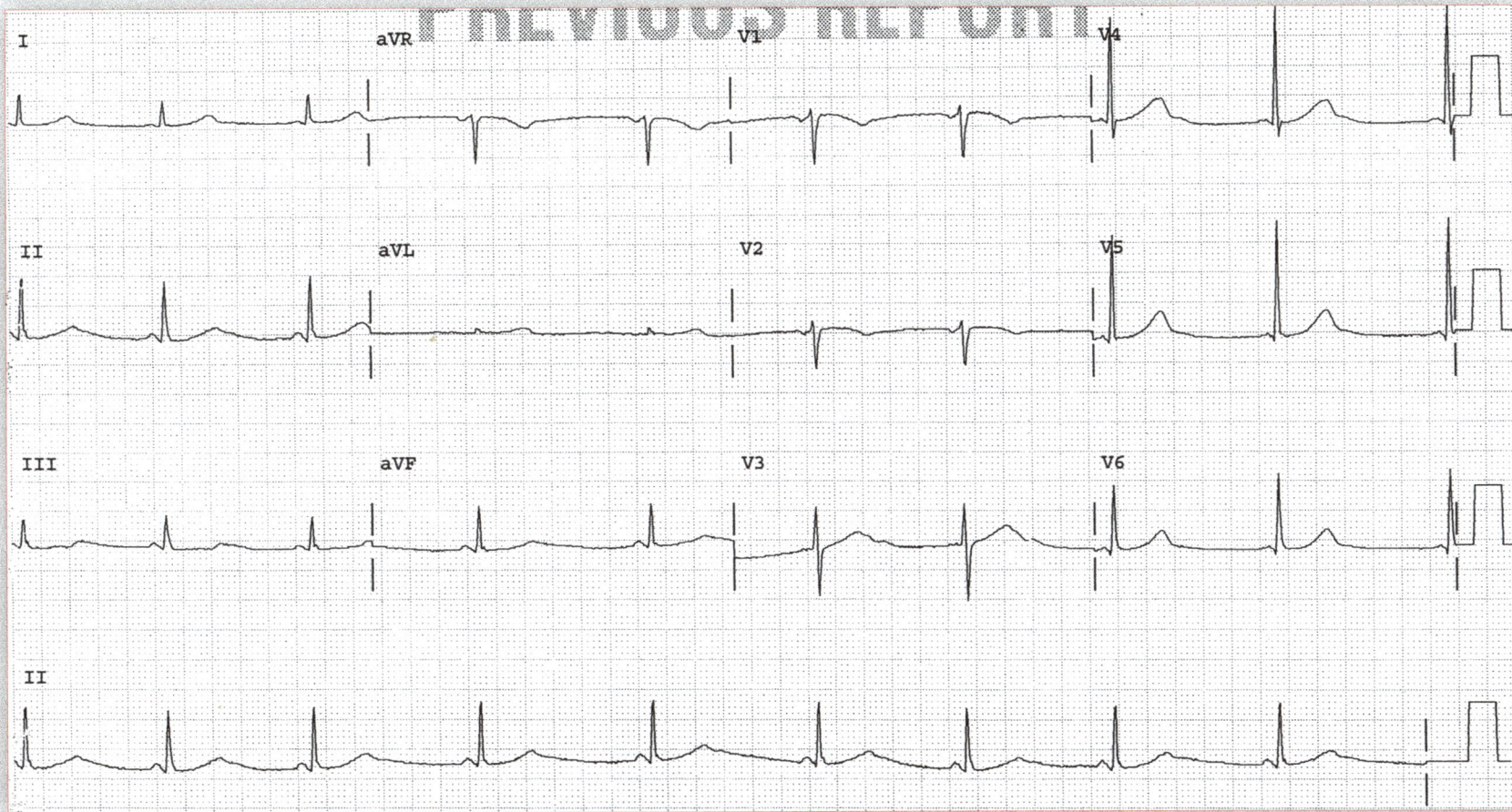

193

I aVR V1 V4

II aVL V2 V5

III aVF V3 V6

II

ECG 44 Analysis: **Sinus bradycardia, Lown-Ganong-Levine (LGL) pattern (preexcitation, accelerated AV conduction)**

There is a regular rhythm at a rate of 54 bpm. The QRS complex duration is normal (0.08 sec), and the axis is normal, between 0° and +90° (positive QRS complex in leads I and aVF). The QT/QTc intervals are normal (400/380 msec). There is a P wave (+) before each QRS complex, and the interval is stable but very short (‖) at 0.10 second (normal, 0.14–0.20 sec). The P waves are upright in leads I, II, aVF, and V4-V6, indicating that this is a sinus bradycardia.

The short PR interval indicates enhanced AV conduction, which has two etiologies. One is accelerated AV nodal conduction and the other is a preexcitation condition known Lown-Ganong-Levine (LGL) pattern. The LGL pattern on the ECG is due to an accessory pathway, known as the bundle of James, which originates in the atrial myocardium and bypasses the AV node, connecting directly to the bundle of His. As the AV node is bypassed (the AV node being the site of slowest conduction in the heart), AV conduction time is fast. Since the activation of the ventricles is via the normal His-Purkinje system, the QRS complexes are narrow and normal in morphology. As there are two pathways that link the atrium to the ventricles (ie, the normal AV node and the bundle of James), LGL is associated with a specific form of a reentrant arrhythmia known as AV reentrant tachycardia, which results from antegrade conduction to the ventricles via one of the pathways and retrograde conduction back to the atria via the other pathway. Other atrial arrhythmias, such as atrial tachycardia, atrial flutter, and atrial fibrillation, may also occur in association with LGL. However, these arrhythmias are not the result of the two pathways; instead, they occur independently, generated within the atrial myocardium, but use the accessory pathway to transmit the impulses to the ventricles. In this situation the ventricular response rate may be very rapid, as the AV node (which controls the ventricular response rate with atrial arrhythmias) is bypassed. When arrhythmias occur in association with the LGL pattern, this is known as the LGL syndrome. ■

A 32-year-old man with diabetes comes to your clinic with complaints of intermittent lightheadedness. He denies any episodes of chest pain, chest pressure, or shortness of breath. His exercise tolerance has been stable, but he does admit to living a sedentary lifestyle. Another health care provider was concerned about his having a myocardial infarction and recommended cardiac catheterization. He is in your clinic for a second opinion. You obtain an ECG.

What is the most likely cause of this patient's symptoms?

Does he need a cardiac catheterization?

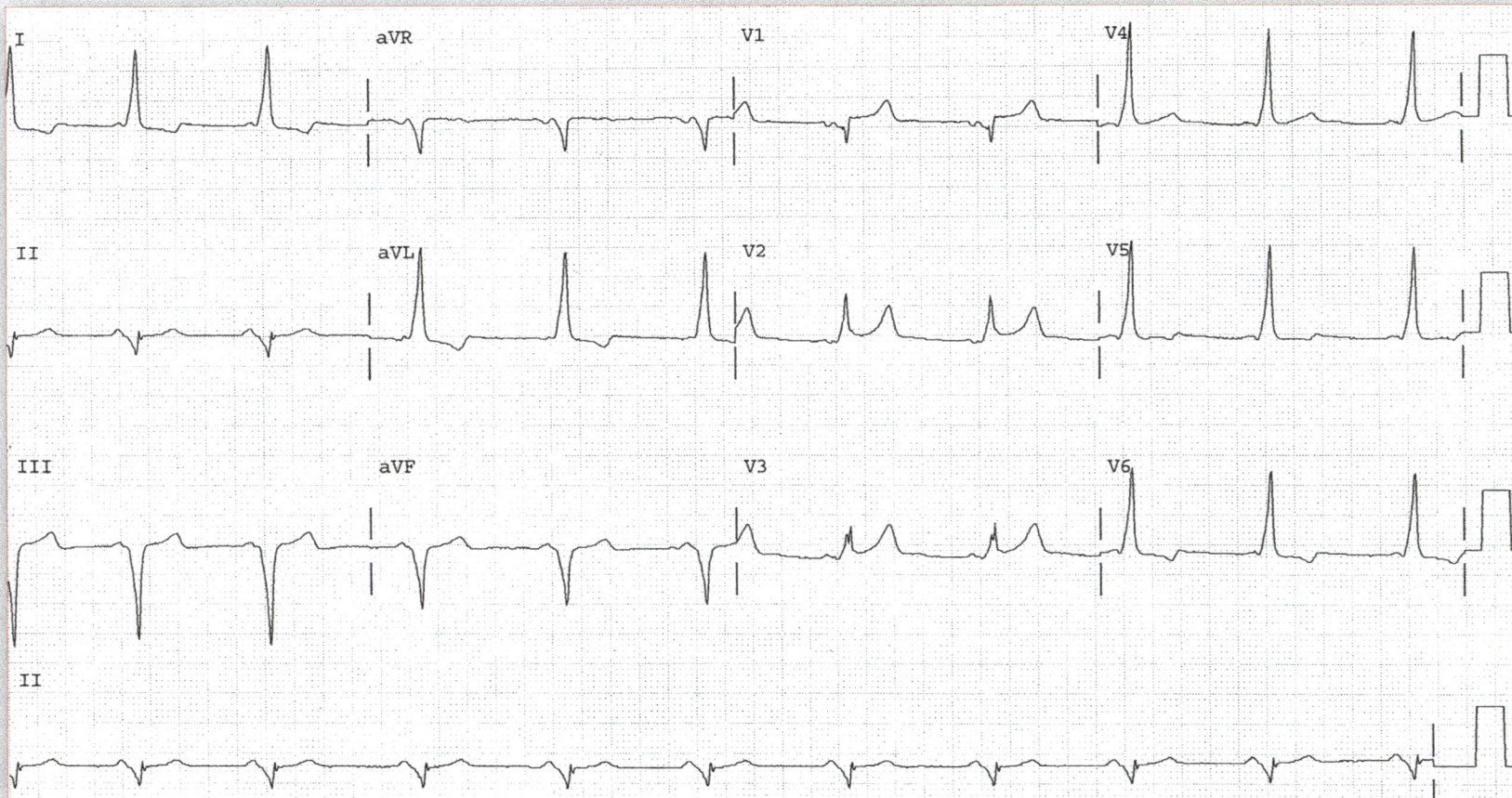

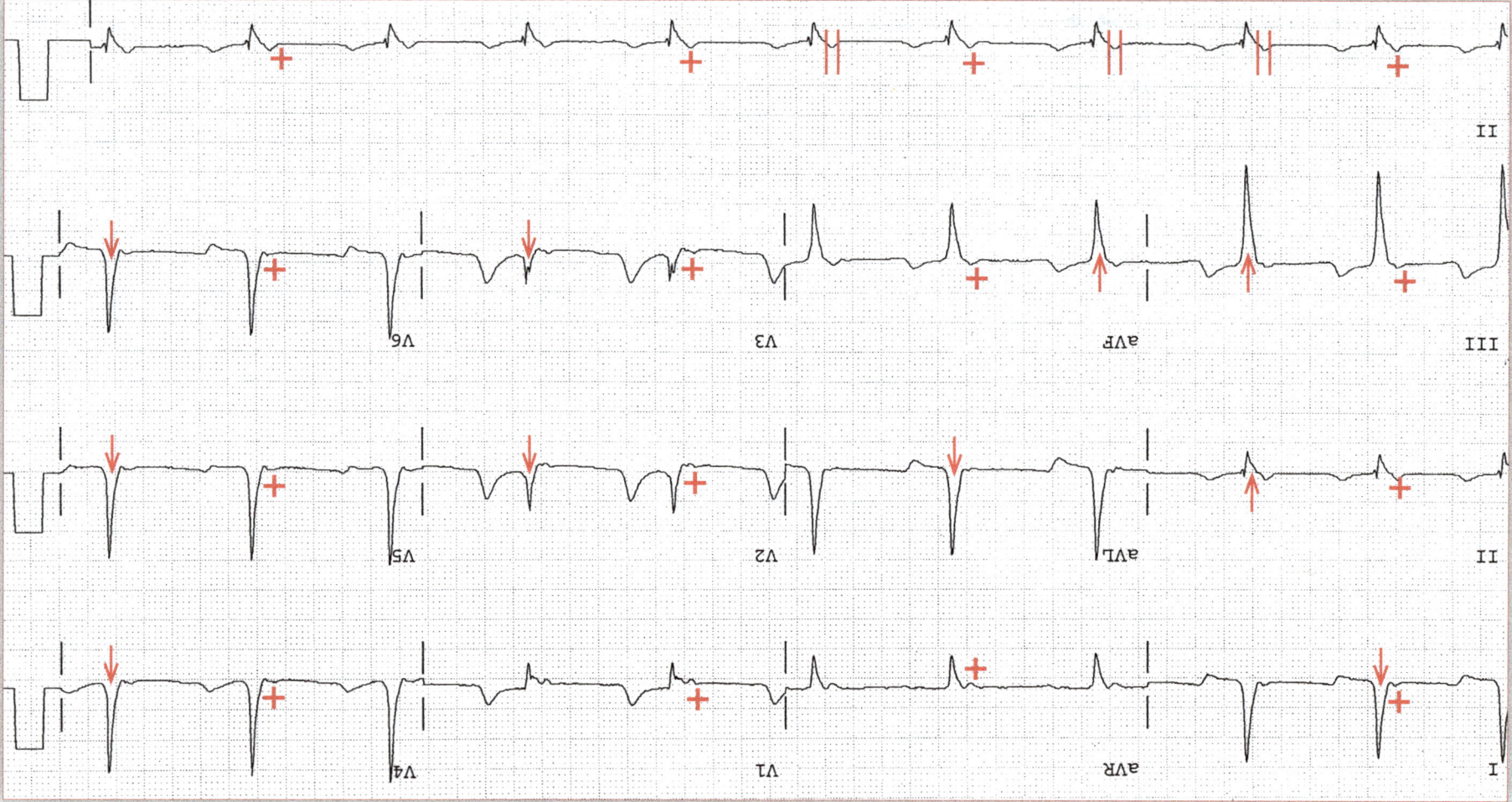

Wolff-Parkinson-White (preexcitation) pattern

ECG 45 Analysis: Normal sinus rhythm,

II

III   aVF   V3   V6

II   aVL   V2   V5

I   aVR   V1   V4

The ECG shows a regular rate of 60 bpm, and a P wave (+) of normal morphology (upright in leads I, II, aVF, and V4-V6) can be seen in front of each QRS complex. Hence this is a normal sinus rhythm. Although the PR interval is stable, it is very short (‖) (0.12 sec). In addition, the QRS complex is widened to 0.14 second and there is a slow or slurred upstroke to the QRS complex; this is called a delta wave (↑,↓). As a result of the delta wave the base of the QRS complex is widened while the peak is narrow.

The QT/QTc intervals are normal (400/400 msec and 340/340 msec when adjusting for the prolonged QRS duration). The presence of a short PR interval and a wide QRS complex (due to a delta wave) is termed Wolff-Parkinson-White (WPW) pattern. It is the result of an accessory pathway, called the bundle of Kent, that links the atrium directly to the ventricle and bypasses the AV node, accounting for the short PR interval. Since the initial activation of the ventricle is via the fast-conducting accessory pathway and not the normal His-Purkinje system, the initial portion of the QRS complex is slow in upstroke and the complex is widened due to the abnormal left ventricular activation that is directly through the ventricular myocardium; hence the widened base of the QRS complex. This initial slowed ventricular activation produces the slurred QRS upstroke, which is termed a delta wave. However, WPW is due to a fusion complex resulting from left ventricular activation via two different pathways. The initial part of the QRS complex is due to early activation (preexcitation) via the accessory pathway, and later activation (terminal portion of the QRS complex) is via the normal AV node–His-Purkinje system. The impulse via these two pathways "fuses," resulting in a fusion complex. Therefore, the terminal portion of the QRS complex is the result of activation via the normal AV node–His-Purkinje pathway; the peak of the QRS complex is narrow.

The PR interval, the duration of the delta wave, and hence the QRS width are dependent on the relative balance of conduction via the two pathways. This is related to AV nodal conduction as the accessory pathway is similar to Purkinje fibers and conduction through this pathway is "all or none" and hence not variable. If conduction via the normal nodal His-Purkinje pathway is relatively slow compared with conduction via the accessory pathway, there is more myocardial activation via the accessory pathway and the PR interval is shorter, the delta wave

continues

and QRS complexes are wider, and the QRS complex is more abnormal. In contrast, if conduction via the normal AV node–His-Purkinje system is more rapid, less myocardium is activated via the accessory pathway and the PR interval is longer, the delta wave is less prominent, and the QRS complex is narrower and more normal in morphology.

Since left ventricular activation (to a greater or lesser extent) is initiated by conduction via an accessory pathway directly through the ventricular myocardium and not via the normal His-Purkinje pathway, abnormalities of the left ventricular myocardium (*ie*, infarction, ischemia, left ventricular hypertrophy, inflammation such as pericarditis or myocarditis) cannot be diagnosed reliably on ECG. The ECG has inferior Q waves and diffuse nonspecific ST-segment and T-wave abnormalities. In the presence of a WPW pattern this is a pseudo inferior infarction pattern and is the result of a posteroseptal bypass tract. It is not an inferior wall MI but is actually a negative delta wave. In the absence of any other clinical evidence suggesting ischemia, there is no indication for cardiac catheterization.

The short PR interval, delta wave, and widened QRS complex are diagnostic for a WPW pattern. Since there are two pathways linking the atria to the ventricles (the bundle of Kent and the normal AV node–His-Purkinje system), a large (macro) circuit is formed, linked proximally by the atrial myocardium and distally via the ventricular myocardium. The presence of this macro-circuit predisposes to a reentrant form of supraventricular tachycardia called AV reentrant tachycardia. Other supraventricular tachyarrhythmias, such as atrial tachycardia, atrial flutter, and atrial fibrillation, may also occur; however, they are not dependent on the presence of this circuit but rather use the accessory pathway as an alternative pathway for activation of the ventricles. In this situation the ventricular response rate may be very rapid, as the AV node (which controls the ventricular response rate with atrial arrhythmias) is bypassed. The presence of arrhythmias in a patient with a WPW pattern on the ECG defines the WPW syndrome. ■

A 44-year-old woman with schizophrenia and a history of narcotic dependence presents to your clinic with dysuria. A urinalysis is positive for white blood cells, and a urine culture reveals a gram-negative bacterium that is sensitive to ceftriaxone and levofloxacin. The patient has a known allergy to cephalosporins. Her medications include quetiapine and methadone. She is otherwise healthy and has a normal physical examination.

Why do you need an ECG before you start this patient on antibiotics?

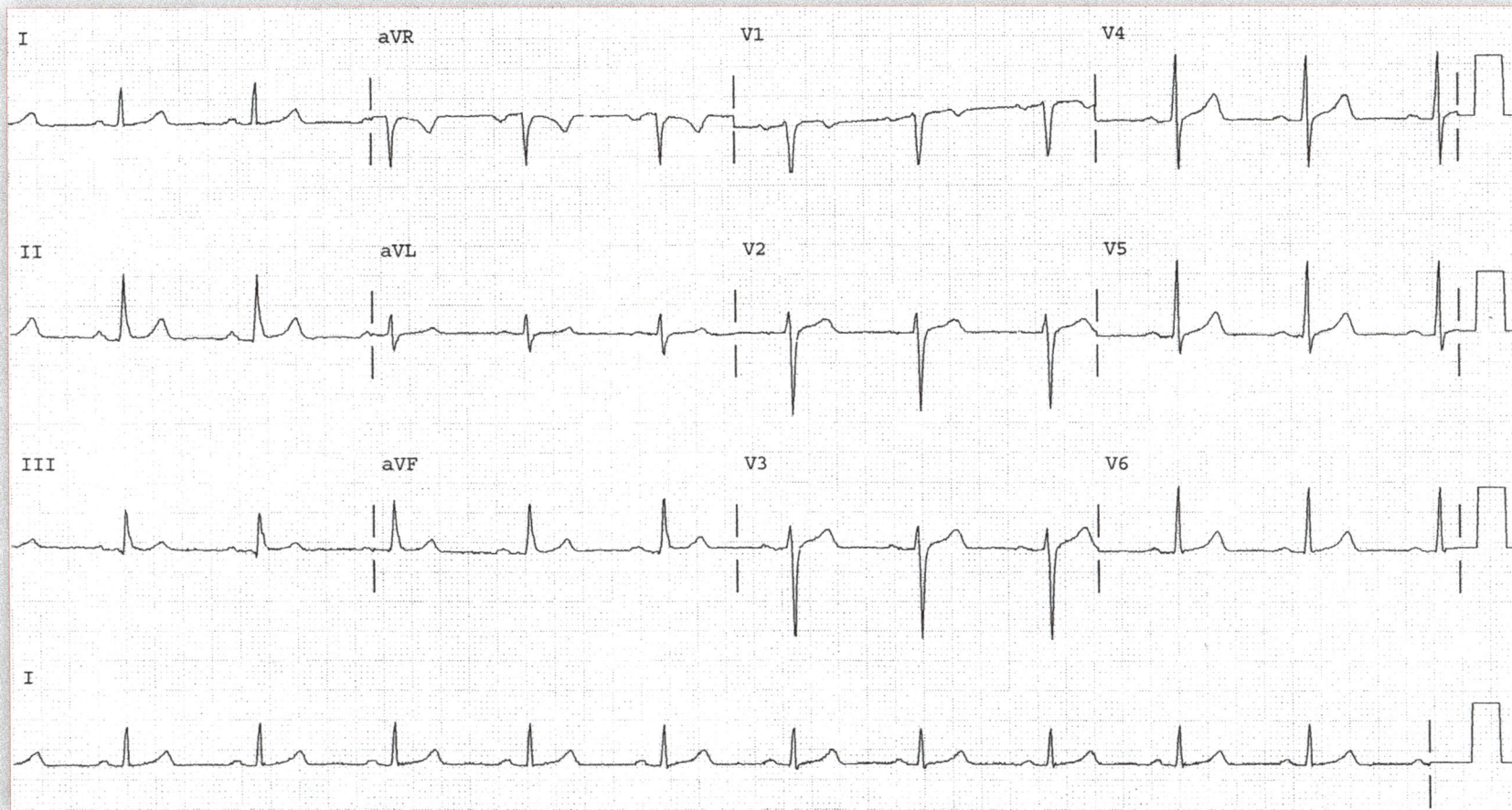

ECG 46 Analysis: Normal sinus rhythm, normal ECG

The ECG shows a regular rhythm at a rate of 64 bpm. The P wave (+), which has a normal duration of 0.12 second, is upright in leads I, II, aVF, and V4-V6; the P wave is biphasic in lead V1 (+), which is normal. This is, therefore, a normal sinus rhythm.

Each QRS complex is preceded by a P wave, and each P wave is followed by a QRS complex. The axis in the frontal plane is normal as the QRS complex is positive in leads I and aVF, thereby indicating that the axis is between 0° and +90°. The PR interval (↔) is normal at 0.20 second and it is constant, the QRS width is normal at 0.08 second, and the QT/QTc intervals (⊓) are normal at 360/370 msec. There is normal R-wave progression across the precordium (*ie*, the R waves become progressively higher in amplitude and the S waves have less depth going from leads V1 to V6). The transition point (R/S > 1) occurs between leads V3 and V4. The ST segments, which have a normal concave morphology (^), are at baseline (determined by the TP segment [↑]). The T waves have a normal morphology (▼); they are upright in leads with a positive QRS complex and are asymmetric, with a slower upstroke and a more rapid downstroke. Lead aVR, being the mirror image of all the other limb leads, shows a negative P wave, QRS complex, and T wave, all of which are normal in this lead. Hence this is a normal ECG.

This patient needs a baseline ECG prior to starting her on a quinolone in order to document her QT/QTc intervals. She is already chronically taking two agents known to prolong the QT/QTc intervals. The antipsychotics, including haloperidol and quetiapine, are a family of compounds known to cause QT prolongation. Methadone is the one narcotic that also can cause significant QT prolongation. Among the antibiotics, quinolones and macrolides are known to prolong the QT interval. Prolongation of the QT interval is more likely to occur when multiple drugs that can cause this change are prescribed. Therefore, it is essential to check baseline and follow-up QT intervals. Prolongation of the QT interval puts a patient at risk for a serious ventricular tachyarrhythmia called torsade de pointes. ◼

A 56-year-old man with hypertension and hyperlipidemia underwent cardiac catheterization earlier in the day in the setting of progressive anginal symptoms and was found to have a 95% distal left anterior descending artery lesion. The stenosis was successfully stented. No other coronary lesions were identified. Later in the day, he becomes tachycardic and the following ECG is obtained. His vital signs are otherwise stable and he is asymptomatic.

Which of the following is the most likely cause of this patient's tachycardia?

A. In-stent restenosis

B. Acute stent thrombosis

C. Acute bleed

D. Infected stent with sepsis

E. New stenosis of the right coronary artery

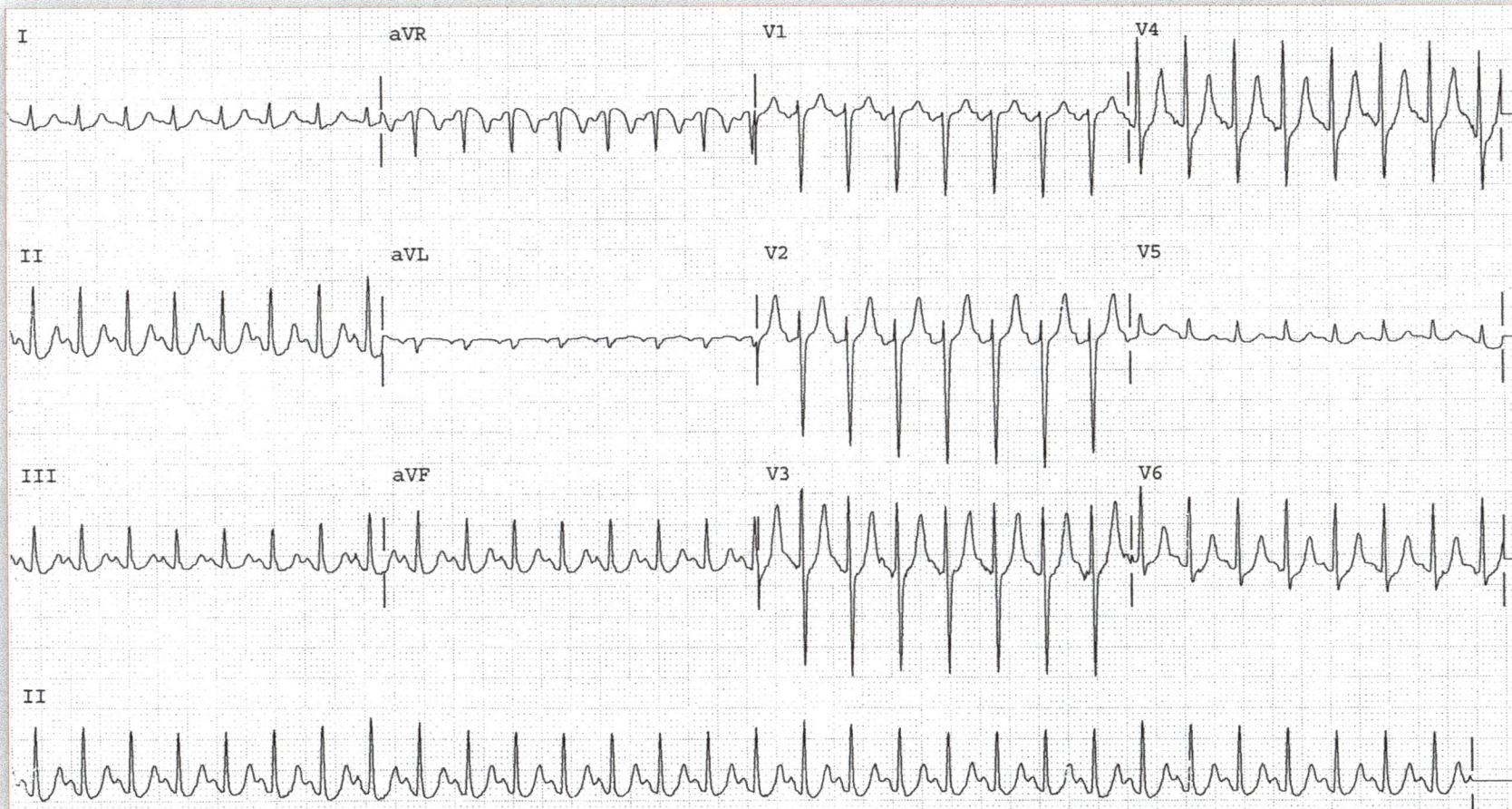

ECG 47 Analysis: Sinus tachycardia, upsloping ST-segment depression

The ECG shows a regular rhythm at a rate of 200 bpm. Any heart rate over 100 bpm is defined as a tachycardia. The P wave (+) is upright in leads I, II, aVF, and V4-V6; it appears to be biphasic in lead V1. Hence this is a sinus tachycardia. Each QRS complex is preceded by a P wave, and each P wave is followed by a QRS complex. It should be pointed out that the P wave may not be seen clearly in every lead; for example, it is not well seen in leads V2-V3, but it can be seen clearly in lead V1 (▼). Because every column is simultaneous, the P wave is present in leads V2-V3 but is just not obvious because it is superimposed at the end of the T wave in these leads (^). The axis in the frontal plane is normal, between 0° and +90° (the QRS complex is upright in leads I and aVF).

The PR interval is 0.12 second (‖), which is short as a result of the rapid sinus rate. This is due to an increase in conduction velocity through the AV node as a result of sympathetic stimulation, which is the usual cause of a sinus tachycardia. The QRS width is 0.08 second (normal), and the QT/QTc intervals are normal (220/400 msec). There is normal R-wave progression across the precordium (R wave becomes progressively higher in amplitude and S wave less deep going from lead V1 to lead V6), with the transition point (R/S > 1) between V3 and V4. The ST segments have a normal concave morphology (↑), and while they are at baseline in most leads (in the presence of a sinus tachycardia during which the TP segment cannot be seen, the PR segment [▲] is used to define baseline) there is some J-point and upsloping ST-segment depression in leads V4 and V6 (↓). In the presence of a tachycardia, J-point and ST-segment depression may be a normal finding as it is due to atrial repolarization (T wave of the P wave).

continues

With sinus tachycardia and the shortening of the PR interval, the T wave of the P wave, which normally occurs during ventricular depolarization and is within the QRS complex, moves out from the QRS complex and is superimposed on the J point, which now becomes depressed. As a result, the ST segment slopes upward toward baseline. Therefore, in the presence of upsloping ST segments, the presence of actual ST-segment depression, which is the marker of ischemia, is established by evaluating the ST segment at 0.08 second (two small boxes) beyond the J point. If at this time the ST segment is more than 1.5 mm below the baseline, it is considered to be abnormal ST-segment depression, suggestive of ischemia. An ST segment that is at baseline at this time is considered to be normal. Such is the case on this ECG. Although the T waves are tall and peaked (a frequent finding during a tachycardia), they are still asymmetric with a slower upstroke and more rapid downstroke. Noted is that lead aVR, which is the mirror image of the other limb leads, has a negative P wave, QRS complex, and T wave.

Tachycardia in the setting of a cardiac catheterization should always be evaluated urgently for potential procedural complications. The most worrisome complications include acute stent thrombosis, pericardial tamponade, aortic dissection, a ventricular arrhythmia, or a serious bleed such as a retroperitoneal bleed, all of which can be associated with tachycardia and hemodynamic instability. In this case, the patient's ECG does not suggest acute stent thrombosis, which is total occlusion of the stent and results in signs and symptoms of an acute ST-segment elevation myocardial infarction. In-stent restenosis, which results from smooth muscle cell migration, proliferation, and hyperplasia within stents, is unlikely given that it is a chronic process, occurring several months after stent insertion and not within 1 to 2 days. Similarly, coronary artery disease is a chronic process, so a new stenosis in the right coronary artery developing within a day is unlikely. Infection of stents is an extremely rare phenomenon. However, bleeding often occurs due to the antiplatelet therapy and anticoagulation administered in the setting of a percutaneous coronary intervention. This can either be from a retroperitoneal bleed, gastrointestinal bleed, or an expanding groin hematoma.

The following ECG is obtained from a sleeping patient with complaints of daytime sleepiness and morning headaches.

What are the most likely diagnosis and treatment?

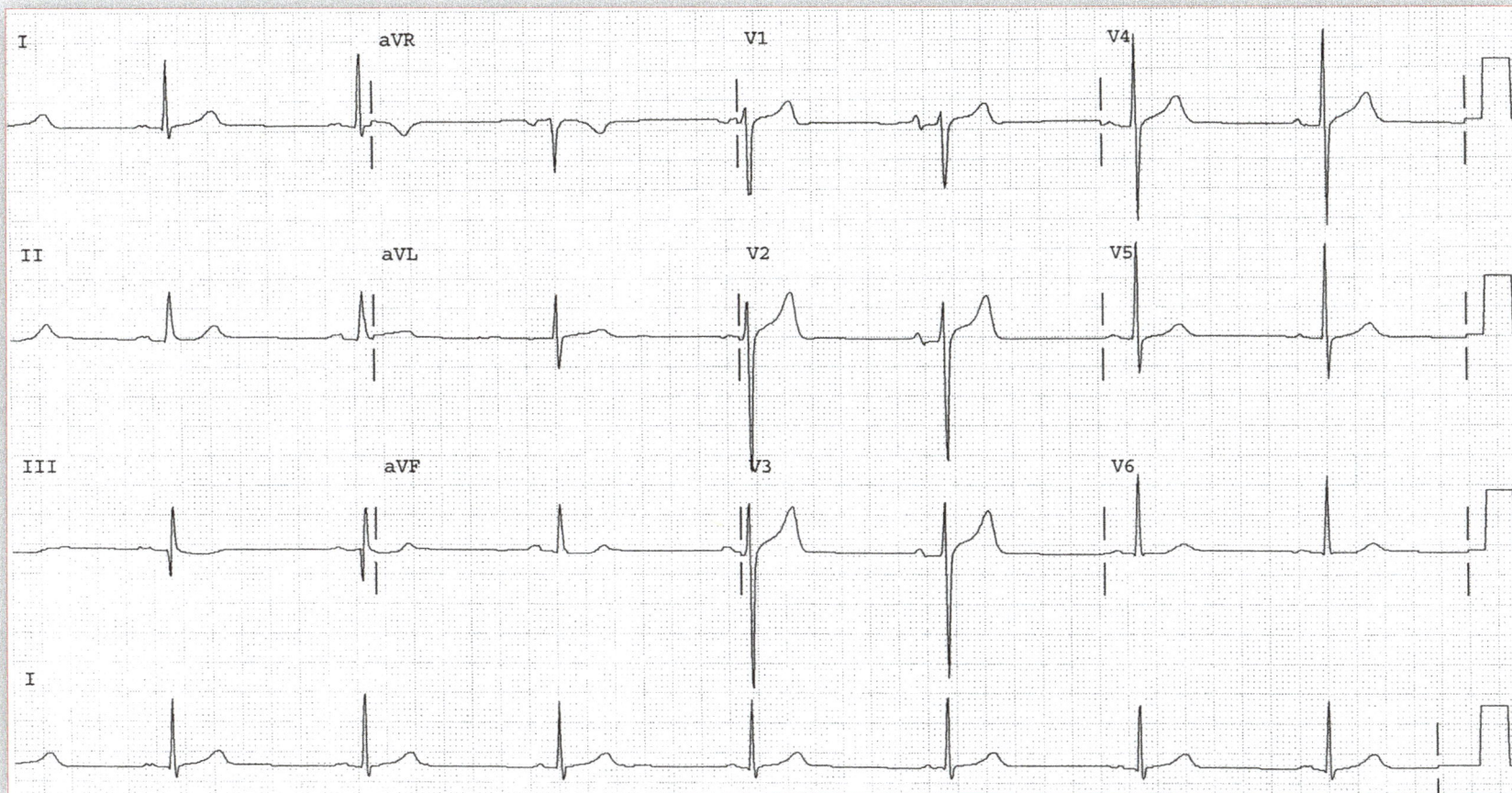

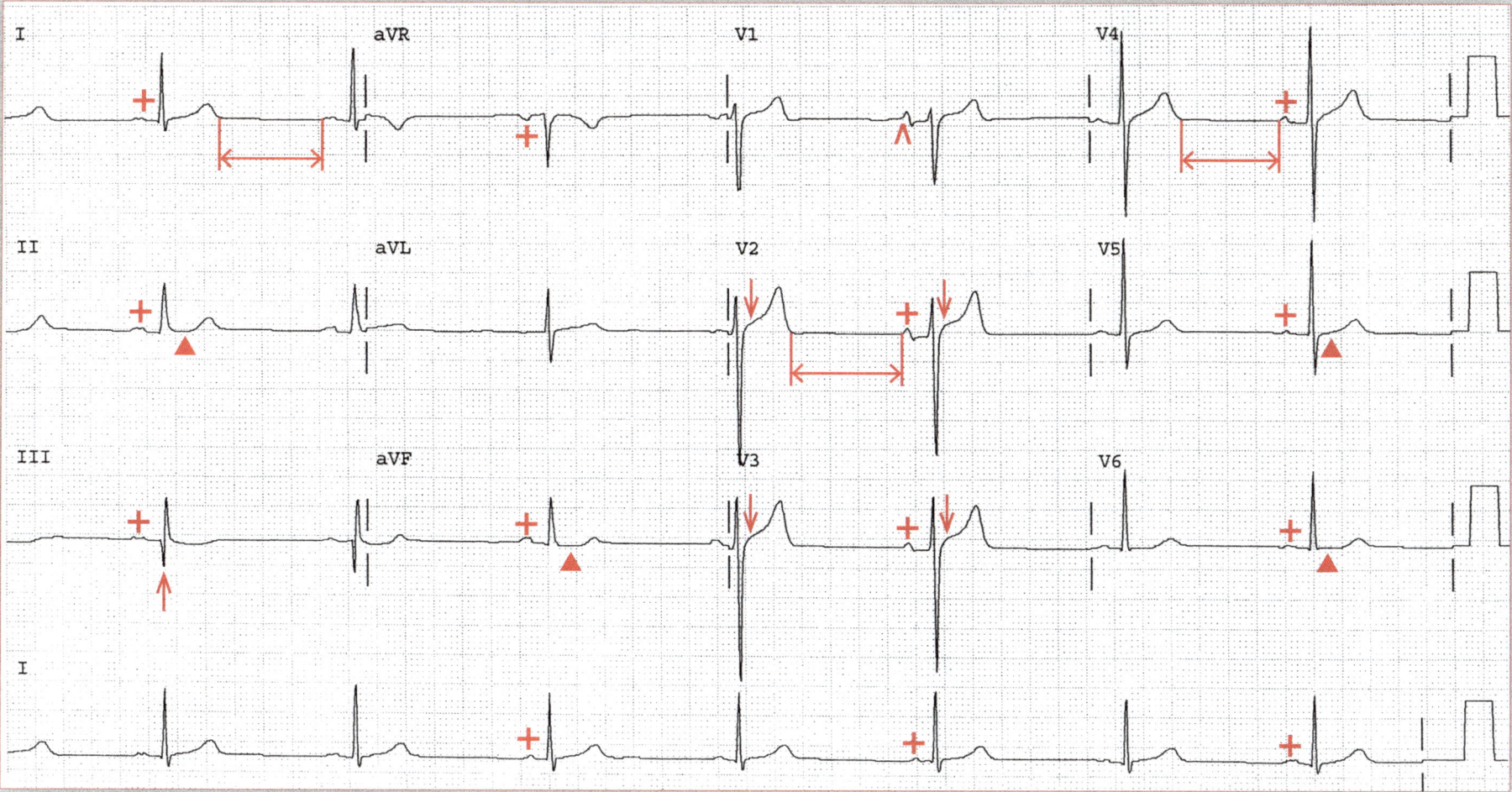

ECG 48 Analysis: **Sinus bradycardia**

The rhythm is regular at a rate of 44 bpm, defined as a bradycardia. The P wave (+) is upright in leads I, II, aVF, and V4-V6; it is biphasic in lead V1 (^), which is normal. Hence this is a sinus bradycardia. Each QRS complex is preceded by a P wave, and each P wave is followed by a QRS complex. The P-wave duration is normal at 0.12 second, and the PR interval is constant at 0.20 second.

The axis in the frontal plane is normal, between 0° and +90° (the QRS complex is positive in leads I and aVF). There is a deep but narrow Q wave in lead III (↑). However, lead III is an indeterminate or ambiguous lead and hence abnormalities that are present in only this lead are nondiagnostic. The QRS complex duration is 0.08 second, the QT interval is 440 msec, and the QT interval corrected for heart rate (*ie*, QTc) is 380 msec, all of which are normal. The ST segments have a normal concave morphology and are at baseline (defined as the TP segment [↔]) in most leads. However, a slight ST-segment elevation (↓) can be seen in leads V2-V3, which represents early repolarization and is a normal variant seen in young individuals who have tall QRS complexes as well as in those with left ventricular hypertrophy. There is flattening of the ST segment in leads II, aVF, and V5-V6 (▲), which is a nonspecific change. The R-wave progression from leads V1 to V6 is normal (R-wave amplitude progressively increases while S-wave depth progressively decreases). The T waves have a normal morphology (*ie*, they are upright in all leads and are asymmetric with a slower upstroke and faster downstroke). Noted is that lead aVR, which is the mirror image of the other limb leads, has a negative P wave, QRS complex, and T wave.

Sinus bradycardia is often seen in situations with enhanced vagal tone, such as during sleep or in young well-conditioned individuals, and does not represent a pathologic process. However, bradyarrhythmias during sleep can also be observed with sleep apnea, particularly if they correlate with episodes of oxygen desaturation. Daytime sleepiness and morning headaches are common symptoms of sleep apnea, and the treatment is nocturnal continuous positive airway pressure. ■

This ECG is obtained from a 20-year-old marathon runner.

What is the diagnosis?

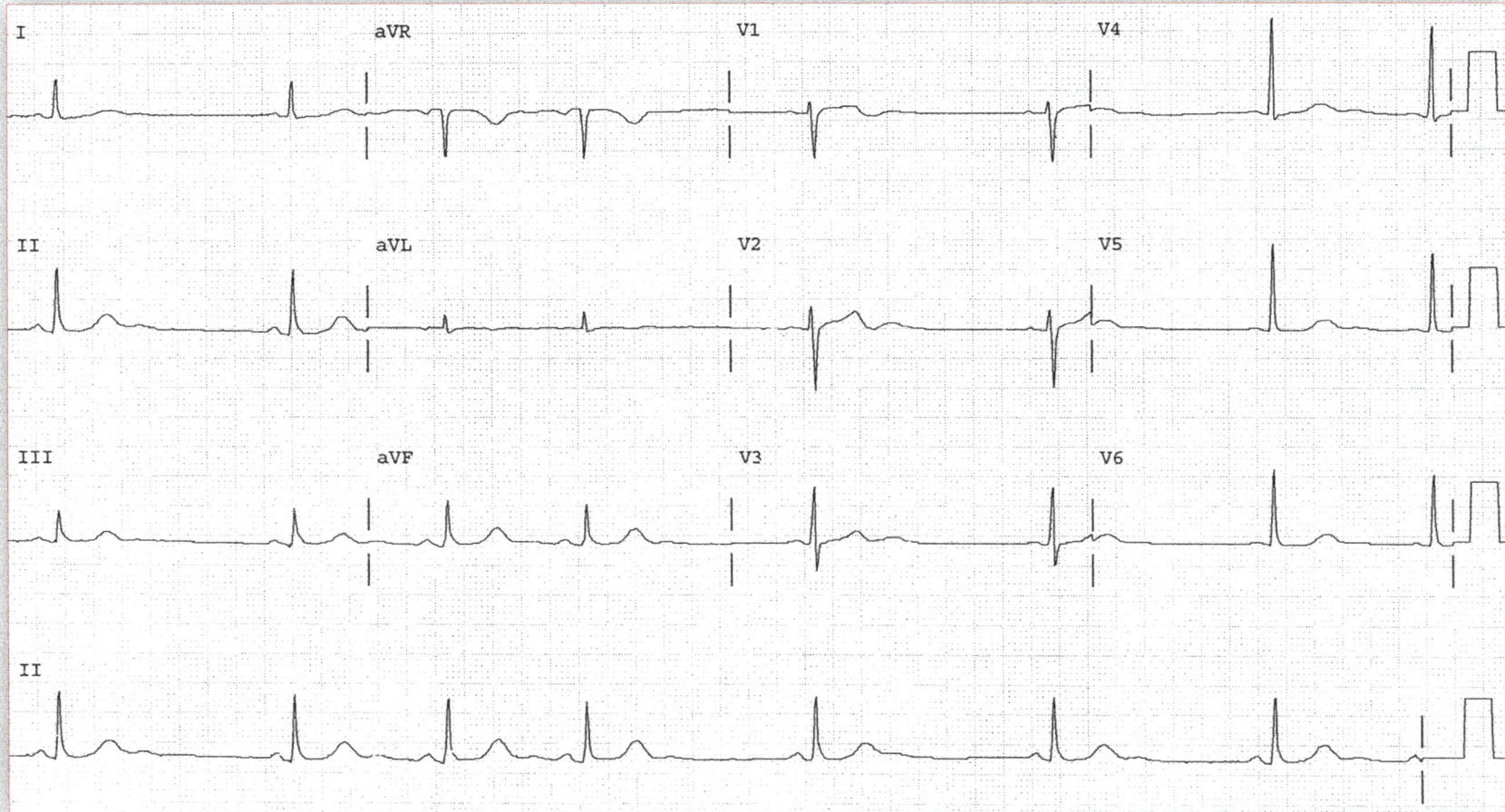

I aVR V1 V4

II aVL V2 V5

III aVF V3 V6

II

ECG 49 Analysis: Sinus arrhythmia

The ECG shows a sinus rhythm with P waves (+) of uniform morphology before each QRS complex. The P waves are upright in leads I, II, aVF, and V4-V6. The PR interval is constant (↔) at 0.16 second. However, the rhythm is not regular (⊔) and the heart rate (RR intervals) ranges from 36 to 62 bpm. There is no pattern to the irregular heart rate (*ie*, it is irregularly irregular). The QRS complex duration is normal (0.08 sec), as is the morphology. The axis is normal, between 0° and +90° (positive QRS complex in leads I and aVF), and the QT/QTc intervals are normal (400/370 msec). Also noted are prominent but normal U waves (^) in leads V2-V3.

Only three supraventricular rhythms are irregularly irregular: 1) sinus arrhythmia in which there is one P-wave morphology and a stable PR interval, 2) multifocal atrial rhythm or wandering atrial pacemaker (rate < 100 bpm) or multifocal atrial tachycardia (rate > 100 bpm) in which there are three or more different P-wave morphologies and PR intervals without one dominant P wave, and 3) atrial fibrillation in which there is no organized atrial activity or P waves. Atrial flutter and atrial tachycardia may be irregular, but there will be a pattern based on the degree of AV block; hence these rhythms will be regularly irregular.

The etiology for this arrhythmia is sinus arrhythmia and it is a respirophasic rhythm (*ie*, the changes in the sinus rate are the result of respiration). Heart rate increases with inspiration and decreases with expiration. These fluctuations in heart rate are mediated by changes in vagal tone and are a normal finding. It may be more apparent in patients with high vagal tone, such as athletes or other well-conditioned people. Respiratory sinus arrhythmia serves to increase pulmonary blood flow during lung inflation. As it is a normal physiologic change in heart rate related to respiration, no further evaluation or therapy is warranted. ■

A 44-year-old woman with anxiety presents with the frequent sensation of "skipped heartbeats." She otherwise denies chest pain, dyspnea, syncope, or lightheadedness. She smokes two packs of cigarettes per day and drinks three glasses of wine per day to calm her nerves. She takes clonazepam and was recently started on a β-blocker for the palpitations. Her physical examination is normal. An ECG is obtained.

What is the etiology of her symptoms?

How would you treat her?

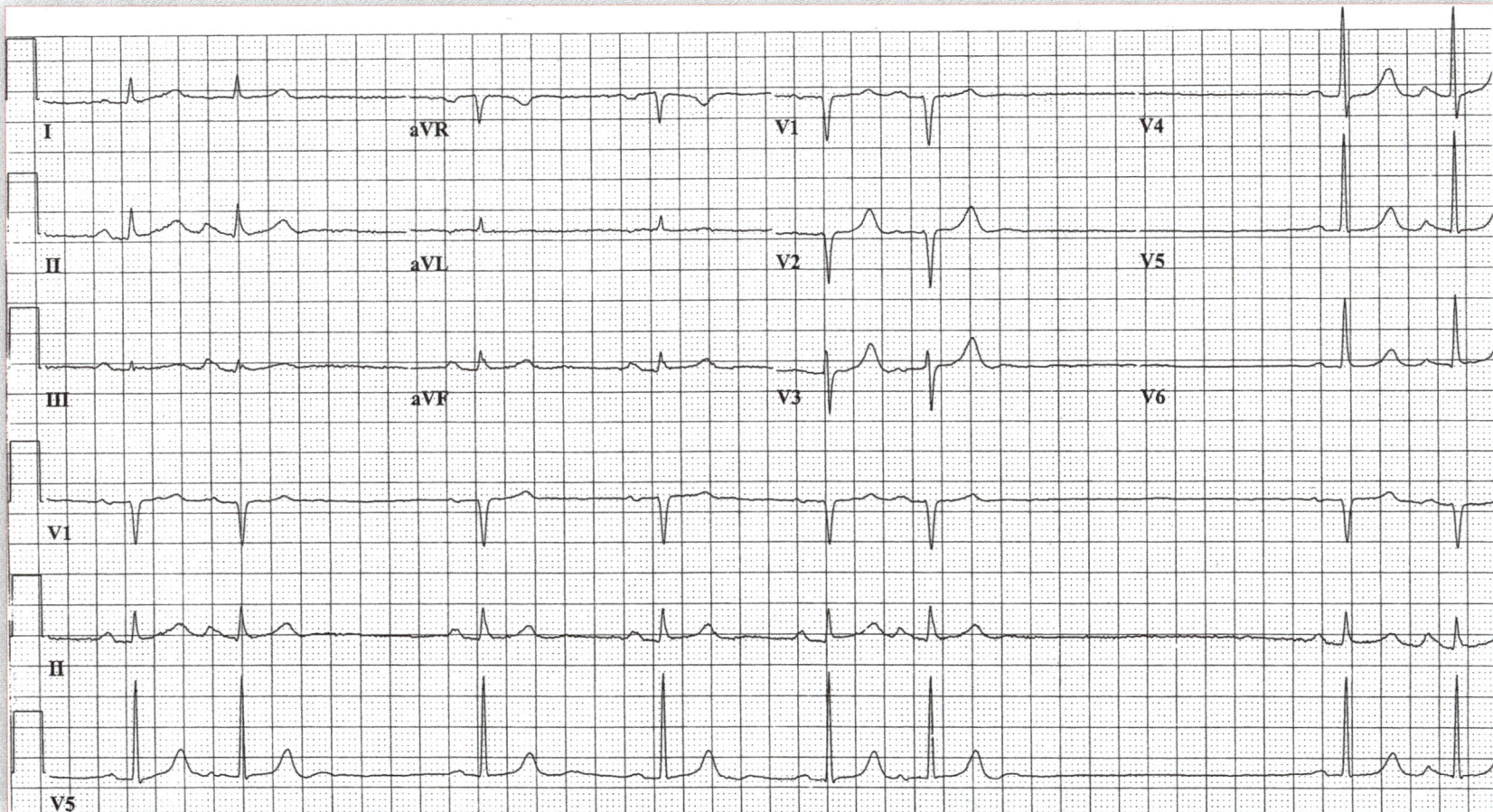

I   aVR   V1   V4

II   aVL   V2   V5

III   aVF   V3   V6

2PP   PP   >2PP

V1

II

V5

0.26 sec   0.24 sec   0.24 sec   0.26 sec

ECG 50 Analysis: Sinus bradycardia, first-degree AV block, low-voltage limb leads, premature atrial complexes

The ECG shows an irregular rhythm at a rate of 50 bpm. The QRS complex duration is normal (0.08 sec), and the axis is normal, between 0° and +90° (positive QRS complex in leads I and aVF). There is low voltage in the limb leads (< 5 mm in each limb lead). The QT/QTc intervals are normal (400/370 msec).

The rhythm is irregular as a result of several complexes that are early (↓) (second, sixth, and eighth). There is a P wave (+) before each QRS complex, but there are different PR intervals. The PR interval before the first, third, fourth, fifth, and seventh QRS complexes is constant at 0.24 second (↔) (ie, a first-degree AV block or prolonged AV conduction). The P wave is positive in leads I, II, aVF, and V4-V6. Hence these are sinus complexes with a first-degree AV block. The three QRS complexes that occur early (↓) (complexes 2, 6, and 8) are also preceded by an early P wave (▼), but the P-wave morphology and PR interval (⊔) (0.26 second) are different from those of the sinus QRS complexes. The QRS complexes have the same duration and morphology as the sinus complexes. These are premature atrial complexes. As a result the rhythm is irregular, but the premature atrial complexes have a fixed coupling interval (⊓) with the sinus beats and hence there is an underlying pattern to the QRS complexes; thus the rhythm is regularly irregular.

Premature atrial complexes are identified by the following:

- An early (premature) P wave preceding a premature QRS complex. The P-wave morphology and/or the PR interval differ from that of sinus rhythm.

- Premature atrial complexes may be unifocal (each premature atrial complex has the same P-wave morphology) or multifocal (the premature atrial complexes have different P-wave morphologies).

- Following the premature atrial complex there is a pause of variable duration; the PP interval surrounding the premature atrial complex may be less than, the same as, or greater than two PP intervals. The variability reflects the effect that the premature atrial complex has on the sinus node; that is, it may not alter the sinus rate, it may reset the sinus node, or it may depress sinus node activity.

The pause associated with the first premature atrial complex (⊓) (ie, second QRS complex) is equal to two PP intervals; hence the premature atrial complex did not affect sinus node automaticity. However, the

continues

pause after the second premature atrial complex (⊔) (*ie*, sixth QRS complex) is much greater than two PP intervals; this is the result of sinus node depression by the premature atrial complex with a longer time before sinus node impulse generation recurred. This is probably due to depression of sinus node automaticity as a result of the β-blocker. However, it may also be a manifestation of underlying sinus node dysfunction.

Premature atrial complexes are often asymptomatic but can be associated with symptoms of palpitations or the sensation of skipped heartbeats. The sensation of a skipped beat is due to the fact that the stroke volume of the premature beat is small because there is less time for ventricular filling. However, the beat after the premature beat has an increased stroke volume due to the pause that results in increased ventricular filling. This increased stroke volume results in an increase in left ventricular contractility, due to the Starling effect. The increased volume and force of left ventricular ejection cause a sensation of palpitations.

Reassurance should be given to this patient that the rhythm is benign and can often go untreated as long as there are no major symptoms. Indeed, premature atrial complexes occur in up to 70% of normal healthy people, although they are infrequent in most. However, given the patient's symptoms, a reasonable initial approach would be to remove potential triggers of the premature beats by reducing alcohol or caffeine intake or quitting smoking. These factors have been associated with increased frequency of premature atrial complexes. If this is unsuccessful, β-blockers can be used to reduce the associated symptoms (*ie*, the sensation of palpitations due to reduction in left ventricular inotropy). Although β-blockers are not likely to reduce the frequency of premature atrial complexes because they do not affect the atrial myocardium directly, they may reduce the frequency if there is an associated sympathetic influence to the premature complexes. Antiarrhythmic agents that do have a direct effect on the atrial myocardium include the class IA (quinidine, disopyramide), class IC (propafenone, flecainide), and class III (amiodarone, sotalol, and dofetilide) agents. ◼

A 24-year-old pregnant woman presents with palpitations. She has no past medical history and is only taking prenatal vitamins. She denies any caffeine or alcohol intake and does not smoke. The following ECG is obtained.

What are your next steps in management?

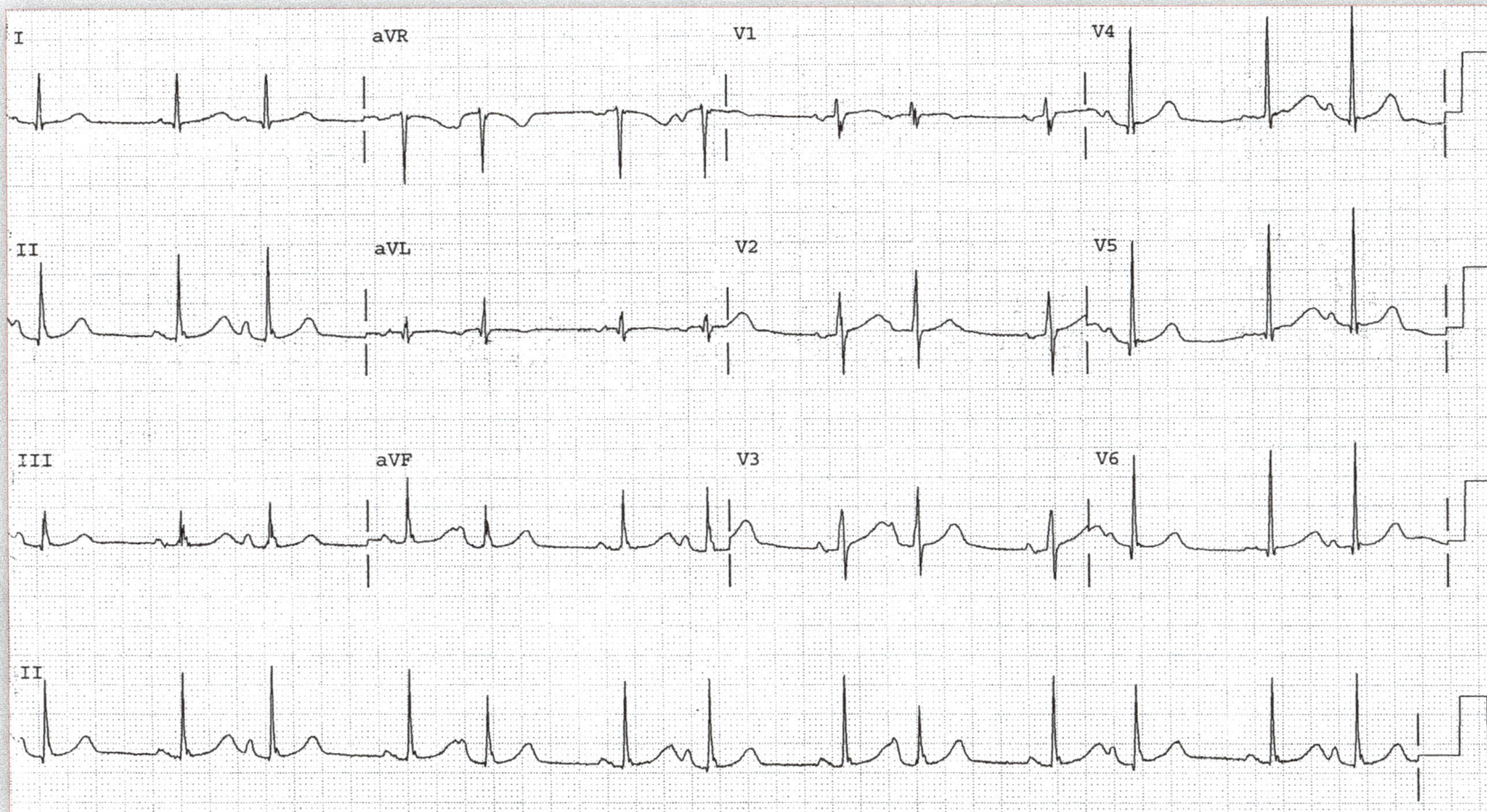

ECG 51 Analysis: Normal sinus rhythm, premature atrial complexes in a bigeminal pattern (atrial bigeminy)

The ECG shows an irregular rhythm at a rate of 84 bpm. Although it is irregular, there is a repeating pattern of long (⊔) and short (⊓) RR intervals; hence the rhythm is regularly irregular.

The QRS complex duration is normal (0.08 sec), and there is a normal morphology. The axis is normal, between 0° and +90° (positive QRS complex in leads I and aVF). The QT/QTc intervals are normal (380/440 msec). Every other QRS complex (*ie*, third, fifth, seventh, ninth, 11th, and 13th) is early (↓) or premature. A P wave (+) precedes each of these QRS complexes, and it is positive in leads I, II, aVF, and V4-V6. The PR interval is stable (0.16 sec) (⊓). However, the QRS complexes that follow the longer RR interval have a different P-wave morphology (*) and PR interval (0.20 sec) (⊔). Hence the complexes after the pause are sinus complexes and they are followed by premature atrial complexes that have a constant relationship to the preceding P wave (hence a fixed coupling interval [↔]).

When every other QRS complex is a premature atrial complex in a repeating pattern, the rhythm is called atrial bigeminy. When every third QRS complex is a premature atrial complex the term used is atrial trigeminy. Bigeminy and trigeminy indicate a repeating pattern; otherwise there are no important clinical implications. It should be noted that on occasion the premature P wave is superimposed on the preceding T wave, altering its morphology.

Reassurance should be given to the patient that this is a benign rhythm of pregnancy. Premature atrial complexes may occur as a result of the increased plasma volume during pregnancy, which results in stretch of the atria and the development of enhanced automaticity. It is likely that the symptoms are also due to the increased plasma and stroke volume associated with pregnancy. In the absence of any history of heart disease or cardiac symptoms, it is unnecessary to pursue any further workup. No specific medical therapy is necessary as long as the patient can tolerate her symptoms. Indeed, drugs should be avoided during pregnancy; in this case they should be used only if there is a symptomatic or potentially serious sustained arrhythmia. ■

The following resting ECG is obtained as part of a routine evaluation of a healthy 28-year-old medical student.

What is the most likely mechanism for the abnormal finding?

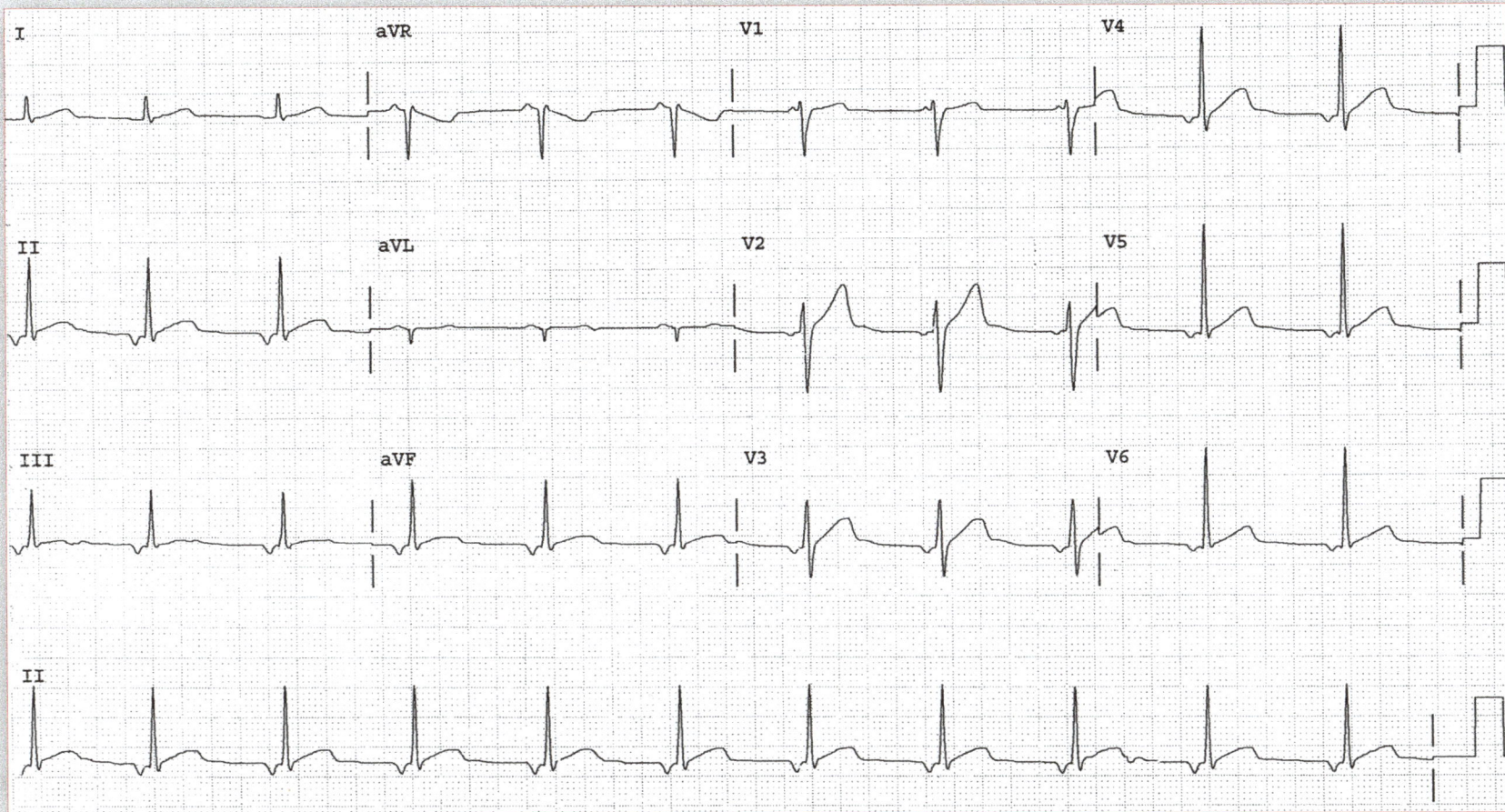

ECG 52 Analysis: Atrial rhythm

The ECG shows a regular rhythm at a rate of 64 bpm. The QRS complexes are normal in duration (0.08 sec) and morphology. The axis is normal, between 0° and +90° (positive QRS complex in leads I and aVF). The QT/QTc intervals are normal (400/410 msec). Although there is a P wave (+) in front of each QRS complex with a stable PR interval (‖) (0.10 sec), the P wave is abnormal as it is inverted or negative in leads II, aVF, and V4-V6. Therefore, this is not a sinus rhythm in which the P wave is positive in leads I, II, aVF, and V4-V6. Rather, the P wave is the result of an impulse generated by some other focus within the atrial myocardium, but not the sinus node. This is an ectopic atrial rhythm that is identified by the presence of a distinct P wave of uniform morphology before each QRS complex, but it is negative or biphasic in leads in which it should be positive (*ie*, leads I, II, aVF, and V4-V6). As atrial activation is no longer via the normal conduction pathway, abnormalities of the right or left atrium cannot be established reliably based on P-wave morphology. The PR interval is constant and may be the same or different from that of sinus rhythm. The QRS intervals are regular.

The presence of negative P waves in the inferior leads means that the ectopic focus is in the low part of the atrium; this has on occasion been termed a coronary sinus rhythm. The short PR interval indicates that the ectopic atrial focus is close to the AV node. The most likely mechanism for this rhythm is enhanced automaticity, in which the ectopic focus has accelerated activity and takes over the pacemaker function from the sinus node. It is also possible that the atrial rhythm is an escape rhythm, a result of a very slow sinus rate. Often, but not always, exercise will increase the sinus node rate and the sinus node can resume dominant pacemaker function because it is more susceptible to sympathetic regulation than the ectopic atrial focus. This is more likely to occur if the atrial rhythm is an escape rhythm. Atropine, which will increase the sinus node rate but not the rate of the ectopic atrial focus, may also be useful; however, this is only of short-term benefit. ■

Case 53

56-year-old man with hypertension and paroxysmal atrial fibrillation who takes hydrochlorothiazide, digitalis, and Coumadin now presents with acute-onset intermittent palpitations. He has also been taking a significant amount of NSAIDs over the past 2 weeks after injuring his knee. His initial laboratory analysis reveals acutely elevated blood urea nitrogen and creatinine levels. An ECG is obtained.

What potential mechanisms are underlying this rhythm disturbance?

Which of these mechanisms is most likely in this patient?

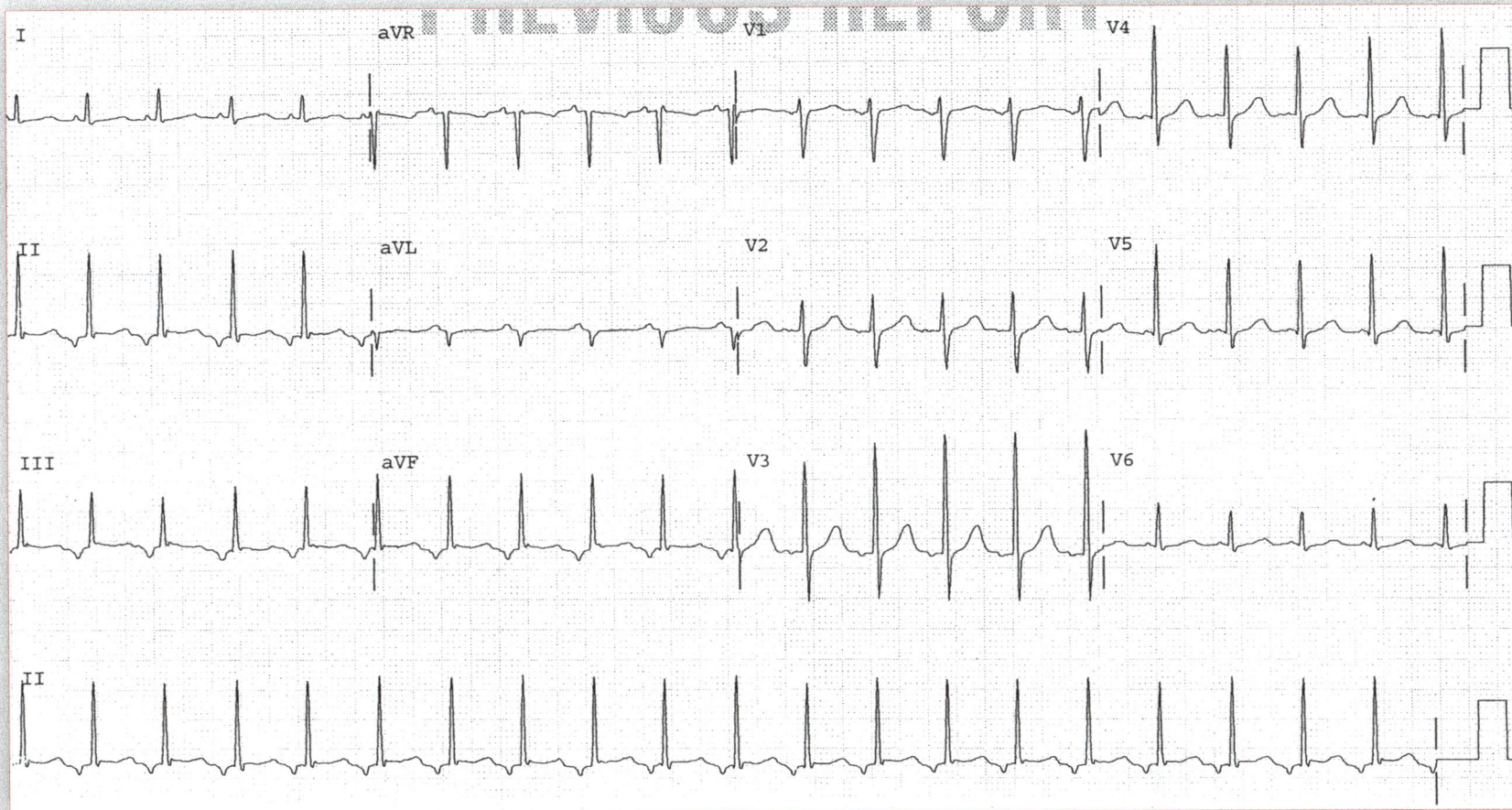

ECG 53 Analysis: Atrial tachycardia

The ECG shows a regular rhythm at a rate of 120 bpm. The QRS complex duration is normal (0.08 sec), and there is a normal morphology and axis, between 0° and +90° (positive QRS complex in leads I and aVF). The QT/QTc intervals are normal (310/440 msec). Although there are P waves (+) in front of each QRS complex, they are negative in leads II and aVF. Therefore, they are not originating from the sinus node but from a low atrial focus within the right atrium, as the P waves are still upright in leads I and V5-V6. As atrial activation is no longer via the normal conduction pathway, abnormalities of the right or left atrium cannot be established reliably based on P-wave morphology. All of the P waves have the same morphology, and there is a short PR interval (‖) (0.12 sec). This is classified as a long RP tachycardia since the RP interval (↔) is longer than half the RR interval (ie, the P wave is closer to the QRS complex that follows it than to the QRS complex that precedes it).

Etiologies for a long RP tachycardia include sinus tachycardia, atrial tachycardia, atrial flutter with 2:1 AV block, ectopic junctional tachycardia, atypical AV nodal reentrant tachycardia (AVNRT) (ie, fast-slow) or, uncommonly, AV reentrant tachycardia (AVRT) associated with a preexcitation syndrome. The negative P waves exclude sinus tachycardia, and there is no second atrial waveform seen, excluding atrial flutter. The most common etiology for this would be an atrial tachycardia with 1:1 AV conduction. This could be confirmed by blocking the AV node (ie, via vagal maneuver or adenosine). The occurrence of AV block with a stable PP interval or atrial rate would confirm atrial tachycardia. If the arrhythmia abruptly terminated, a reentrant mechanism (AVNRT or AVRT) would be the etiology.

Tachycardias, including atrial tachycardia, have three possible mechanisms: enhanced automaticity, triggered activity, and reentry:

- With enhanced automaticity, the tachycardia is produced by an ectopic focus within the myocardium that has enhanced pacemaker function, which may be a result of catecholamines. The tachycardia often has a warm-up period in which the atrial rate gradually speeds up. There may also be a cool-down phase, or a gradual slowing of the rate, before the tachycardia terminates.

- The mechanism of triggered activity is delayed after-depolarizations of the myocardium that occur at the very end of the action potential (ie, these low-amplitude depolarizations are triggered by the preceding action potential). These delayed after-depolarizations are the result of calcium currents. If the magnitude of these calcium currents increases, such as with catecholamine stimulation, and the depolarizations generated are of sufficient amplitude, they may provoke another spontaneous action potential. This mechanism is most often seen in the setting of excessive digitalis levels enhanced by sympathetic stimulation and catecholamines. It may also be seen in dilated cardiomyopathy. This patient has acute renal insufficiency, likely the result of excessive NSAID use. Digoxin levels usually increase in the presence of renal insufficiency and hence the atrial tachycardia may be a digoxin-toxic arrhythmia.

continues

231

- The third mechanism is reentry, which results from an electrical circuit (micro or macro) within the myocardium. The circuit consists of two distinct pathways with different electrophysiologic properties. The pathways, which are capable of antegrade and retrograde conduction, are linked proximally and distally through the normal myocardial tissue. Often these circuits are the result of fibrosis or scar in the myocardium (structural block); they may also be caused by changes in refractoriness of the tissue (functional block), such as with autonomic inputs. The reentrant tachycardia results from antegrade (unidirectional) block in one pathway (pathway 1) while the impulse conducts through the other pathway (pathway 2). If the impulse reaches the terminal portion of pathway 2 and is able to enter pathway 1 in a retrograde fashion, it is conducted back to the proximal portion of the circuit and then may reenter pathway 2 in an antegrade direction. If this process continues, a reentrant rhythm is established. These tachycardias typically have an acute onset without a warm-up period and acute termination without a cool-down period. Hence the ventricular rate abruptly increases and decreases.

The treatment for atrial tachycardia when there is a rapid ventricular rate associated with symptoms is AV nodal blocking agents (β-blockers, calcium-channel blockers, or digoxin). These agents will reduce the ventricular response rate by slowing or blocking conduction through the AV node. In addition, a β-blocker might actually suppress the ectopic atrial focus in the setting of digoxin toxicity, although often Digibind is used as therapy. Long-term therapy for atrial tachycardia generally requires the use of a class IA (quinidine, disopyramide), class IC (propafenone, flecainide), or class III (amiodarone, dronedarone, sotalol, dofetilide) antiarrhythmic agent. In some cases, ablation of the atrial focus may be used. ■

A long-term-care facility sends one of its residents urgently to the emergency department after receiving the following ECG report: "Patient complains of intermittent palpitations. No lightheadedness or dizziness.

Stable vital signs. However, ECG with evidence of heart block. Send to EW for a pacemaker." On physical examination, you note intermittent cannon A waves and are concerned about heart block.

Does this patient need a pacemaker?

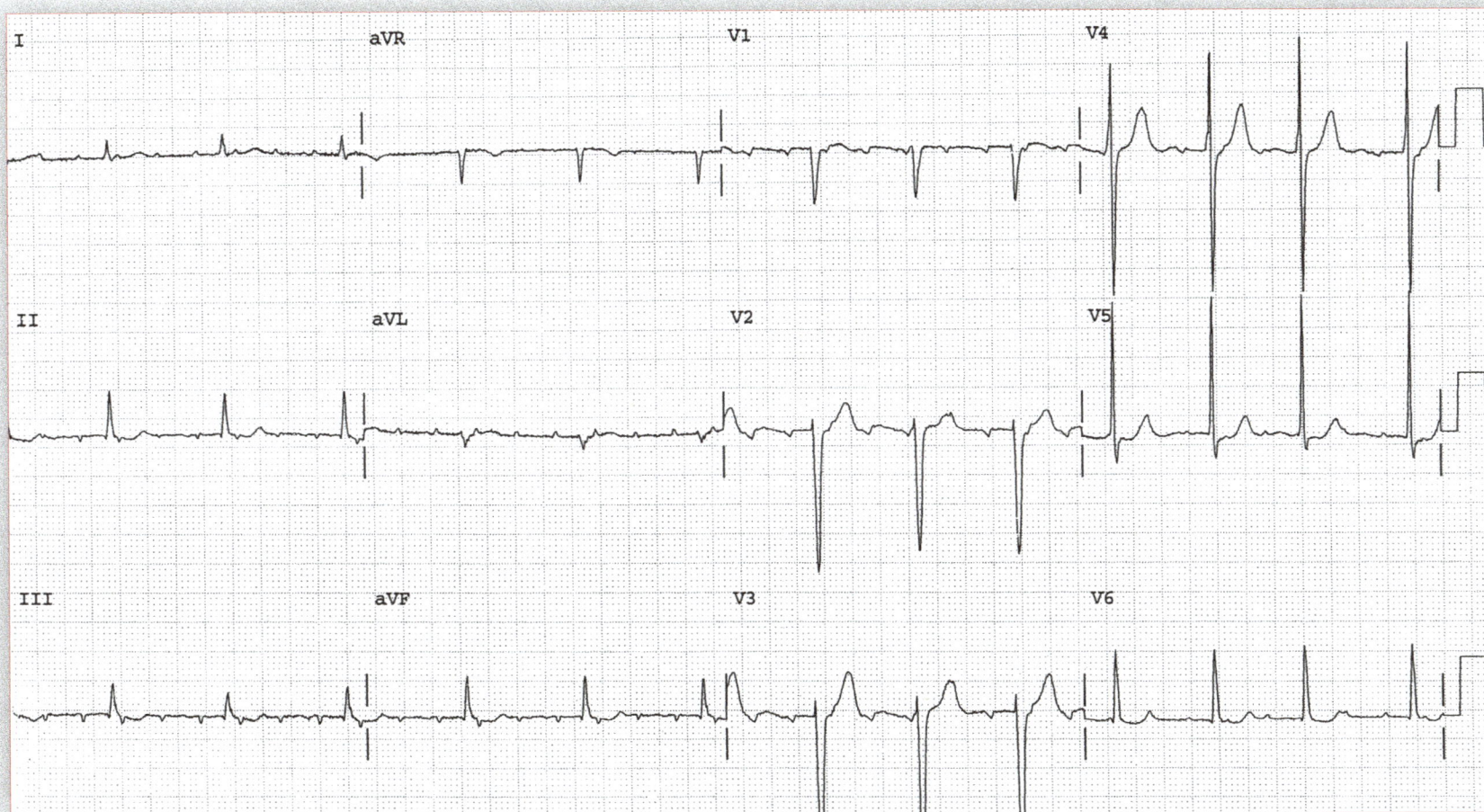

ECG 54 Analysis: Atrial tachycardia with AV block

The QRS complexes are occurring at a rate of 70 bpm, and they are slightly irregular. The QRS complex duration is normal (0.08 sec), and there is a normal morphology and axis, between 0° and +90° (positive QRS complex in leads I, II, aVF, and V4-V6). The QT/QTc intervals are normal (320/350 msec). Atrial activity (+) is easily seen in leads II, III, and aVF. The atrial rate is regular (⊔) at 210 bpm. Atrial activity can also be seen in leads V1-V3, although some P waves are within the ST segment (^) and not obvious. The P waves are inverted in leads II, aVF, and V1-V4. They are originating not from the sinus node but from an ectopic atrial focus. Hence there is an underlying atrial tachycardia. However, there is one QRS complex for every three P waves, and hence there is 3:1 AV block. An isoelectric baseline can be seen between each P wave (↑).

An atrial tachycardia is identified by the following:

- Distinct P waves of uniform morphology before each QRS complex. The mechanism is most often an ectopic focus that fires and stops, resulting in a distinct P wave. When two sequential P waves are seen, there is an isoelectric baseline between the P waves. The P wave is distinct even when the mechanism is a small reentrant circuit (micro-reentry) since only a small area is involved with the reentrant circuit that then stimulates the rest of the atrium.

- The atrial rate is typically between 100 and 220 bpm.

- P waves differ from those of sinus rhythm (ie, they are inverted or biphasic in any or all of leads I, II, aVF, and V4-V6).

- Although the PR intervals are usually constant, some variability of the PR intervals (∥) (and hence the QRS intervals) may also be seen as a result of antegrade concealed AV nodal conduction. At the rapid atrial rate, some of the atrial impulses completely penetrate the AV node, resulting in a QRS complex; some impulses do not penetrate the AV node (ie, they are blocked). Some impulses may penetrate the AV node, but they are blocked within this structure and so do not conduct through the entire node. However, such impulses, which are called concealed, partially depolarize the AV node and alter (and slow) the conduction of the subsequent atrial impulse through the node. This results in variability of the PR interval and hence the QRS intervals, as is seen in this patient.

- QRS intervals are regular (or may have a slight irregularity as discussed above) when there is a fixed degree of AV block (eg, 2:1, 3:1, 4:1) or regularly irregular if there is a variable degree of AV block present; Mobitz type I AV block (Wenckebach) may also be present.

continues

This patient does not need a pacemaker for the atrial tachycardia with AV block. Rapid atrial rates (*ie*, atrial flutter or atrial tachycardia) are often accompanied by varying degrees of AV block that are stable with adequate ventricular rates. This block is due to the intrinsic refractory period of the AV node. A ventricular pacemaker would only be indicated if the patient were having extremely slow ventricular rates or symptomatic bradycardia, due to a high degree of AV block or even complete heart block. The first line of therapy for this rhythm when associated with 1:1 conduction is often a β-blocker or a calcium-channel blocker (verapamil or diltiazem), which slows conduction through the AV node, creating AV block and slowing the ventricular response rate without affecting the atrial rate.

The cannon A waves are the result of the variable relationship between the P waves and QRS complexes, very similar to the situation seen with complete heart block. In addition, there is 3:1 AV block and hence several P waves do not result in a ventricular complex but instead result in an atrial contraction. Hence there is occasional right atrial contraction against a closed tricuspid valve, resulting in an increased amplitude of the A wave of the jugular pulsation.

Treatment for the atrial tachycardia requires the use of an antiarrhythmic drug that affects the atrial myocardium; these include the class IA (disopyramide or quinidine), class IC (flecainide or propafenone), and class III (amiodarone, dronedarone, sotalol, dofetilide) antiarrhythmic agents. Alternatively, electrophysiologic mapping of the atria can be performed to localize the ectopic focus (or reentrant circuit). If identified, radiofrequency ablation may be effective as therapy. ▪

You are called in the middle of the night to see a hospitalized patient who has acutely developed an irregular rhythm. The patient is asymptomatic and sleeping. He is a 63-year-old man without a known cardiac history who was admitted a few days ago with hypoxemia as a result of exacerbation of severe chronic obstructive lung disease. His clinical status has been improving with antibiotics.

What is the rhythm on ECG?

What are your next steps in management?

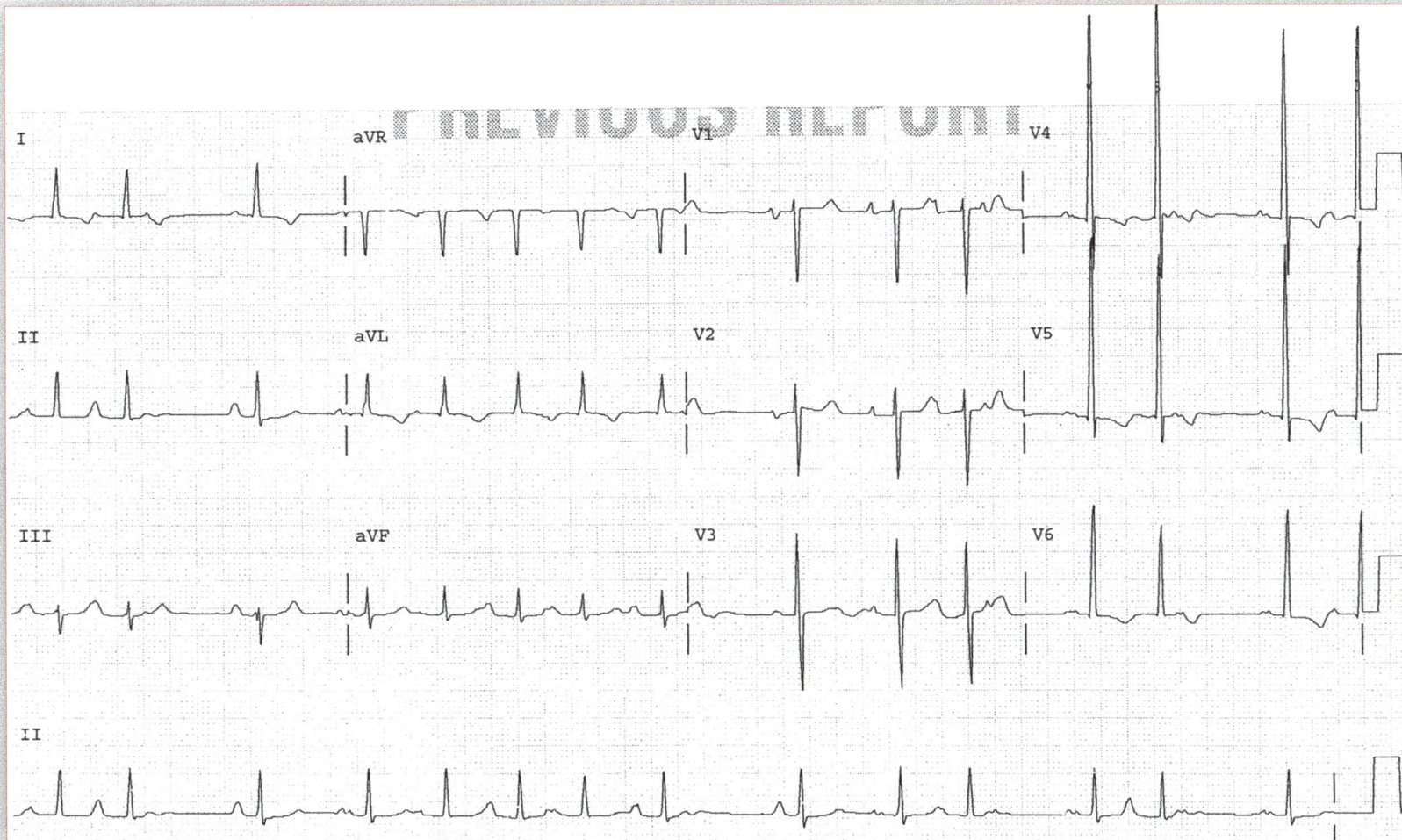

I aVR V1 V4

II aVL V2 V5

III aVF V3 V6

II

1 2 3 4 5 6 7

ECG 55 Analysis: Wandering atrial pacemaker (multifocal atrial rhythm), left ventricular hypertrophy (LVH) with associated ST-T wave changes

The QRS intervals are irregular (⊓), and there is no pattern present; hence the rhythm is irregularly irregular. The average heart rate is 84 bpm. The QRS complex duration is normal (0.08 sec), and the axis is normal, between 0° and +90° (positive QRS complex in leads I and aVF). The QT/QTc intervals are normal (360/430 msec). The QRS (R-wave) amplitude is at least 30 mm in leads V4-V5 ([ ). This meets one of the criteria for left ventricular hypertrophy (LVH) (*ie*, S-wave depth or R-wave amplitude in any precordial lead ≥ 25 mm). The typical ST-T wave changes associated with LVH (^) are also present.

Only three supraventricular rhythms are irregularly irregular: 1) sinus tachycardia in which there is one P-wave morphology and a stable PR interval, 2) multifocal atrial rhythm or wandering atrial pacemaker (rate < 100 bpm) or multifocal atrial tachycardia (rate > 100 bpm) in which there are three or more different P-wave morphologies and PR intervals without a dominant P wave, and 3) atrial fibrillation in which there is no organized atrial activity or P wave. There is a P wave (+) before each QRS complex, but there is variability of the P-wave morphology as well as the PR intervals (↔); there are three or more different P-wave morphologies (and possibly as many as six). This is most apparent on the lead II rhythm strip. This is known as a wandering atrial pacemaker or multifocal atrial rhythm, which is identified by the following:

- Average heart rate < 100 bpm; when the rate is > 100 bpm, the rhythm is called a multifocal atrial tachycardia

- Distinct P wave before each QRS complex

- Presence of three or more different P-wave morphologies; inability to identify a stable or dominant P wave

- Variable PR intervals

- PP and QRS intervals that are irregularly irregular

Wandering atrial pacemaker represents multiple foci of atrial activity that compete with the sinus node for pacemaker function. As there are multiple foci in the right and left atrium, the P-wave morphology and PR intervals are variable.

continues

Wandering atrial pacemaker can be a benign rhythm that occurs in normal individuals, often during sleep. It is a very common arrhythmia seen in association with pulmonary disease. It is, however, also associated with other conditions, including electrolyte disturbances, digitalis intoxication, or organic heart disease. Not uncommonly, wandering atrial pacemaker (multifocal atrial rhythm) or multifocal atrial tachycardia can degenerate into atrial fibrillation.

In this patient, the exacerbation of chronic obstructive lung disease is likely the underlying process. At this point it would be reasonable to confirm that the patient has normal electrolyte levels. Treatment of the underlying process is the mainstay of therapy. An echocardiogram to assess for structural heart disease is only necessary if an abnormality is found on cardiac examination or if the rhythm persists despite adequate treatment of the chronic obstructive lung disease ■

A 72-year-old man with known chronic obstructive pulmonary disease and a 100-pack-year history of smoking presents to the emergency department with significant respiratory distress. His past medical history is only significant for hypertension. On physical examination, he has pronounced wheezes and profound use of accessory muscles for respiration. His cardiac examination reveals tachycardia with an irregular rhythm. An ECG is obtained.

What is the diagnosis?

How would you manage this ECG abnormality?

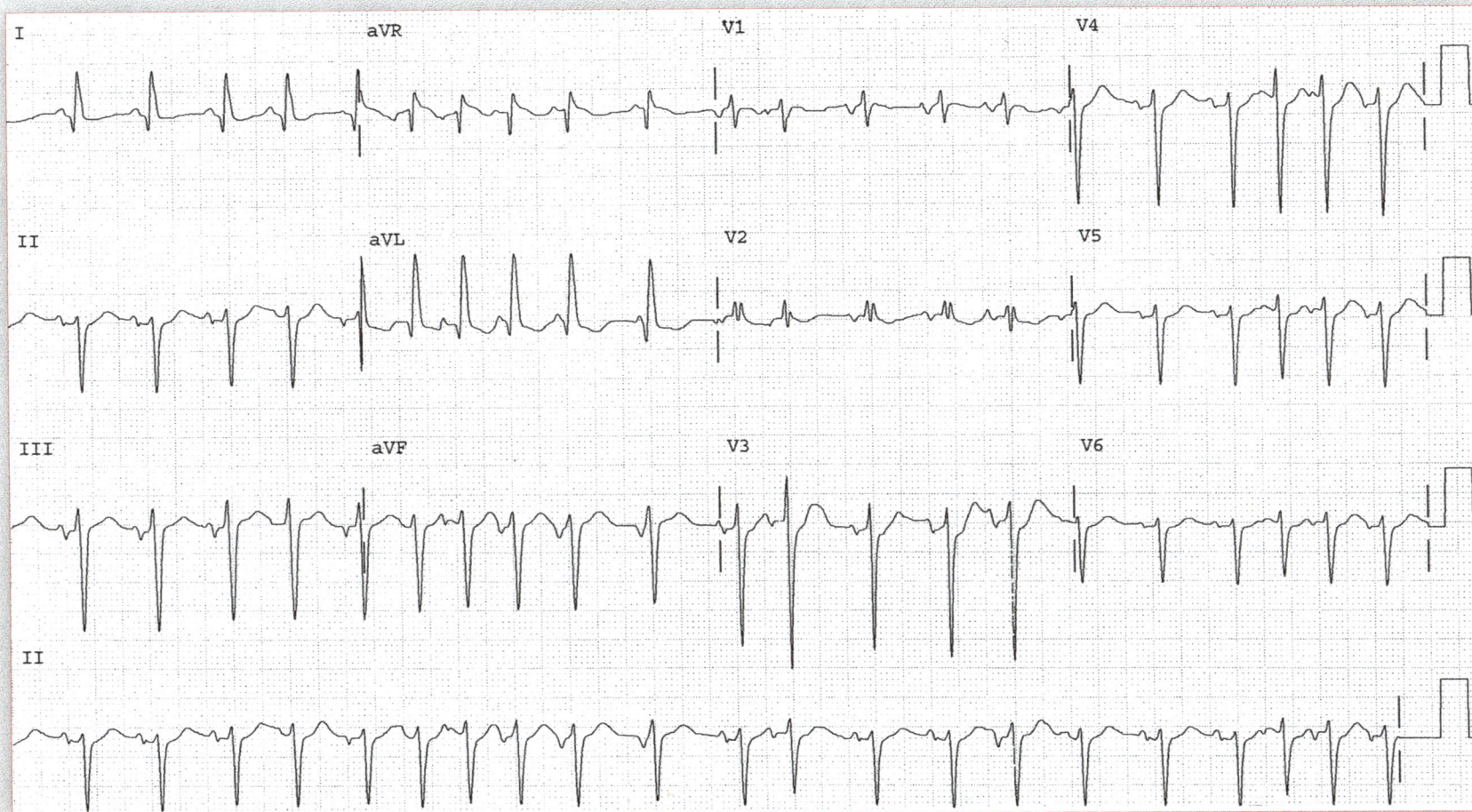

ECG 56 Analysis: Multifocal atrial tachycardia, left anterior fascicular block (LAFB), old lateral wall myocardial infarction, clockwise rotation

The QRS complexes (RR intervals) are irregular (⊓), and there is no pattern present; hence the rhythm is irregularly irregular. The average heart rate is 126 bpm. The QRS complex duration is normal (0.08 sec), and the axis is extremely leftward, between −30° and −90° (positive QRS complex in lead I and negative QRS complex in leads II and aVF with an rS morphology). This is a left anterior fascicular block (LAFB).

The QT/QTc intervals are slightly prolonged (320/460 msec). Only three supraventricular rhythms are irregularly irregular: 1) sinus tachycardia in which there is one P-wave morphology and a stable PR interval, 2) multifocal atrial rhythm or wandering atrial pacemaker (rate < 100 bpm) or multifocal atrial tachycardia (rate > 100 bpm) in which there are three or more different P-wave morphologies and PR intervals without a dominant P wave, or 3) atrial fibrillation in which there is no organized atrial activity or P wave. There is variability of the P-wave (+) morphology (at least seven different P-wave morphologies) and PR intervals, most apparent in the lead II rhythm strip. This is known as a multifocal atrial tachycardia, which is identified by the following:

- Average heart rate > 100 bpm
- Distinct P wave seen before each QRS complex
- Presence of three or more different P-wave morphologies; inability to identify a stable and dominant P wave.
- Variability of the PR intervals
- Irregularly irregular PP and QRS intervals

continues

Q waves are noted in leads I and aVL (^), diagnostic for an old lateral wall myocardial infarction. Also noted is poor R-wave progression across the precordium (*ie*, the amplitude of the R waves does not progressively increase from leads V1 to V6). This is often the result of clockwise electrical rotation of the heart in the horizontal plane, which is determined by imagining the heart as viewed from under the diaphragm. In this situation the right ventricle is in front and the left ventricle is to the left. With clockwise rotation, the left ventricular forces are more laterally and posteriorly directed and occur later in the precordial leads (*ie*, poor R-wave progression and late transition). With counterclockwise electrical rotation, the left ventricular forces are more anteriorly directed and appear earlier in the precordial lead (*ie*, early transition with a tall R wave in lead V2). LAFB is sometimes associated with poor precordial R-wave progression. Another cause for the poor R-wave progression is right ventricular hypertrophy, suggested by the deep S waves in leads V5-V6. Poor R-wave progression may also be seen with severe lung disease.

Multifocal atrial tachycardia is often associated with pulmonary disease, particularly chronic obstructive pulmonary disease or acute pulmonary embolism, as well as cardiac conditions including heart failure, valvular heart disease, and coronary artery disease. Management focuses on treating the underlying precipitant, in this case the exacerbation of chronic obstructive lung disease. Caution should be used in administering β-agonists for chronic obstructive lung disease, as this can worsen the tachycardia. Treatment of multifocal atrial tachycardia initially involves slowing the ventricular rate; calcium-channel blockers (verapamil or diltiazem) or β-blockers are often used as well (although β-blockers may worsen the underlying lung disease if there is a significant asthmatic component). Therapy of the arrhythmia itself involves administration of antiarrhythmics, primarily the class IC (propafenone or flecainide) or class III (amiodarone, dronedarone, or sotalol) agents. There is some evidence that magnesium may be of some benefit. Not uncommonly, multifocal atrial tachycardia degenerates into atrial fibrillation. ■

A 56-year-old woman with known mitral regurgitation from mitral valve prolapse presents with acute-onset palpitations and lightheadedness.

What is the diagnosis?

What would be the best treatment?

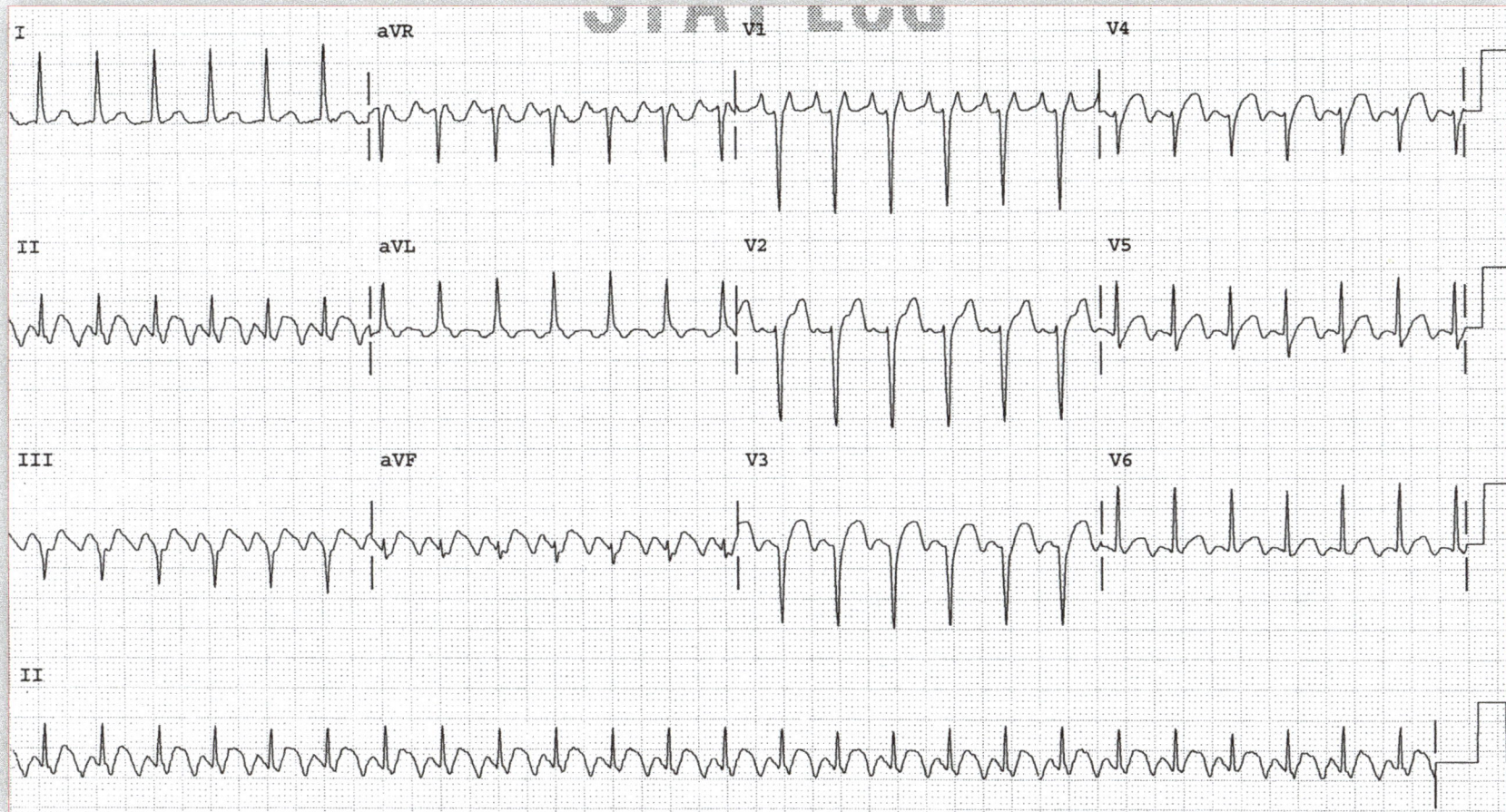

ECG 57 Analysis: Atrial flutter, left axis, clockwise rotation

The ECG shows a regular rhythm at a rate of 150 bpm. The QRS complex duration is normal (0.08 sec), and the axis is physiologically leftward, between 0° and −30° (positive QRS complex in leads I and II and negative QRS complex in lead aVF). The QT/QTc intervals are normal (240/380 msec). There is also poor R-wave progression from leads V1 to V4, with transition (R/S > 1) occurring at lead V5, characteristic of clockwise rotation of the heart in the horizontal plane. This is determined by imagining the heart as viewed from under the diaphragm. In this situation the right ventricle is in front and the left ventricle is to the left. With clockwise rotation, the left ventricular forces are more posteriorly directed and occur later in the precordial leads (*ie*, poor R-wave progression and late transition).

Although no distinct P waves can be seen, there is a continuous undulation of the baseline between each RR interval, particularly evident in leads II, III, and aVF. Two distinct atrial waveforms can be seen for each QRS complex in lead V1. These atrial waveforms (+) are occurring at a regular rate of 300 bpm. This identifies the underlying rhythm as atrial flutter with 2:1 AV block or 2:1 AV conduction. The only regular atrial arrhythmia that occurs at a rate of 260 bpm or higher is atrial flutter. Importantly, close examination of leads II, III, and aVF demonstrates that there is one atrial waveform before the QRS

complex (^) and a second flutter wave that can be seen at the end of the QRS complex (↑), giving the appearance of an S wave. The waveforms are negative-positive in the inferior leads, consistent with a typical atrial flutter.

Typical atrial flutter is identified by the following characteristics:

- Flutter waves (with negative-positive morphology in leads II, III, and aVF from a counterclockwise reentrant pathway in the right atrium) are uniform in morphology, amplitude, and interval.

- There is no isoelectric baseline between flutter waves (*ie*, the baseline between the waveforms is continuously undulating, giving the appearance of a saw-tooth pattern). This is due to the fact that atrial flutter results from a reentrant circuit located within the right atrium. There is then subsequent left atrial depolarization; therefore, there is continuous electrical activity. By contrast, atrial tachycardia is due to an ectopic focus (or micro-reentrant circuit) that fires and stops, in which there is an isoelectric baseline between each atrial waveform.

- The atrial rate is between 260 and 320 bpm. Flutter rate may be slower as a result of antiarrhythmic drugs or disease of the atrial myocardium; however, waveforms maintain typical flutter morphology.

continues

- The QRS intervals are regular when there is a stable pattern of AV conduction (*eg*, 2:1, 3:1, 4:1) or may be regularly irregular if there is a variable pattern of AV conduction, including second-degree Mobitz type I AV block (Wenckebach).

- There may be a variable relationship between the flutter wave and QRS complex due to antegrade concealed AV nodal conduction, similar to what may be seen with atrial tachycardia. As a result of the rapid atrial rate some of the atrial impulses completely penetrate the AV node, resulting in a QRS complex. Some impulses do not penetrate the AV node (they are blocked). Other impulses may penetrate the AV node, but instead of conducting through the entire AV node they are blocked within this structure. However, such impulses, which are called concealed, partially depolarize the AV node and alter (and slow) conduction of the subsequent atrial impulse through the node. This results in variability of the PR interval and hence the QRS intervals.

Atrial flutter is associated with multiple conditions, including mitral valve prolapse, rheumatic heart disease, sick sinus syndrome, left ventricular dysfunction (diastolic or systolic), pulmonary embolism, and pulmonary disease; it is also associated with cardiac surgery. The initial treatment for atrial flutter is rate control, which involves AV nodal blockade with a β-blocker, calcium-channel blocker (verapamil or diltiazem), or digoxin. Subsequent reversion of the arrhythmia may be achieved with electric cardioversion or with an antiarrhythmic drug that affects atrial myocardium (*ie*, class IA, IC, or III antiarrhythmic agents). Long-term therapy to prevent recurrence is with antiarrhythmic agents or radiofrequency ablation. ■

An 85-year-old man presents with new-onset symptoms of heart failure. An echocardiogram demonstrates an ejection fraction of 30% with diffuse hypokinesis and no regional wall motion abnormalities; there is mild left ventricular hypertrophy (LVH). No valvular disease is seen. Coronary angiography reveals only mild, non-obstructive coronary artery disease. Evaluation for non-ischemic causes of his systolic dysfunction, including thyroid dysfunction, infiltrative diseases, autoimmune disorders, and hemochromatosis, has been unrevealing. He does report feelings of palpitations over the past 5 or 6 months. His past medical history is significant for hypertension, for which he takes atenolol; he has otherwise been healthy. The following ECG is obtained.

What is the diagnosis?
How would you manage this patient?

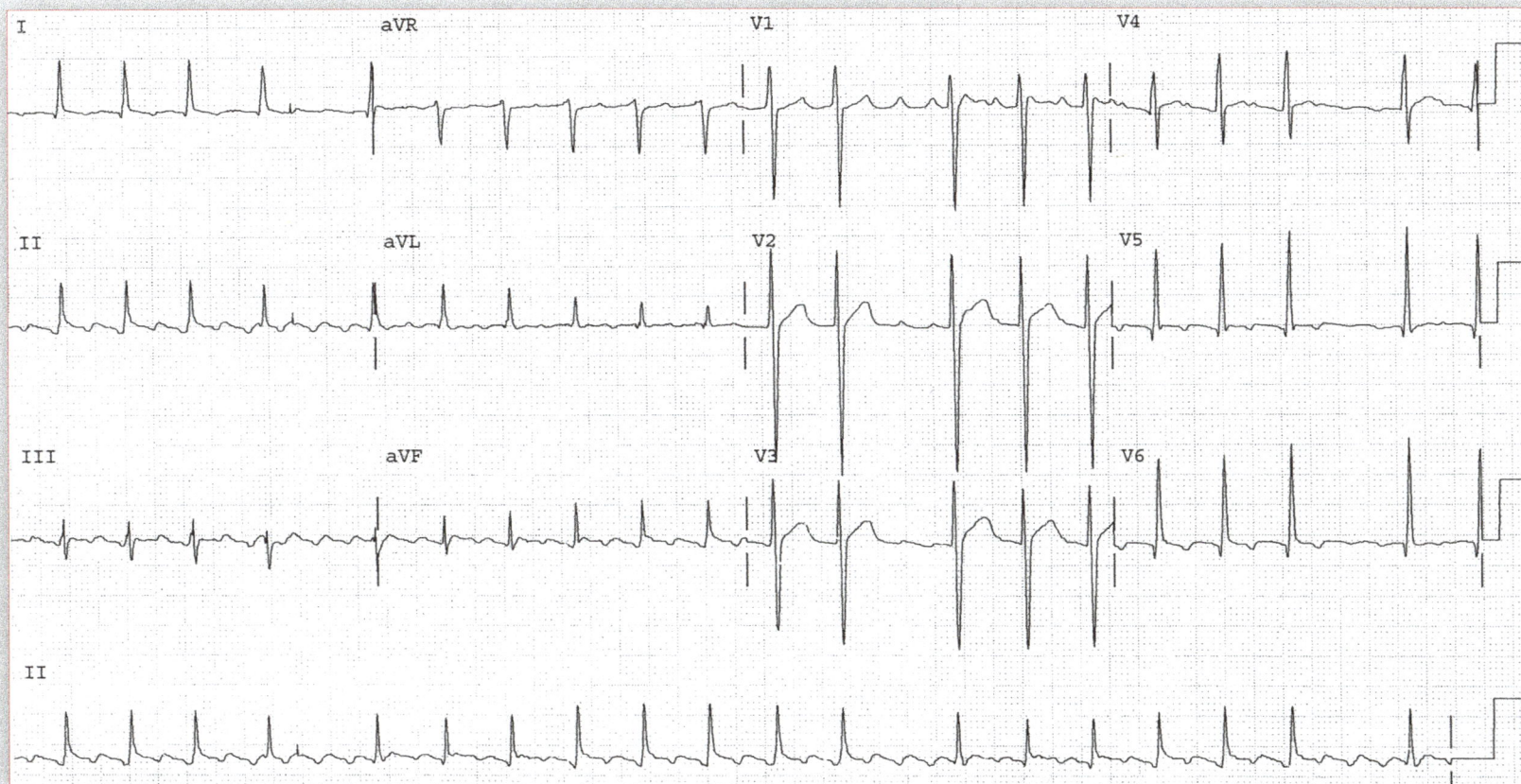

ECG 58 Analysis: Atrial flutter, LVH, nonspecific ST-T wave changes

The ECG shows a rhythm that is irregular, but with a pattern to the irregularity: The short RR intervals (⊔) are the same, and the long RR intervals (⊓) are the same. Hence the rhythm is regularly irregular. The average heart rate is 130 bpm. During the longer RR intervals, typical atrial flutter waves (+) (that are negative-positive in the inferior leads) can be seen at an atrial rate of 280 bpm. The irregularity of the rhythm is due to various degrees of AV conduction block: 2:1 (⊔) and 4:1 (⊓) (which accounts for the shorter and longer RR intervals). There is a variable relationship between the flutter wave and QRS complex (‖) due to antegrade concealed AV nodal conduction, similar to what may be seen with atrial tachycardia.

With the rapid atrial rate some of the atrial impulses completely penetrate the AV node, resulting in a QRS complex. Some impulses do not penetrate the AV node (*ie*, they are blocked). Other impulses may penetrate the AV node, but they do not conduct through the entire AV node because they are blocked within this structure. However, such impulses, which are called concealed, partially depolarize the AV node and alter (and slow) the conduction of the subsequent atrial impulse through the node. This results in variability of the "PR" interval and hence the QRS interval. This can be observed between the third and fourth QRS complexes. This RR interval (↔) is slightly longer than the other intervals, and there is a longer interval between the flutter wave and the QRS complex. Variability in the interval between the flutter wave and QRS complex is also seen between the fourth and fifth QRS complexes.

The QRS complex duration is normal (0.08 sec), and the axis is normal, between 0° and +90° (positive QRS complex in leads I and aVF). The QRS complex morphology is normal, but left ventricular hypertrophy (LVH) is present, with an S-wave depth in lead V2 ([ ) of 25 mm and an R-wave amplitude in lead V5 ( ]) of 15 mm. This meets one of the criteria for LVH (*ie*, S-wave amplitude in lead V1 or V2 + R-wave amplitude in lead V5 or V6 ≥ 35 mm). There are nonspecific ST-T wave changes in leads I, aVL, and V4-V6 (^) that are secondary to LVH and represent chronic repolarization abnormalities, likely due to subendocardial ischemia. The QT/QTc intervals are normal (280/410 msec).

continues

The initial treatment for heart failure includes diuresis, angiotensin-converting enzyme inhibitors, β-blockers, and maintenance of AV synchrony. This patient has a cardiomyopathy of unclear etiology, since coronary artery disease, valvular disease, and other non-ischemic causes have been ruled out. However, the presence of palpitations for many months, likely the result of the atrial flutter, is concerning for a tachycardia-mediated cardiomyopathy. Persistent atrial tachyarrhythmias have been associated with systolic dysfunction. This is commonly seen with atrial flutter, which is often at a persistent ventricular rate of 130 to 160 bpm (due to 2:1 AV block). With physical activity, 1:1 flutter may occur with ventricular rates of 260 to 320 bpm. It is often difficult to achieve adequate rate control with atrial flutter as rates will often increase dramatically with any sympathetic activation; the ventricular rates are related to the underlying atrial rate of 300 bpm (ie, 60, 75, 100, 150, and 300 bpm) depending on the degree of AV block.

In addition to the acute management of heart failure, management of atrial flutter in this patient includes rate control with an AV nodal blocking agent followed by restoration of sinus rhythm with direct current or chemical cardioversion. Since the atrial flutter was of several months duration, 3 to 4 weeks of adequate anticoagulation would be required prior to reversion to reduce the potential for an embolic event after reversion. Although this is less common with atrial flutter than atrial fibrillation, any small risk should be reduced. An alternative if earlier reversion is important, particularly if management of heart failure is difficult or if heart rate control is not adequately achieved, would be a transesophageal echocardiogram prior to reversion in order to assess for left atrial appendage thrombus, which is usually the site of thrombus formation and is associated with an increased risk for arterial embolism. Anticoagulation for at least a month thereafter would be indicated as there is a period of time during which atrial contraction remains depressed as a result of atrial stunning from the arrhythmia and only slowly returns to normal. The addition of an antiarrhythmic to prevent recurrence of atrial flutter would be reasonable. If this were unsuccessful, then radiofrequency catheter ablation of the reentrant circuit is an option. ■

This patient presented to the emergency department with a narrow complex rhythm at a rate of 150 bpm. After a diagnosis of supraventricular tachycardia was made, 6 mg of intravenous adenosine was administered. This ECG was obtained immediately thereafter.

What is the diagnosis?

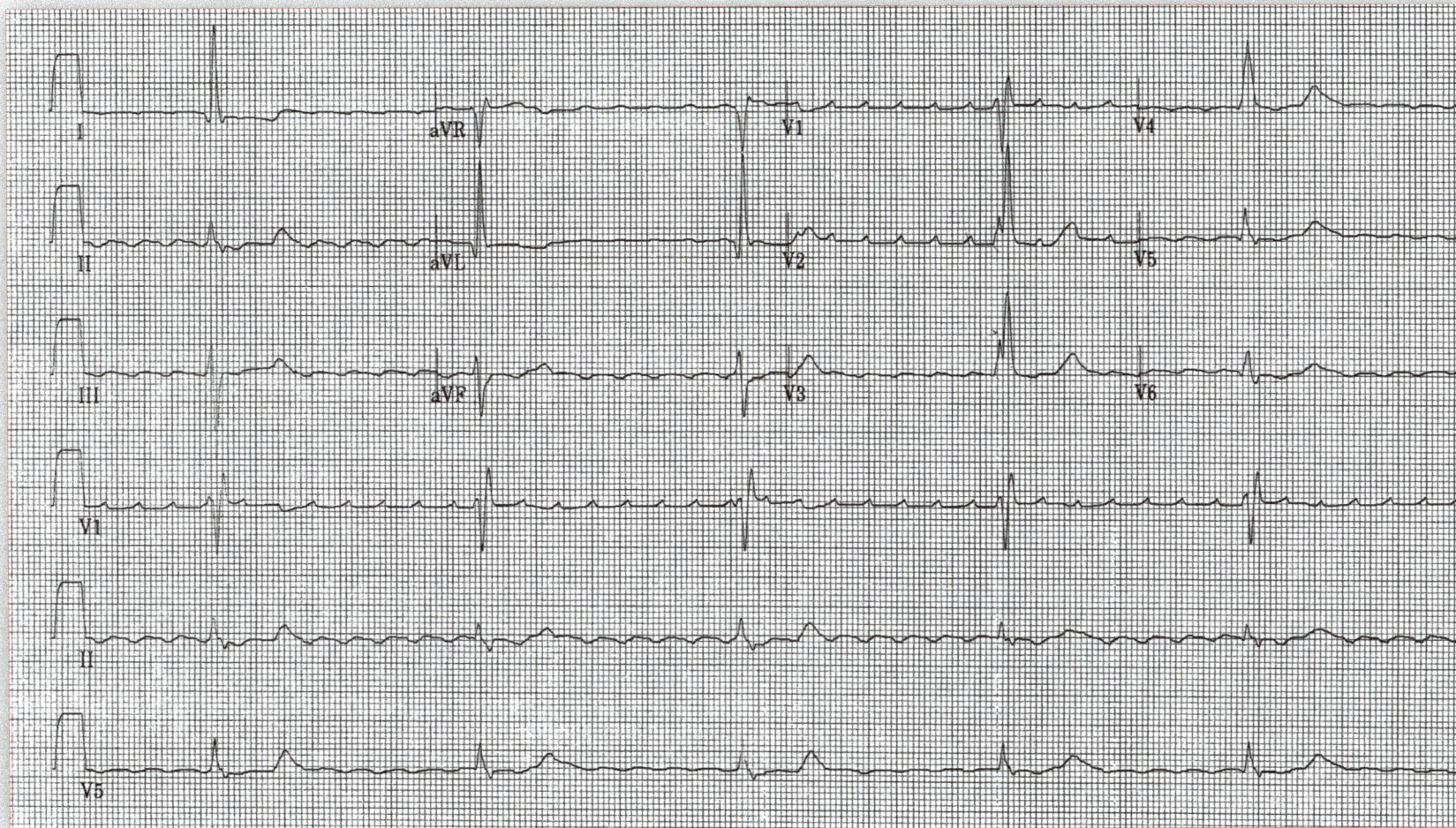

ECG 59 Analysis: Atrial flutter, third-degree AV block, right bundle branch block

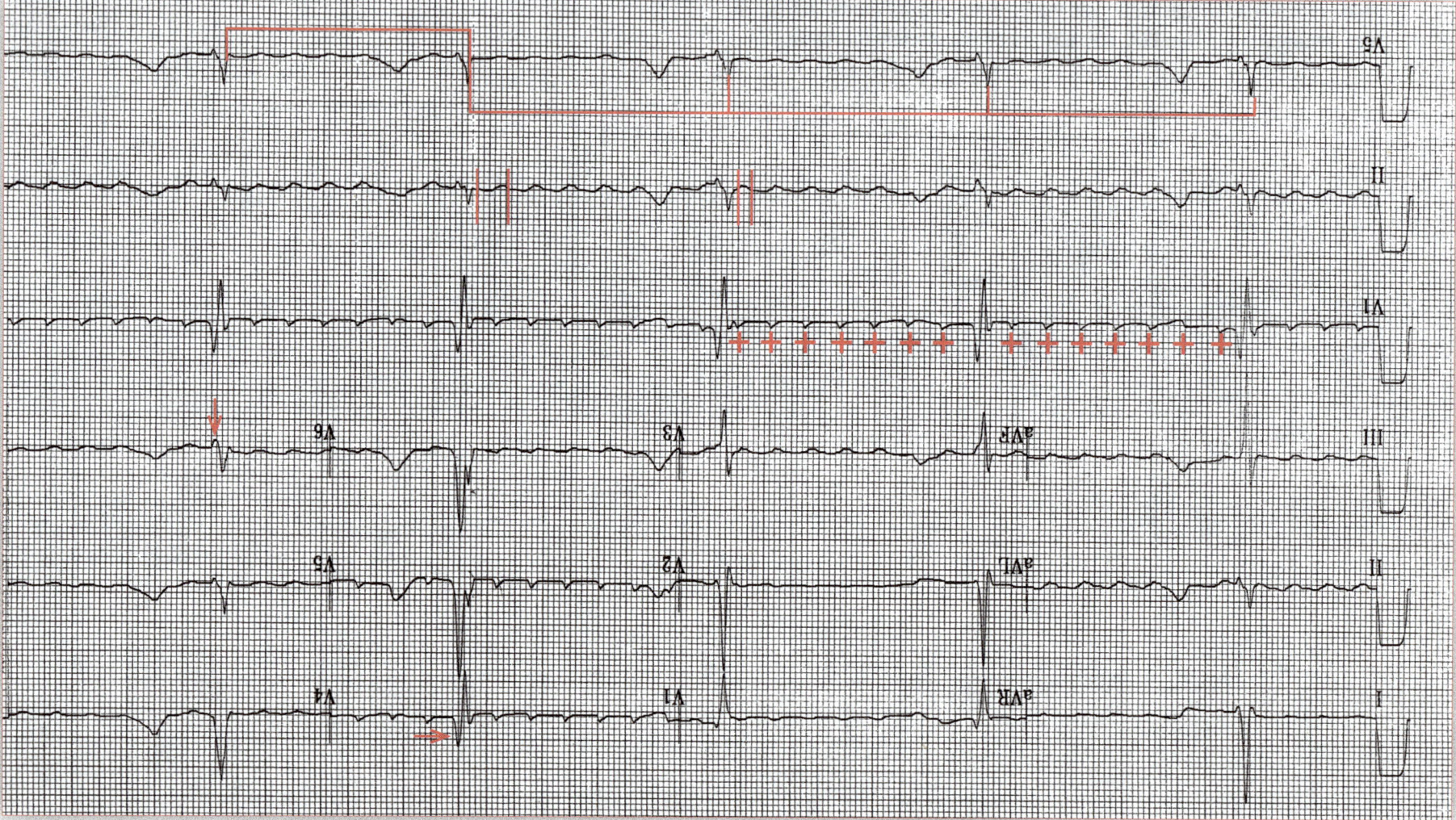

The ECG shows a fairly regular rhythm (⊓) at a rate of 32 bpm; however, the last RR interval is slightly shorter (⊔). The atrial rate (+) is regular at 280 bpm. The slow ventricular rate is a result of a high degree of AV block (8:1). Given the high degree of AV block, it is possible that complete or third-degree AV block is present with an underlying escape rhythm. As a result, the atrial flutter waves (+) are well seen. The flutter waves are negative-positive inferiorly and uniform in morphology, amplitude, and interval; there is no isoelectric baseline between them (ie, the baseline between the waveforms is continuously undulating, giving the appearance of a saw-tooth pattern). This is due to the fact that atrial flutter results from a reentrant circuit located within the right atrium; therefore, there is continuous electrical activity activating the right and then the left atrium. The interval between the flutter wave and QRS complex is variable (‖), which is a result of antegrade concealed AV nodal conduction. With the rapid atrial rate some of the atrial impulses completely penetrate the AV node, resulting in a QRS complex. Some impulses do not penetrate the AV node (ie, they are blocked). Other impulses may penetrate the AV node, but they do not conduct through the entire AV node because they blocked within this structure. However, such impulses, which are called concealed, partially depolarize the AV node and alter (and slow) the conduction of the subsequent atrial impulse through the node. This probably also accounts for the slight difference in the last RR interval.

In addition, the QRS complexes are wide (0.16 sec) and there is an RSR' morphology in lead V1 (←) and a broad S wave (↑) in lead V6. This is a pattern of a typical right bundle branch block, which results in late forces to the right ventricle directed in a left-to-right direction, accounting for the R' in lead V1 and the small but broad terminal S wave in lead V6. The axis is physiologically leftward (positive QRS complex in leads I and II and negative QRS complex in lead aVF). The QT/QTc intervals are prolonged (680/500 msec) but are normal when accounting for the prolonged QRS complex (600/440 msec).

Adenosine can be administered safely in the setting of any narrow complex tachycardia to terminate the arrhythmia or help identify the underlying rhythm by blocking the AV node and exposing atrial waveforms. When the complex is narrow, the impulse is conducted normally through the AV node and His-Purkinje system to activate the ventricle. Adenosine, which blocks AV nodal conduction, is safe in this situation since the AV node is involved with the arrhythmia. Reentrant rhythms in which the AV node is a necessary part of the circuit, such as AV nodal reentrant tachycardia and AV reentrant tachycardia, will be converted to a normal rhythm or will not be altered. There will be transient slowing of the ventricular rate of other supraventricular tachycardias originating in the atrial myocardium and using the AV node for conduction to the ventricles, such as atrial flutter, atrial tachycardia, and atrial fibrillation. This is a result of transient AV nodal block. Although this does not affect the underlying arrhythmia, the transient slowing may be useful for exposing the P waves (or atrial waveforms), determining the atrial rate, and hence establishing the etiology of the atrial arrhythmia. ■

This ECG was obtained from a 52-year-old man with diabetes, hypertension, and ischemic cardiomyopathy with an ejection fraction of 40%. He has no history of stroke or thromboembolic disease. He has normal renal function. A transthoracic echocardiogram reveals trace mitral regurgitation without evidence of mitral stenosis.

What is the diagnosis?

How would you assess his future risk for thromboembolic stroke?

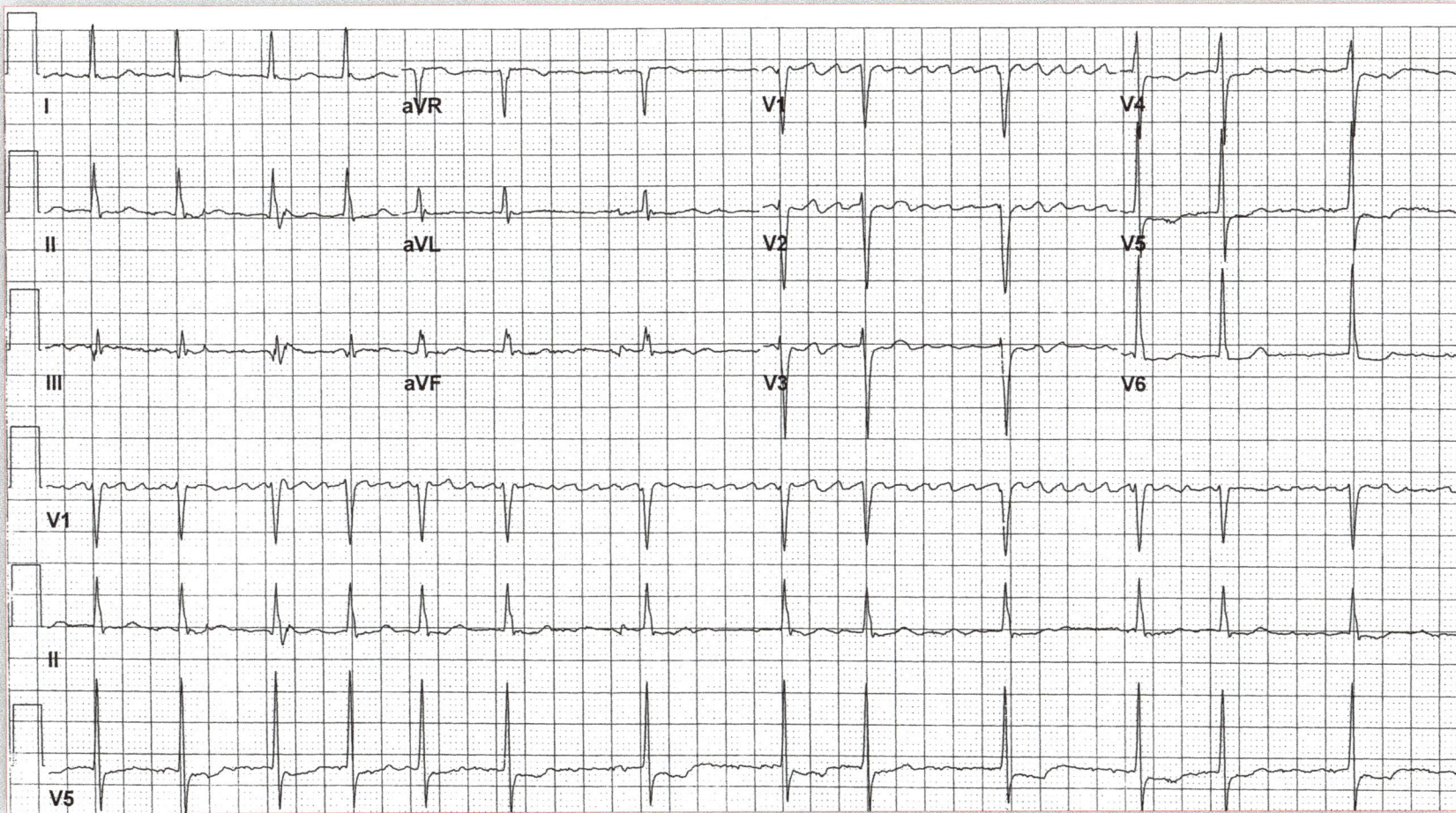

ECG 60 Analysis: Atrial fibrillation, nonspecific ST-T wave changes

The rhythm is irregularly irregular (⊓), with an average rate of 78 bpm. The QRS complex duration is normal (0.08 sec), and there is a normal morphology and axis, between 0° and +90° (positive QRS complex in leads I and aVF). The QT/QTc intervals are normal (360/410 msec). Diffuse nonspecific ST-T wave changes are present, especially in leads V4-V6 (↑). There are no organized P waves. However, prominent atrial waveforms (^) are noted in leads V1-V2. Although these waveforms look similar to atrial flutter, they are not uniform and vary in morphology, amplitude, and interval. As a reentrant arrhythmia within the right atrium, flutter waves are completely uniform in morphology, amplitude, and interval. Thus this is coarse atrial fibrillation, which generally implies a more recent onset. In contrast to atrial flutter (in which the rhythm is either regular or regularly irregular), the ventricular rate in atrial fibrillation is irregularly irregular.

The features of atrial fibrillation include the following:

- The atrial rate ranges from 320 to 450 bpm or even faster.

- There is no organized atrial activity or distinct P wave; fibrillatory waves are present.

- Fibrillatory waves are irregular in morphology, amplitude, and interval. They may be coarse (resembling atrial flutter waveforms) when atrial fibrillation is recent in onset or fine when atrial fibrillation is of longer duration. When atrial fibrillation is present longer, there is electrical and structural remodeling with dilation of the left atrium and the development of fibrosis, which results in finer fibrillatory waveforms.

- QRS intervals are irregularly irregular due to the irregular atrial rate and hence the irregularity of impulse conduction through the AV node. The ventricular rate depends entirely on AV nodal conduction. It is generally up to 170 bpm when the AV nodal conduction properties are normal, as this is the maximum rate that the normal AV node will conduct in the absence of a sympathetic stimulus. When ventricular rates exceed 200 bpm, sympathetic activation is likely enhancing AV nodal conduction. Hence conditions that are associated with elevated sympathetic tone should be considered as the cause for the atrial fibrillation. When ventricular rates in atrial fibrillation are less than 100 bpm, increased vagal tone, intrinsic AV nodal disease or the presence of AV nodal blocking agents (digoxin, β-blockers, or calcium-channel blockers such as verapamil or diltiazem) should be considered.

continues

Patients with atrial fibrillation are at risk for thromboembolic stroke due to clot formation in the noncontractile or hypocontractile left atrial appendage. The atrial fibrillation in this patient is not the result of a valvular abnormality, particularly mitral stenosis or significant mitral regurgitation. Nonvalvular atrial fibrillation carries a 4.5% risk per year for thromboembolic stroke, whereas the risk is much higher with valvular atrial fibrillation. The CHADS2 scoring system can be used to quantify stroke risk in nonvalvular atrial fibrillation, with 1 point each for heart failure, hypertension, age over 75, and diabetes and 2 points for prior stroke or other embolic event. A score of 2 or more requires warfarin for anticoagulation. Treatment with aspirin is sufficient for a score of 0. A score of 1 is intermediary and can be treated with either aspirin or warfarin. This patient's CHADS2 score is 3, placing him at high risk for thromboembolic stroke. ◼

A 46-year-old man with a history of coronary artery disease and a small inferior wall myocardial infarction who had a stent placed in the right coronary artery 2 years ago has the following ECG in the setting of palpitations. The patient has no history of hypertension, diabetes, stroke, or thromboembolic disease and has normal renal function.

What is the diagnosis?

If this arrhythmia were paroxysmal, which of the following would be the most appropriate suppressive antiarrhythmic therapy for this patient?

A. Amiodarone   **B.** Flecainide   **C.** Propafenone   **D.** Sotalol

Would anticoagulation with Coumadin be necessary if the rhythm were chronic?

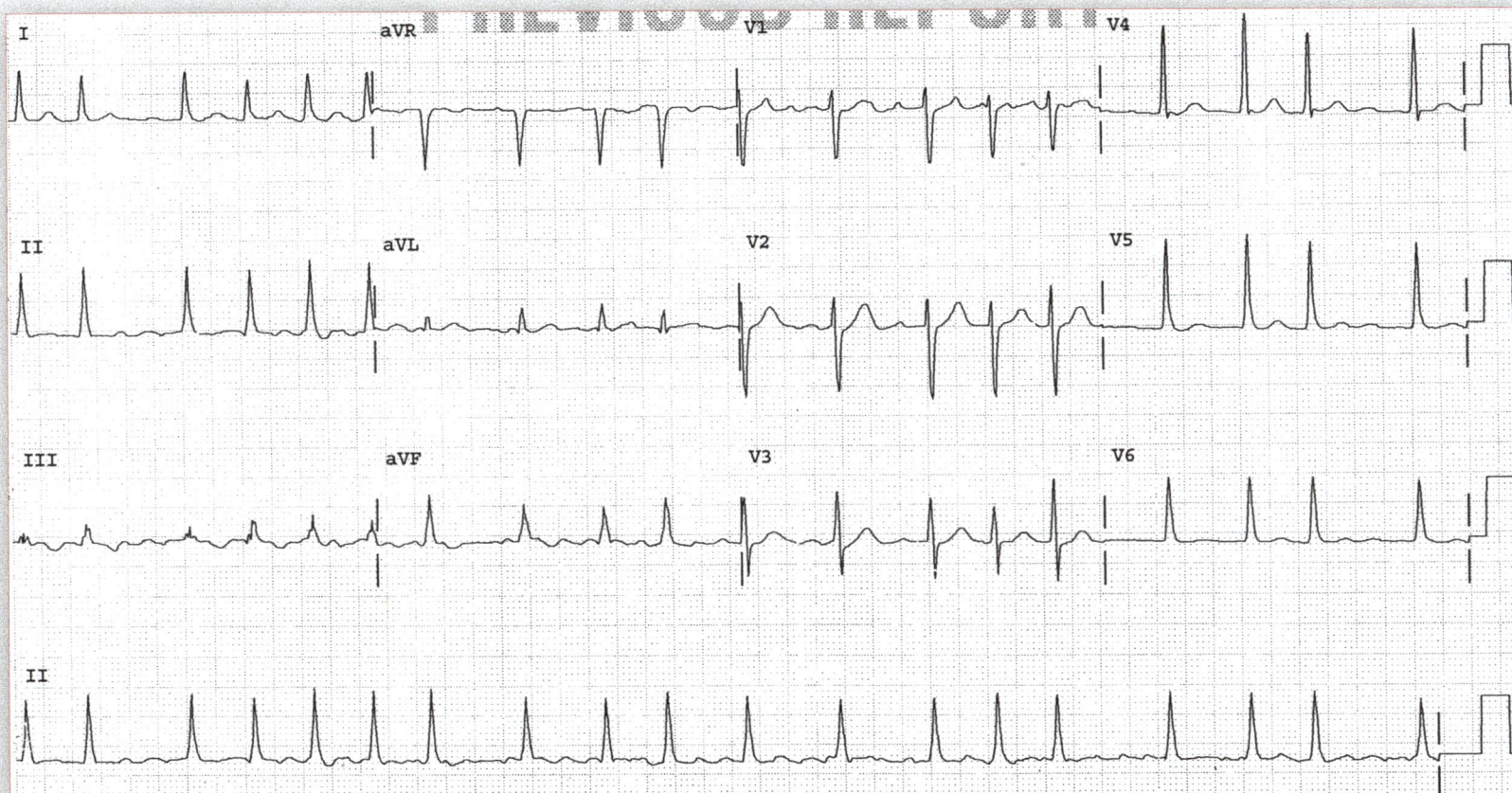

I   aVR   V1   V4

II   aVL   V2   V5

III   aVF   V3   V6

II

ECG 61 Analysis: Atrial fibrillation

The ECG shows a rhythm that is irregularly irregular (⊓), with an average heart rate of 114 bpm. The QRS complex duration is normal (0.08 sec), and there is a normal QRS morphology and axis, between 0° and +90° (positive QRS complex in leads I and aVF). The QT/QTc intervals are 320/420 msec. Although there is no evidence of organized atrial activity, irregular atrial waveforms (^) can be seen in leads II, III, aVF, and V1; these waveforms are not uniform in morphology, amplitude, or interval, and they are not present in front of each QRS complex. There is no obvious atrial activity in other leads. Hence this is atrial fibrillation with fine fibrillatory waves, implying that the atrial fibrillation has been present for a long period of time.

The features of atrial fibrillation include the following:

- The atrial rate ranges from 320 to 450 bpm or even faster.

- There is no organized atrial activity or distinct P wave; fibrillatory waves are present.

- Fibrillatory waves are irregular in morphology, amplitude, and interval. They may be coarse (resembling atrial flutter waveforms) when atrial fibrillation is recent in onset or fine when atrial fibrillation is of longer duration. When atrial fibrillation is present longer, there is electrical and structural remodeling with dilation of the left atrium and the development of fibrosis, which results in finer fibrillatory waveforms.

- The QRS complex intervals are irregularly irregular due to the irregular atrial rate and hence the irregularity of impulse conduction through the AV node. The ventricular rate depends entirely on AV nodal conduction. It is generally up to 170 bpm when the AV nodal conduction properties are normal, as this is the maximum rate that the normal AV node will conduct in the absence of a sympathetic stimulus. When ventricular rates exceed 200 bpm, sympathetic activation is likely enhancing AV nodal conduction. Hence conditions that are associated with elevated sympathetic tone should be considered as the cause for the atrial fibrillation. When ventricular rates in atrial fibrillation are less than 100 bpm, increased vagal tone, intrinsic AV nodal disease, or the presence of AV nodal blocking agents (digoxin, β-blockers, or calcium-channel blockers such as verapamil or diltiazem) should be considered.

continues

Long-term antiarrhythmic therapy for prevention of atrial fibrillation typically consists of class IA agents such quinidine and disopyramide, class IC agents such as propafenone or flecainide, and class III agents such as amiodarone, sotalol, or dofetilide. The class III agent ibutilide is only available for intravenous administration and hence it is used for acute termination of the arrhythmia. However, the class I agents in general and the class IC agents specifically are felt to be contraindicated in patients with structural heart disease, which includes a previous myocardial infarction and myocardial scar, cardiomyopathy, or left ventricular hypertrophy. The class IA agents are infrequently used because of the side effects associated with these drugs. Amiodarone is the best agent available to maintain sinus rhythm; however, long-term therapy is associated with side effects, some of which are serious (*eg*, pulmonary fibrosis, thyroid and hepatic abnormalities). It would not be a preferred first-line agent in this relatively young patient. Sotalol would be the most ideal antiarrhythmic for this patient because it tends to be well tolerated and is only contraindicated in patients with significant renal insufficiency (the drug is excreted renally) or a prolonged QT interval.

As discussed previously, the need for long-term anticoagulation therapy for chronic or permanent atrial fibrillation when there is no attempt made to restore sinus rhythm is based on the CHADS2 scoring system. This patient, who is young and does not have heart failure, diabetes, hypertension, or a prior embolic event, is at low risk for an embolism (*ie*, CHADS2 score = 0). Hence anticoagulation with Coumadin would not be necessary. However, aspirin is often prescribed for such patients. This patient, however, is likely already taking aspirin as a result of coronary disease and a previous stent placement. ■

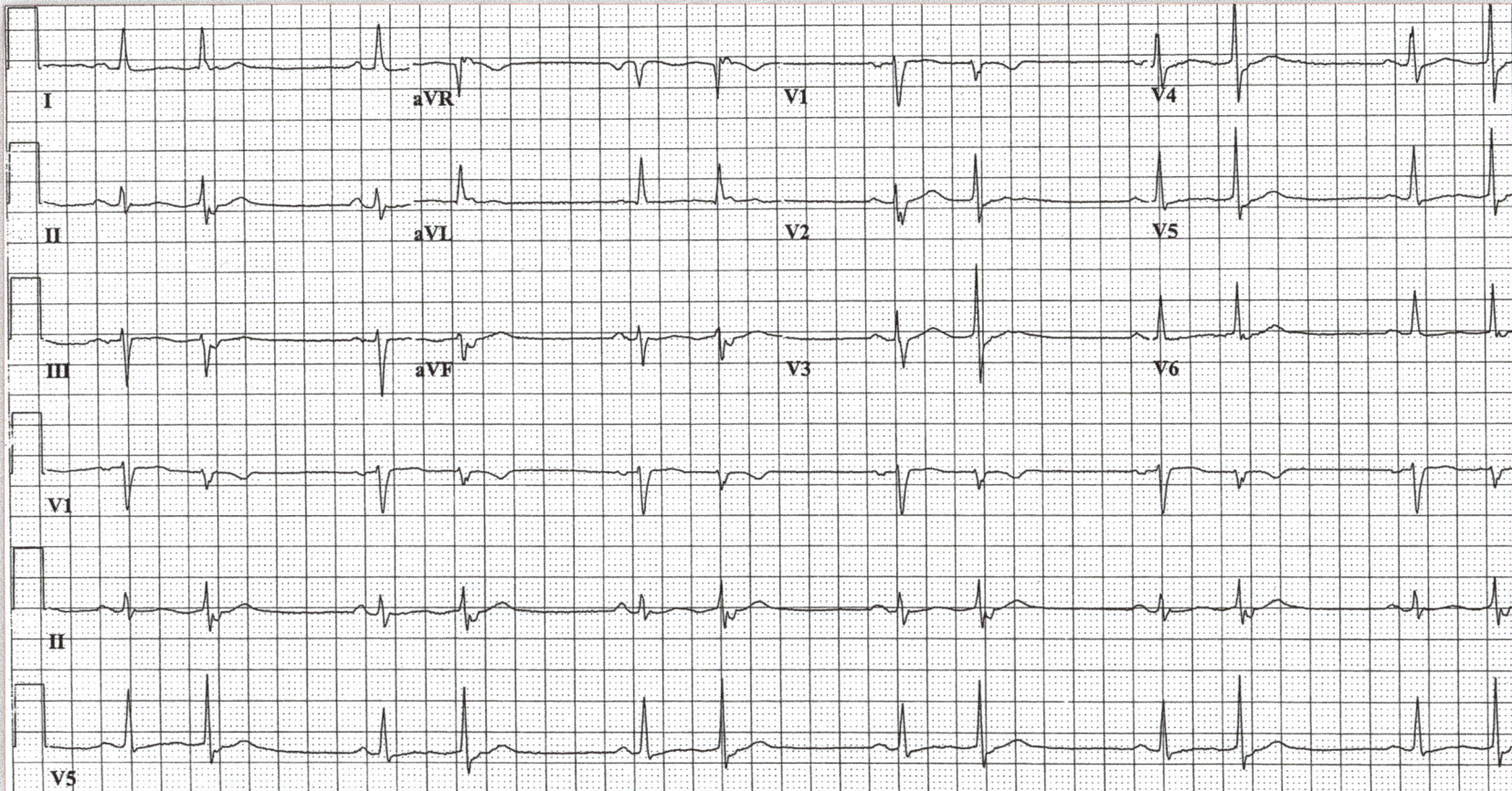

A 57-year-old woman with a history of paroxysmal atrial fibrillation currently on digoxin presents to the urgent care clinic with feelings of extra heartbeats.

What is the diagnosis?

Is any therapy needed?

ECG 62 Analysis: Normal sinus rhythm, premature junctional complexes in a bigeminal pattern

The ECG shows a regularly irregular rhythm, with intermittent long (⊓) and short (⊔) RR intervals. The average heart rate is 72 bpm. The QRS complex duration is normal (0.08 sec), and there is a normal morphology. The axis is physiologically leftward, between 0° and −30° (positive QRS complex in leads I and II and negative QRS complex in lead aVF). The QT/QTc intervals are normal (400/440 msec). There is a P wave (+) before the QRS complex after the long RR interval, and the P wave is positive in leads I, II, aVF, and V4-V6; hence this is a sinus P wave. After each sinus complex there is a premature QRS complex (^), accounting for the short RR interval. Thus the rhythm has a bigeminal pattern.

The early or premature QRS complexes (^) are not preceded by a P wave (*ie*, atrial activation); hence they are not originating from the sinus node or atrial myocardium. However, they are narrow (and hence supraventricular because they are being conducted via the normal His-Purkinje system) and have a morphology that is similar to the sinus complexes, although in some leads their amplitude (↓) is different than that of the sinus complexes. These are premature junctional complexes occurring in a bigeminal pattern (*ie*, junctional bigeminy) and can often be seen in the setting of digoxin therapy, although they can also be seen in normal subjects. The premature junctional complexes have a slight negative notching at the very end of the QRS complex, seen best in the limb leads. This is a retrograde P wave (↑), especially obvious in lead II. However, not all premature junctional complexes will have visible retrograde P waves.

The difference in amplitude reflects the fact that impulses originating in the AV junction, a result of an ectopic focus in this structure, enter the bundle of His (which is composed of a series of conduction pathways or tracks) at a different location compared with impulses that originate in the atrium and are conducted through the AV node. Hence junctional or AV nodal beats are conducted through different tracts within the His-Purkinje system compared with impulses from the atrium conducted through the AV node. Thus they often have an amplitude and/or axis that is different than that seen with the sinus (or atrial) complexes.

continues

Premature junctional complexes have the same clinical implications as premature atrial complexes. Hence they do not require therapy unless they are very symptomatic or are associated with other sustained arrhythmia. The first approach in this patient would be to discontinue the digoxin, as it is not indicated for therapy of paroxysmal atrial fibrillation. Digoxin has antiarrhythmic activity only by increasing vagal tone and does not revert or prevent atrial fibrillation, with the possible exception of atrial fibrillation associated with overt heart failure. In this patient, improvement in left ventricular function and improvement in heart failure may result in atrial fibrillation reversion. However, the major indication for digoxin is to slow conduction through the AV node and hence slow the ventricular response rate during sustained atrial fibrillation. If the premature complexes should continue and are associated with symptoms, a β-blocker might reduce the sensation associated with this arrhythmia. The mechanism for the symptom of palpitations is generally the increased inotropy and stroke volume associated with the post-extrasystolic beat (via the Starling mechanism). By reducing the inotropy of this beat, β-blockers often alleviate the symptoms, although they do not usually suppress the arrhythmia.

A 74-year-old woman with no significant past medical history develops dyspnea and lightheadedness only with exertion. She is on no medications. Echocardiography reveals a structurally normal heart, and cardiac computed tomography shows no evidence of coronary artery disease. During exercise, the following ECG is obtained while the patient is having symptoms.

What is the diagnosis?

How would you manage this patient?

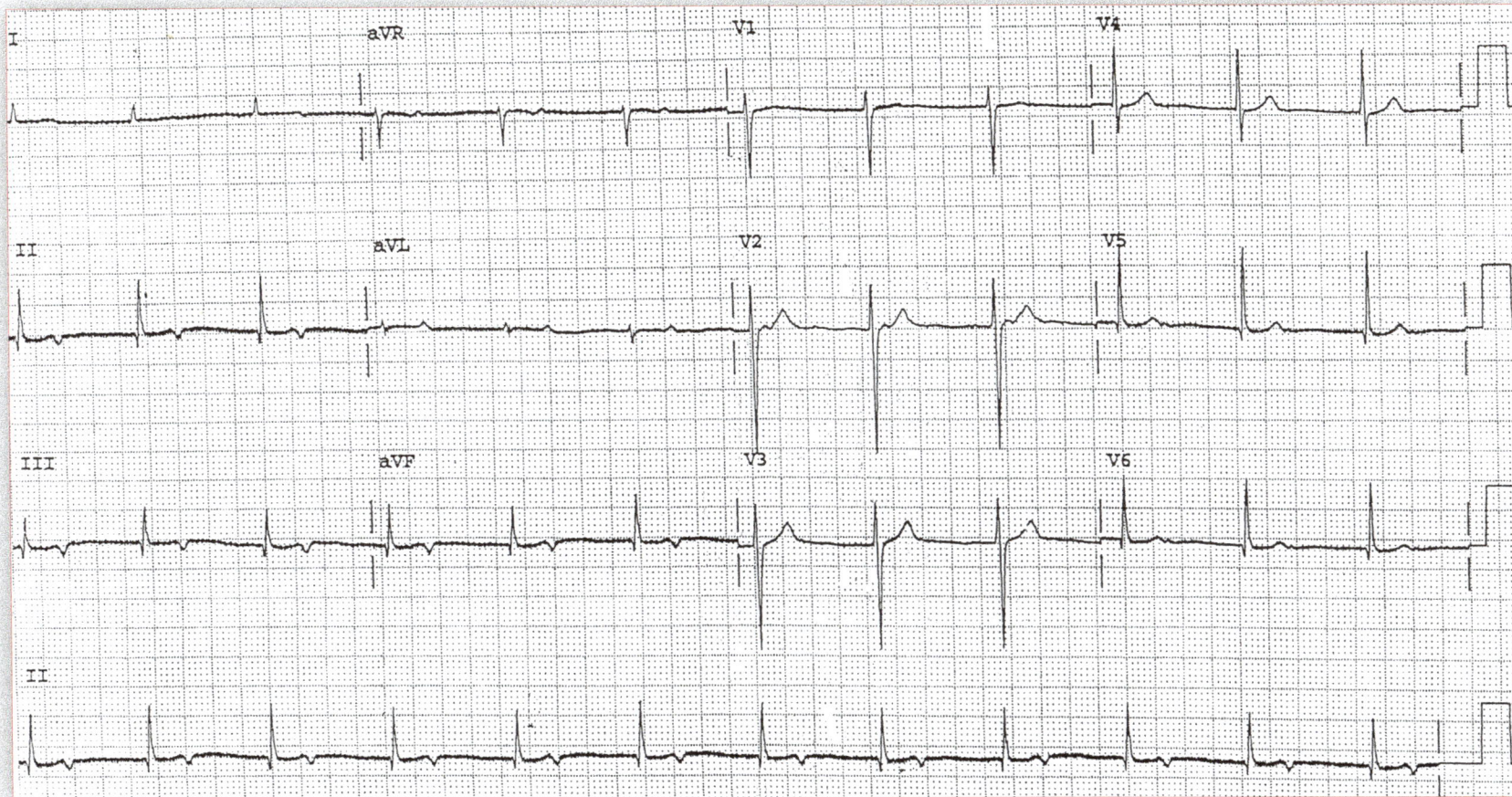

ECG 63 Analysis: Junctional rhythm, retrograde atrial activity

The ECG shows a stable rhythm at a rate of 72 bpm. The QRS complexes are narrow (0.08 sec) and have a normal morphology and axis, between 0° and +90° (positive QRS complex in leads I and aVF). The QT/QTc intervals are normal (320/350 msec). The QRS complexes are supraventricular, conducted through the normal His-Purkinje system. There are no P waves before any of the QRS complexes; therefore, the QRS complexes are not the result of initial sinus or atrial activation. The complexes originate in the AV node or junction, and hence this is a junctional (or AV nodal) rhythm. There is in fact retrograde atrial activity (*ie*, an inverted P wave [+] after the QRS complexes), best seen in leads II, III, and aVF. Although these P waves might be confused for T waves, T waves are generally broader and have a longer duration. Moreover, in leads V5-V6 the retrograde P wave can be seen following the T wave (^). It is common for ectopic junctional rhythms to have retrograde P waves as a result of ventriculoatrial (VA) conduction from the junction back to the atrium. This atrial activation occurs from the bottom of the atrium toward the top; hence the P waves are inverted in the inferior leads, especially lead aVF, which is at 90° and hence is a vertical lead. The RP interval is usually constant, reflecting stable VA conduction time. In this case, the RP interval (↔) is fairly prolonged (0.28 sec), reflecting slow VA conduction.

A junctional rhythm may be an escape rhythm, as a result of complete heart block, or it may be accelerated, with a rate faster than the sinus rate. In this case the junctional rhythm is not an escape rhythm. It is due to an "accelerated" ectopic junctional focus that is faster than the sinus rhythm. As a result the retrograde P wave (retrograde atrial activation) suppresses sinus node activity so that it is not seen on the ECG. Junctional rhythms are often well tolerated and associated with sick sinus syndrome, digoxin toxicity, administration of nodal blocking agents, and cardiac surgery. In this case, the patient is asymptomatic at rest. With exercise, her junctional rhythm occurs at a heart rate of 72 bpm, suggesting that the junction has responded to the increase in catecholamine levels with exercise, but the sinus node has not responded appropriately, as its rate must be less than 72 bpm so that the junctional focus assumes the dominant pacemaker function. This is a marker for sinus node dysfunction, manifest as chronotropic incompetence of sinus node activity. Without any reversible causes of her sinus node dysfunction and given her exertional symptoms, which are likely from an inappropriately slow heart rate with exercise, a rate-responsive permanent pacemaker would be useful. ■

A 45-year-old man has a medical history significant for asthma, for which he uses inhalers, and supraventricular tachycardia, for which he was prescribed digoxin. He now presents with palpitations, which he feels occurred after excessive use of his inhaler for an exacerbation of asthma. His physical examination is normal, without cardiac murmur or evidence of volume overload. The following ECG is obtained.

What is the diagnosis?

Does this patient need cardiac catheterization urgently?

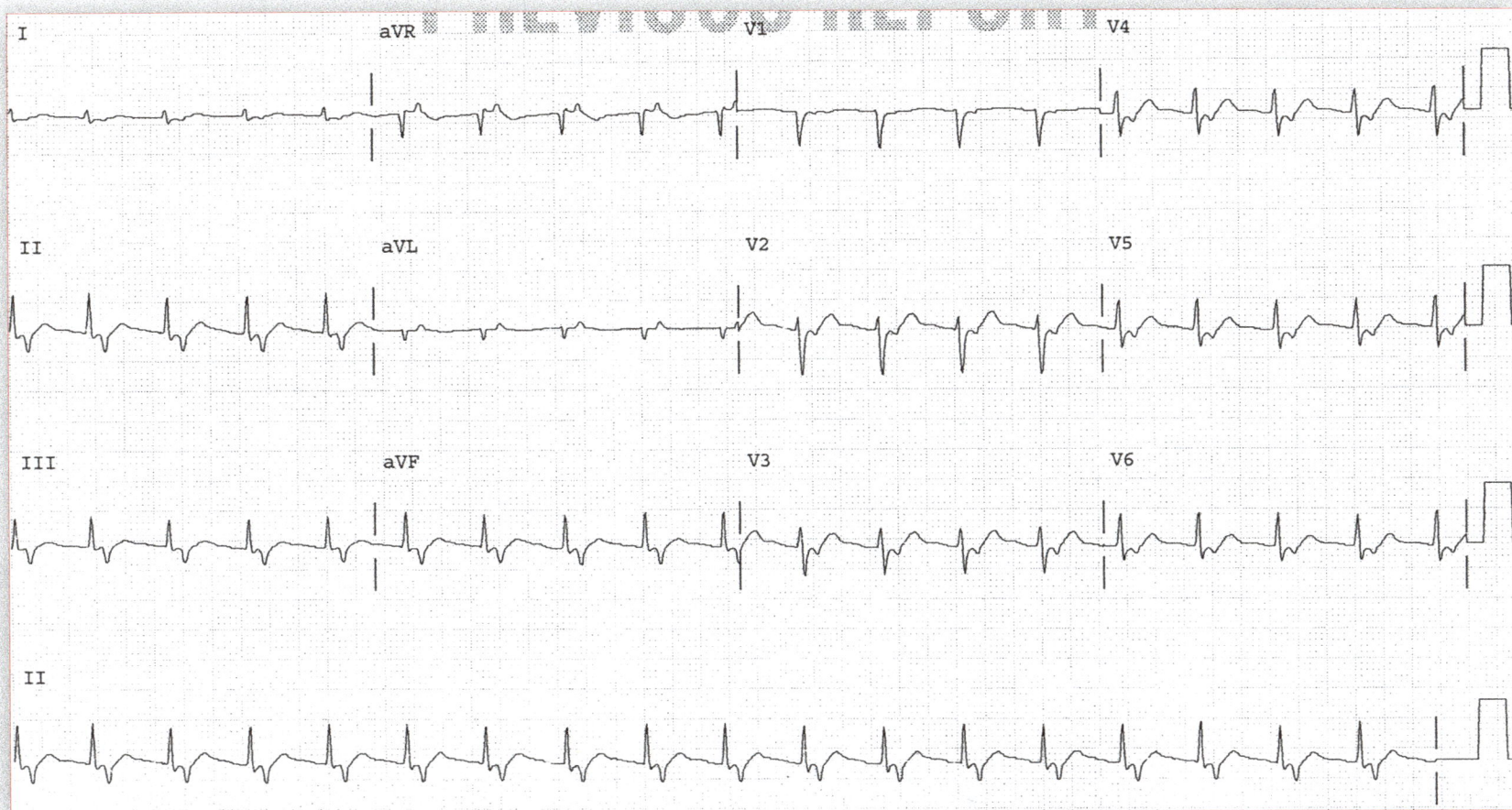

ECG 64 Analysis: Ectopic junctional tachycardia

The ECG shows a regular rhythm at a rate of 120 bpm. The QRS complexes are narrow (0.08 sec), and the axis is normal, between 0° and +90° (positive QRS complex in leads I and aVF); therefore, the complexes are supraventricular (*ie*, conduction to the ventricle is via the normal His-Purkinje system). The QT/QTc intervals are normal (300/420 msec). There are no P waves before any of the QRS complexes. Therefore, the impulse is not originating in the atrium or sinus node but rather is being generated by the AV node or junction. This is a junctional rhythm. Because the rate exceeds 100 bpm, it is termed an ectopic junctional tachycardia. Retrograde (negative) P waves (+) are seen after the QRS complexes in most leads. These retrograde P waves should not be confused with abnormal ST segments. Indeed, the ST segments are normal. The RP interval (‖) is short and constant, reflecting stable ventriculoatrial conduction. This rhythm is termed a short RP tachycardia. Therefore, there is no evidence of coronary artery disease or ischemia and hence catheterization is not indicated.

As the patient has a history of supraventricular tachycardia treated with digoxin, it is likely that the cause of his tachycardia is an ectopic junctional rhythm. This is supported by the fact that the rate is 120 bpm and there is a distinct retrograde P wave with a short RP interval (short RP tachycardia), features typical for an ectopic junctional tachycardia. However, an ectopic junctional tachycardia is the result of an ectopic focus that does not respond to digoxin (digoxin works electrophysiologically by increasing vagal tone). Hence digoxin is effective for reentrant arrhythmias involving the AV node and not for arrhythmias that are due to an ectopic focus. As the mechanism is enhanced automaticity, cardioversion is not effective and indeed should not be performed if the etiology is digoxin toxicity. Initial therapy involves discontinuing agents that may be responsible, such as sympathomimetic drugs. If the arrhythmia persists, therapy with a β-blocker or a calcium-channel blocker might be effective. ◾

A 22-year-old college student presents to the university health services with an episode of sustained palpitations and lightheadedness. This episode occurred when he was playing basketball, but he reports several previous episodes that occurred both during exercise and at rest. Earlier

ECG 65A

episodes were self-limiting, lasting about 1 hour. However, this episode had already lasted 2 hours when he decided to seek medical attention. The following two are ECGs obtained, one during the symptomatic episode (65A) and one after the symptoms resolved (65B).

What is the diagnosis?

What immediate treatment would be useful?

ECG 65B

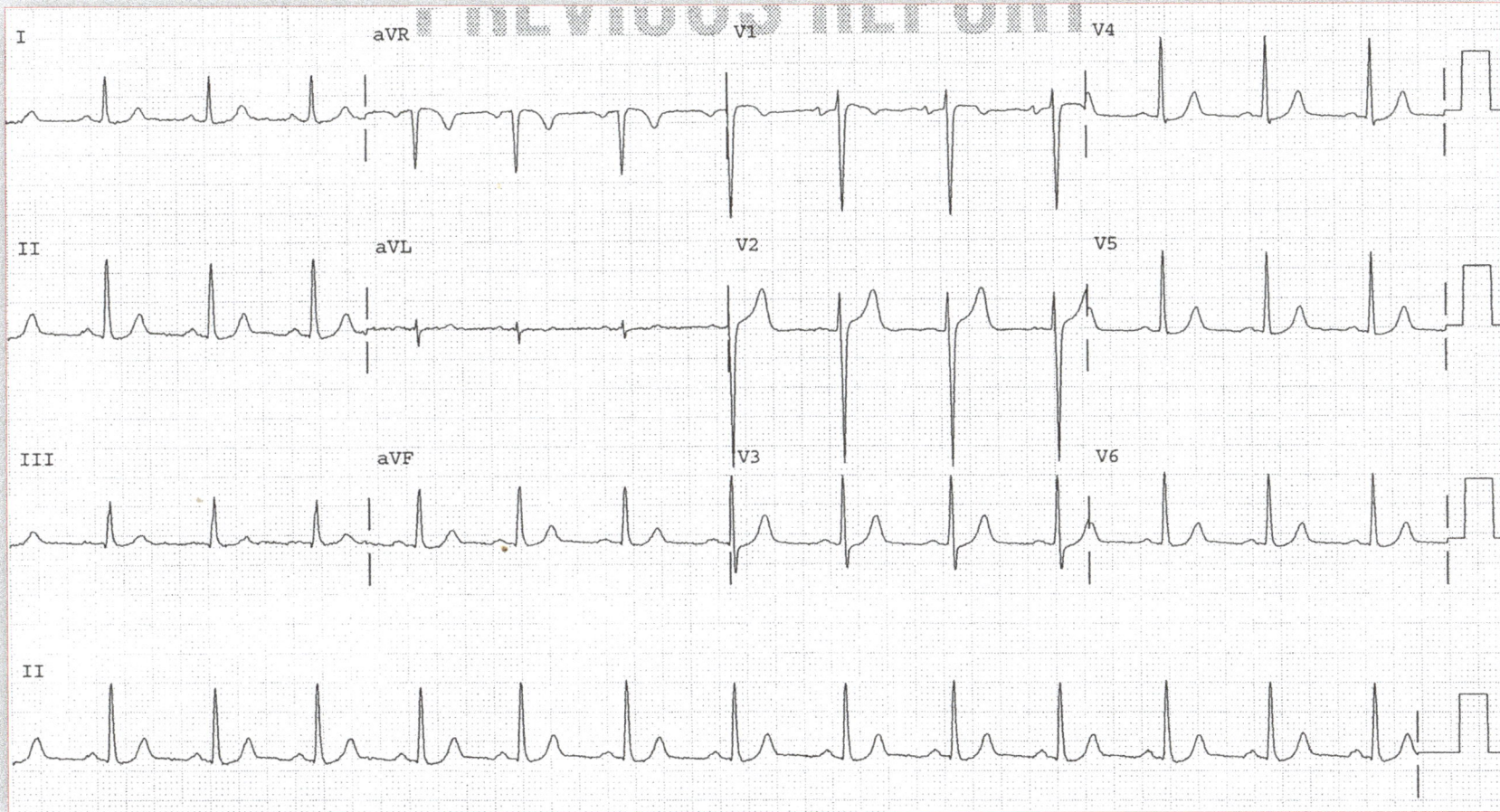

ECG 65A Analysis: AV nodal reentrant tachycardia (AVNRT)

ECG 65A shows a regular rhythm at a rate of 160 bpm; hence this is a tachycardia. No obvious P waves are seen either before or after the QRS complexes. There is, however, a small waveform at the end of the QRS complex, especially seen in leads V1-V2 (↓). Although not an obvious P wave, it is suggestive of atrial activity.

The QRS complexes are narrow (0.08 sec) and have a normal axis, between 0° and +90° (positive QRS complex in leads I and aVF). Hence the QRS complexes are supraventricular in origin. The QT/QTc intervals are normal (240/390 msec). Given the absence of any obvious P waves, this rhythm may be referred to as a no-RP tachycardia. The rhythm is a junctional tachycardia, but in contrast to an ectopic junctional tachycardia in which there are usually retrograde P waves, the absence of atrial activity before or after the QRS complex is characteristic of an AV nodal reentrant tachycardia (AVNRT), which is a type of junctional tachycardia in which the mechanism for the arrhythmia is reentry within the AV node.

By comparison, **ECG 65B** (see next page) shows normal sinus rhythm. There is a regular rhythm at a rate of 78 bpm. P waves (+) can now be seen in front of each QRS complex, with a stable PR interval (0.16 sec). The QRS complexes are identical in duration and axis to those during the AVNRT (**ECG 65A**). The QT/QTc intervals are normal (320/360 msec). However, there is a subtle difference in the QRS morphology in leads V1-V2. During the AVNRT (**ECG 65A**), a small R′ (↓) is noted at the very end of the QRS complex. This R′ is not seen during sinus rhythm (▼) on **ECG 65B**. This waveform is the retrograde P wave, which occurs almost simultaneously with ventricular activation. Hence AVNRT presents without any distinct P wave seen before or after the QRS complex, or the P wave is superimposed at the end of the QRS complex, as can be seen in this case. Only by comparison with an ECG of sinus rhythm is it obvious that this represents a change in the QRS morphology and hence is likely the retrograde P wave.

continues

I aVR V1 V4

II aVL V2 V5

III aVF V3 V6

II

ECG 65B Analysis: Normal sinus rhythm, normal ECG

AVNRT generally results from dual pathways within the AV node. There is a fast pathway that conducts the impulse rapidly but has a long refractory period (*ie*, recovers slowly) and a slow pathway that conducts the impulse slowly but has a short refractory period (*ie*, recovers more quickly). These two pathways are proximally linked in the upper portion of the AV junction (within the atrial tissue) and distally linked at the lower portion of the AV junction (within the bundle of His), forming a circuit. During sinus rhythm the fast pathway predominates and the impulse reaches the His-Purkinje system and hence ventricular myocardium via this pathway. However, if a premature atrial complex reaches the AV node when the fast pathway has not fully recovered, it may be blocked in the fast pathway (unidirectional block) and conducted to the ventricle via the slow pathway, which recovers more quickly. Therefore, the premature atrial complex has a long PR interval. Since conduction through the slow pathway is slow, the impulse may reach the distal portion of the circuit at a time when the fast pathway has recovered, and hence the impulse will enter the fast pathway retrogradely to activate the atrium at the same time there is antegrade conduction to the ventricles. Hence the P wave and QRS complex occur simultaneously (or nearly simultaneously). If the retrograde impulse conducted via the fast pathway reaches the proximal portion of the circuit at a time when the slow pathway has recovered, the impulse also reenters the slow pathway, setting up a reentrant arrhythmia. This is the typical or common form of AVNRT and is called slow-fast (slow to the ventricle and fast back to the atrium). An uncommon (atypical) form of AVNRT in which the circuit is fast-slow (*ie*, fast to the ventricle and slow to the atrium) presents as a long RP tachycardia.

Immediate treatment for an AVNRT involves altering the electrophysiologic characteristics of the AV nodal pathways. The quickest way to do this is through a maneuver that enhances vagal tone (and hence slows conduction and prolongs refractoriness within the AV node), such a carotid sinus pressure or Valsalva maneuver. Another effective therapy is adenosine, which transiently slows or blocks conduction through the AV node. Alternative therapies that can be used are other AV nodal blocking agents, such as intravenous verapamil or diltiazem, a β-blocker, or even digoxin. If these therapies are ineffective, electric cardioversion is usually effective.

Long-term therapy involves oral drugs that affect AV nodal conduction, such as digoxin, verapamil, diltiazem, or a β-blocker. If the AV nodal blocking agents are ineffective, class IA, IC, and III antiarrhythmic drugs can be useful. However, AV nodal ablation is preferred, especially in younger patients, to avoid the toxicity associated with these agents. ■

A 50-year-old lawyer with a history of hypertension who is on a thiazide diuretic presents to the emergency department with acute-onset palpitations and dyspnea. He admits to drinking much more alcohol and caffeine recently due to long business meetings and other stressors at work. He also mentions that he has had several

ECG 66A

similar episodes that always require a visit to the emergency department, where he received some unknown intravenous medication. ECG 66A is obtained while the patient is experiencing palpitations. ECG 66B is the patient's baseline ECG, obtained when he is not symptomatic.

What is the diagnosis?

How would you manage the patient long-term?

ECG 66B

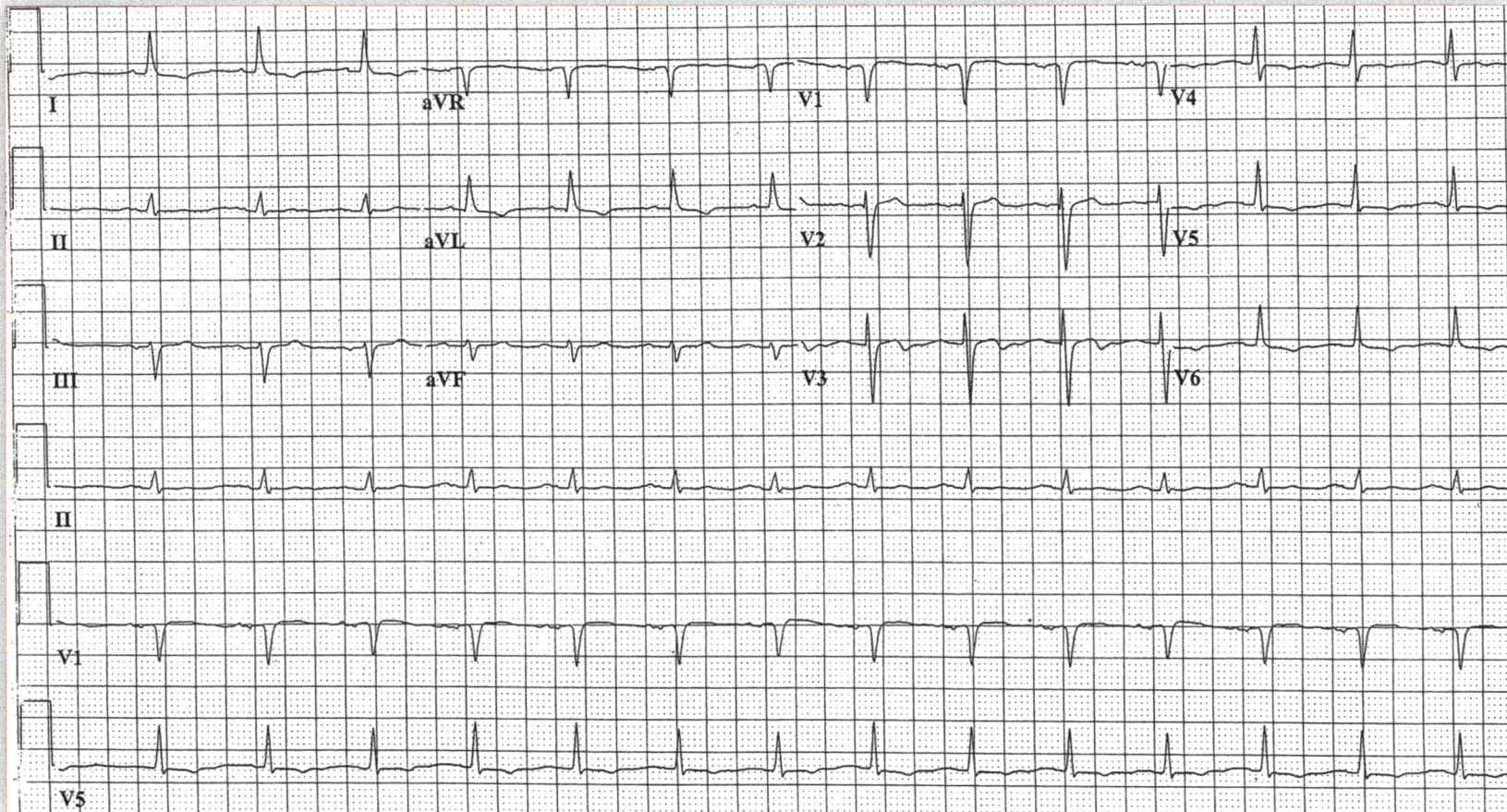

ECG 66A Analysis: AV nodal reentrant tachycardia (AVNRT), left axis, nonspecific ST-T wave abnormalities

ECG 66A shows a regular narrow QRS complex (duration = 0.08 sec) tachycardia at a rate of 160 bpm. The QRS morphology is normal, and the axis is physiologically leftward, between 0° and –30° (positive QRS complex in leads I and II and negative QRS complex in lead aVF). The QT/QTc intervals are normal (260/420 msec). There are nonspecific ST-T wave abnormalities in leads I, aVL, and V3-V6 (^). This is a supraventricular tachycardia. There are no obvious P waves before or after any of the QRS complexes; no R′ is seen in lead V1. Therefore, the origin of the tachycardia is the AV node or junction. The absence of P waves (a no-RP tachycardia) is characteristic of an AV nodal reentrant tachycardia (AVNRT), which is the most common regular narrow complex (supraventricular tachycardia) to present without any obvious P waves.

continues

ECG 66B Analysis: Normal sinus rhythm, nonspecific ST-T wave abnormalities

In **ECG 66B**, the patient's baseline ECG, the QRS complex duration, morphology, and axis and the QT/QTc intervals are identical to those seen during the AVNRT in **ECG 66A**. There is a P wave (+) before each QRS complex, with a stable PR interval (0.16 sec). Hence another typical way for AVNRT to present is with QRS complexes that are identical to those seen in sinus rhythm without a P wave superimposed on the terminal portion of the QRS complex.

Common precipitants of AVNRT include alcohol, stimulants, exercise, and nicotine. Acute termination of the reentrant rhythm can be achieved with vagal maneuvers such as carotid sinus pressure or Valsalva. Increased vagal tone slows conduction through the AV node and by altering the electrophysiologic properties can terminate the reentrant arrhythmia. Another effective approach is the administration of intravenous adenosine, which also slows and blocks conduction through the AV node. β-blockers and calcium-channel blockers such as verapamil or diltiazem can be used for immediate termination. If the patient is unstable or if pharmacologic therapy is ineffective, direct current cardioversion is recommended. If this is unsuccessful, antiarrhythmic therapy with class IA, IC, or III agents is an option. For episodic arrhythmia, a single large dose of an antiarrhythmic drug previously established as being effective for arrhythmia termination may be used for the episode. This approach, termed the "pill in the pocket approach" or "cocktail drug therapy" is used to treat an arrhythmia event when it occurs and avoids the use of long-term drug therapy. Long-term therapy to prevent AVNRT often begins with an AV nodal blocking agent (verapamil, diltiazem, β-blocker, or digoxin given alone or in combination). If these therapies are ineffective, a class IA, IC, or III antiarrhythmic agent can be used. However, given the potential for side effects with antiarrhythmic therapy, catheter ablation of the slow pathway is often used to manage AVNRT, with a success rate of approximately 90%. ■

Notes

An asymptomatic 52-year-old woman whom you see in clinic has the following baseline ECG.

How would you characterize the abnormality?

What is the most likely mechanism for this finding?

How would you manage this patient?

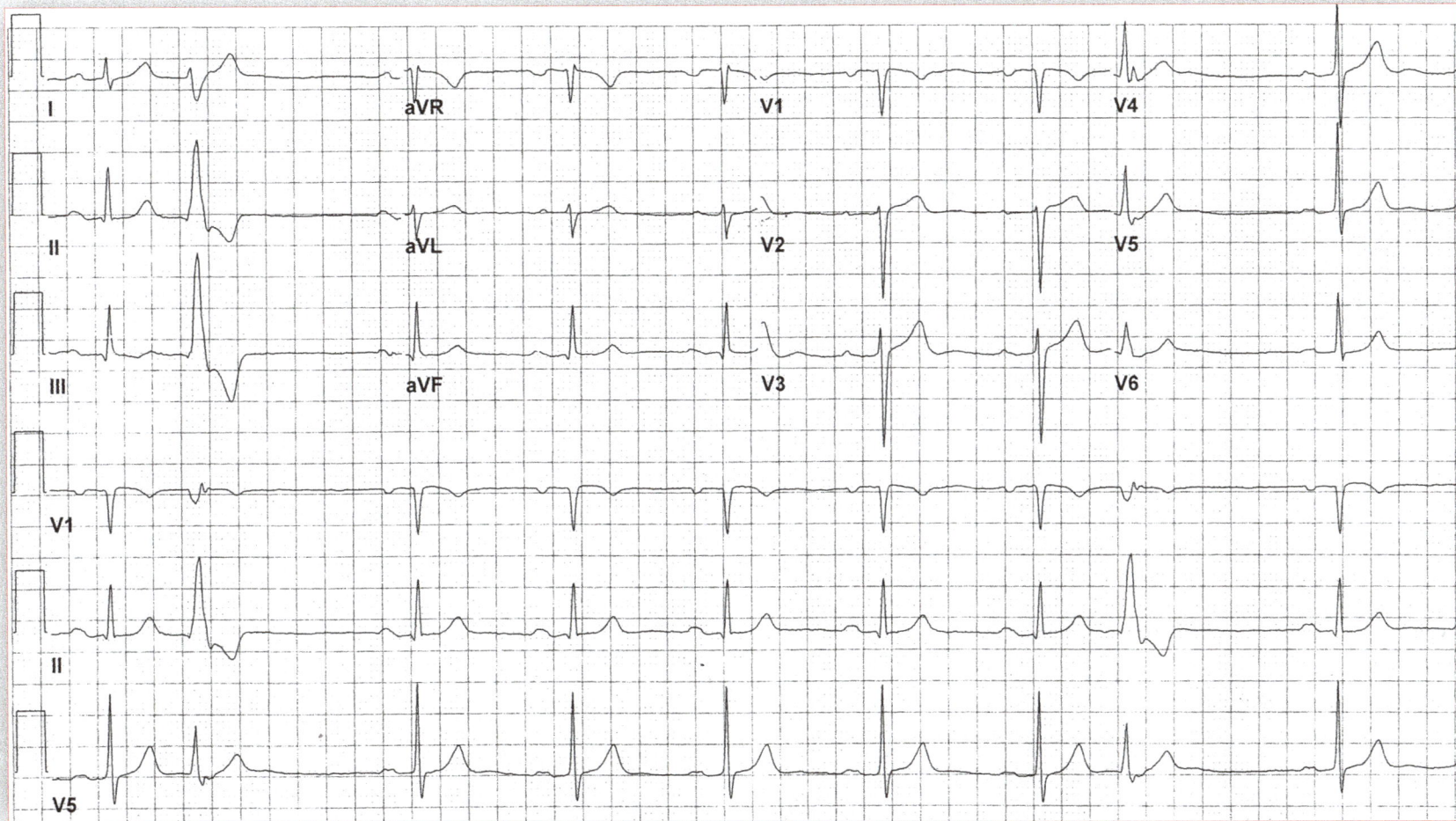

I   aVR   V1   V4

II   aVL   V2   V5

III   aVF   V3   V6

V1   PP   PP

II   2 PP   2 PP

V5

ECG 67 Analysis: Sinus bradycardia, premature ventricular complexes (PVCs) (unifocal)

There is a regularly irregular rhythm at a rate of 56 bpm. The irregularity is due to two wide (duration = 0.16 sec) premature QRS complexes (^) (second and eighth complexes) that are followed by a pause. The PP interval (⊔) around the premature complex is equal to two PP intervals (⊓) and hence is termed a compensatory pause. All other QRS complexes are narrow (0.08 sec) and occur at regular intervals. There is a P wave (+) before each narrow QRS complex, with a stable PR interval (0.30 sec). The P wave is positive in leads I, II, aVF, and V4-V6. Hence there is a sinus bradycardia with a first-degree AV block.

The narrow QRS complexes have a normal morphology and axis, between 0° and +90° (positive QRS complex in leads I and aVF). The QT/QTc intervals are normal (380/370 msec). These complexes are the result of normal conduction through the AV node and His-Purkinje system. The premature complexes are wide with an abnormal morphology and do not have a P wave before them. They are called premature ventricular complexes (PVCs), premature ventricular beats, or ventricular extrasystoles. They may also be called ventricular premature beats or ventricular premature complexes. Since all the PVCs have the same morphology, they are termed unifocal PVCs.

Characteristics of PVCs include the following:

- An early (premature) and wide QRS complex (≥ 0.12 sec) that is without a preceding P wave. A P wave after the QRS complex may be seen. This P wave may be retrograde due to ventriculoatrial conduction or may be an on-time sinus P wave. This can be determined by comparing the interval between the P waves of the sinus complexes prior to the PVC and the P wave following the PVC with the underlying PP interval. If the P wave after the PVC has the same timing as the sinus P waves, it is the on-time sinus P wave. If the P wave after the PVC is early, it is related to the PVC and hence is retrograde.

- Usually the PVC is associated with a full compensatory pause (*ie*, the PP interval surrounding the PVC is twice the baseline PP interval). This is due to retrograde (ventriculoatrial) conduction through the AV node. The PVC causes retrograde activation of the His-Purkinje network and penetrates the AV node in a retrograde fashion. The next on-time sinus impulse finds the AV node refractory and hence there is no AV conduction and the sinus P wave (which is usually not apparent on the ECG as it usually occurs during the PVC) is blocked or nonconducted. The subsequent sinus P wave then conducts through the AV node in normal fashion.

continues

- On occasion the PVC is interpolated (*ie*, there is no pause after the PVC and the PP interval surrounding the PVC is the same as the baseline PP interval). In this situation, the PR interval of the complex following the PVC is often longer than the baseline PR interval. This is the result of concealed retrograde conduction, which is due to the fact that the retrograde conduction through the AV node is only partial. Thus, the AV node is only partially refractory; the subsequent atrial impulse can penetrate the AV node, but it is conducted through the node at a slower rate (longer PR interval) due to the fact that the partially refractory AV node will conduct more slowly.

The PP interval surrounding the PVC (⊔) is twice the underlying PP interval (⊓) or sinus rate; hence there is a full compensatory pause.

The most common mechanism for PVCs is reentry. Therefore, unifocal PVCs usually have a fixed coupling relationship (↔) with the preceding sinus beat (*ie*, with each premature beat the interval between the sinus QRS complex and PVC is the same). PVCs occur frequently both in healthy individuals and in those with heart disease. When they are present in a patient with heart disease they have been associated with an increased risk for morbidity and mortality (due to sudden cardiac death), particularly if they occur frequently or are repetitive (*ie*, two or more sequential PVCs). For this patient, it would be reasonable to obtain an echocardiogram to rule out structural heart disease. Even in the absence of any abnormality, a Holter monitor might also be used to assess the frequency of PVCs and the presence of repetitive forms.

Treatment of unifocal PVCs is usually not needed if there are no symptoms. Therapy is not warranted even for patients with heart disease who may be at an increase risk as there are no data that suppression of PVCs will prevent a sustained ventricular arrhythmia or sudden cardiac death. However, symptoms associated with PVCs, including palpitations, shortness of breath, or even dizziness, may prompt therapy for their suppression. Symptoms of palpitations are often the result of the post-PVC sinus beat, which has increased left ventricular diastolic filling due to the post-PVC pause and an increase in inotropy via the Starling effect resulting in an increased stroke volume. β-blockers may help to alleviate the symptom of palpitations. For more serious symptoms, suppressive therapy with a class IA, IC, or III agent may be needed.

Therapy to suppress asymptomatic PVCs may be necessary in patients with significant left ventricular systolic dysfunction if the PVCs are very frequent or repetitive and impact left ventricular function, causing a worsening of heart failure. The PVCs may result in a dyssynchronous and ineffective contraction, and there may be failure to augment stroke volume with the post-extrasystolic beat. In a patient with underlying sinus bradycardia, frequent PVCs result in a further slowing of the effective heart rate. As PVCs have a suboptimal stroke volume, the effective cardiac output is reduced and this may be associated with development of symptoms related to a bradycardia. ■

A 71-year-old man with known coronary disease, hypertension, and diabetes presents with frequent episodes of an irregular heartbeat. He reports transient sensations of a racing heartbeat followed very quickly by normal heartbeats. An ECG is obtained.

What is the diagnosis?

Anatomically, where would you localize the two abnormalities?

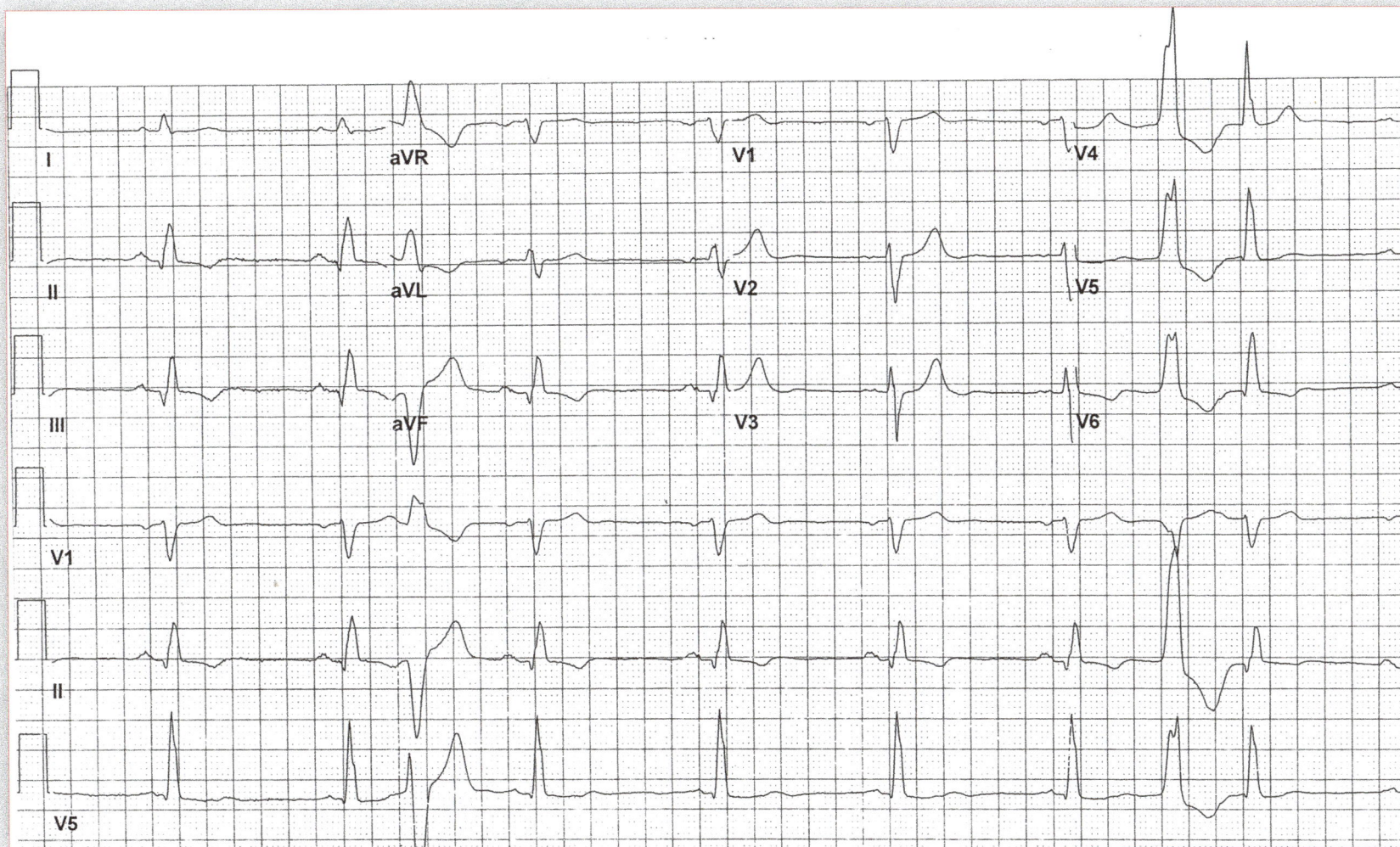

ECG 68 Analysis: Sinus bradycardia, intraventricular conduction delay (IVCD), chronic inferior wall myocardial infarction (MI), premature ventricular complexes (PVCs) (multifocal, interpolated)

The ECG shows a regularly irregular rhythm at a rate of 48 bpm. The irregularity is the result of two premature complexes (^) (third and eighth QRS complexes) that are wide (0.16 sec) and have an abnormal morphology. Each of the narrower QRS complexes (duration = 0.12 sec) have a P wave (+) before them with a stable PR interval (0.20 sec). The P waves are positive in leads I, II, aVF, and V4-V6. Hence this is a sinus bradycardia.

There is no specific pattern to the widening of the sinus QRS complexes (*ie*, it is not a right or left bundle branch block), and hence this is an intraventricular conduction delay (IVCD). The axis is normal, between 0° and +90° (positive QRS complex in leads I and aVF). There are Q waves (↑) in leads II, III, and aVF associated with T-wave inversion (*); this is characteristic of a chronic inferior wall myocardial infarction (MI). The QT/QTc intervals are normal (440/390 msec and 400/360 msec when corrected for the prolonged QRS interval).

The two premature and wide QRS complexes do not have a preceding P wave, and they have an abnormal morphology. These are premature ventricular complexes (PVCs) with different morphologies; hence they are multifocal PVCs. The coupling intervals (↔) between the sinus beat and the PVCs are different (0.44 and 0.70 sec), meaning that there are two distinct locations for the reentrant circuits that are responsible for the two different PVC morphologies. Neither of the PVCs is associated with a pause, and indeed the PP interval surrounding the PVC (⊔) is the same as the sinus PP interval (⊔). Hence these PVCs are interpolated. However, the PR interval of the on-time sinus beat following the PVC (⊓) is slightly longer (0.24 sec) than the baseline PR interval (⊓) (0.20 sec). This is the result of concealed retrograde (ventriculoatrial) conduction; the premature ventricular impulse partially penetrates the AV node in a retrograde direction but does not completely depolarize this structure. Hence the impulse is concealed within the AV node. However, the AV node becomes partially depolarized and is partially refractory. Therefore, the next on-time sinus impulse conducts through the AV node but with a slower conduction velocity (due to slower AV nodal conductivity), accounting for the longer PR interval.

continues

The site of origin of a PVC within the myocardium can be established based on the ECG. This patient has a known inferior infarction that could very easily be the source of a scar-related PVC. In general, the leads in which the PVC is negative identify the site of origin of the PVC (*ie*, the direction of impulse activation is away from the site of origin and hence the impulse is directed away from the lead that is located over the site of origin, thereby producing a Q wave in this lead). The first PVC on this ECG is negative in leads II and aVF, suggesting that it is originating from the inferior wall, activating the ventricle in a direction away from the inferior wall. Since the complex has a right bundle branch–like morphology in lead V1, it is originating in the left ventricle. Thus, this PVC originates from the inferior wall of the left ventricle, correlating with the site of the old infarction. The second PVC, however, has a left bundle branch–like pattern in lead V1 (QS morphology), suggesting that it is originating in the right ventricle. The PVC is positive in lead II and therefore appears to be inferiorly directed. Thus, the second PVC may be coming from the right ventricular outflow tract, a common source of non–infarct-related PVCs. It is possible that there is also a right ventricular infarction associated with the inferior wall MI, and hence the origin of this PVC is the right ventricular free wall. ■

A 52-year-old man with newly diagnosed idiopathic dilated cardiomyopathy (based on the absence of coronary artery disease on previous coronary angiograms) and an ejection fraction of 40% presents with palpitations. The following ECG is obtained.

What is the rhythm diagnosis?

Does this patient need an implantable cardioverter–defibrillator placed?

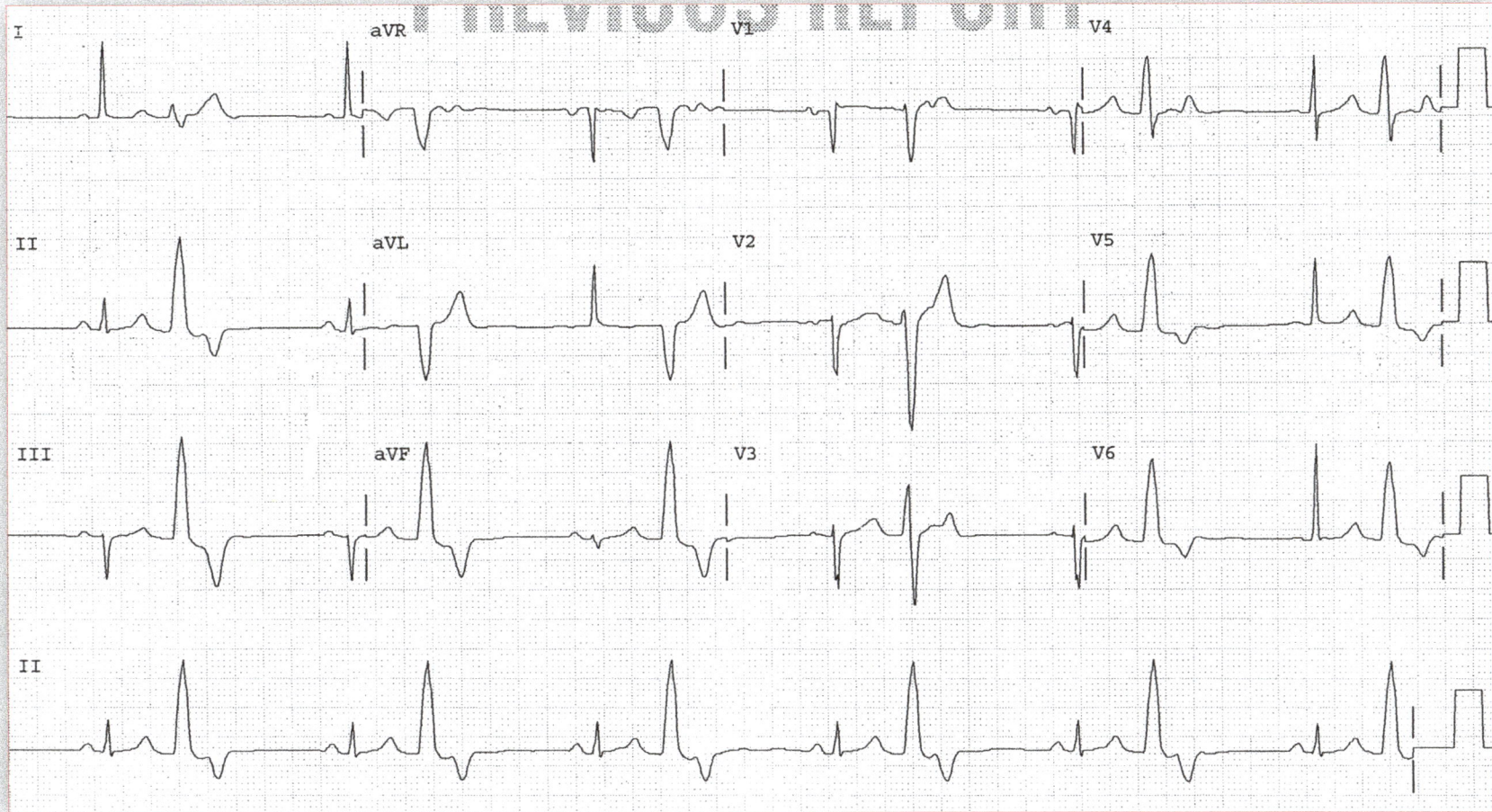

ECG 69 Analysis: Normal sinus rhythm, physiologic left axis, premature ventricular complexes (PVCs) (unifocal) in a bigeminal pattern (ventricular bigeminy)

The ECG shows a regularly irregular rhythm with alternating short (⊔) and long (⊓) RR intervals. There are narrow QRS complexes (^) (duration = 0.08 sec) associated with P waves followed by premature complexes (*) that are not preceded by a P wave. The premature QRS complexes are wide (0.14 sec) and have an abnormal morphology that resembles neither a right nor a left bundle branch block. These are premature ventricular complexes (PVCs). Each of the narrow QRS complexes has a preceding P wave (+) with a stable PR interval (0.16 sec). The P wave is positive in leads I, II, aVF, and V4-V6. Hence these are sinus complexes. The axis is physiologically leftward, between 0° and −30° (positive QRS complex in leads I and II and negative QRS complex in lead aVF). The QT/QTc intervals are normal (380/420 msec).

As there is a PVC after each sinus complex; this is called ventricular bigeminy, which is a term used to identify a repeating pattern (*ie*, every other QRS complex is a PVC). The morphology of the PVCs is uniform, so these are unifocal PVCs. The coupling interval (↔) between the sinus beat and PVC is fixed, meaning that the mechanism is reentry and there is a single reentrant circuit accounting for the one morphology of the PVCs and a fixed relationship (fixed coupling interval) between the sinus complex and the PVC. Noted with each PVC is an alteration of the T wave (↓), and in lead V1 (▲) this is a P wave, which is positive in leads II, aVF, and V5-V6. In addition, the PP interval (⊔⊔) between the P wave of the sinus complex and the P wave after the PVC is the same as the PP interval between the P wave after the PVC and the next sinus P wave. Hence this is the on-time sinus P wave, since the P waves can be marched out (*ie*, the PP intervals are constant). This P wave is blocked and not conducted through the AV node as a result of retrograde

activation and depolarization of the AV node by the PVC, causing this structure to be refractory to the on-time sinus node activation. Hence the patient has an underlying sinus rhythm at a rate of 76 bpm.

The term ventricular bigeminy is of significance only because it means a repeating pattern (*ie*, every other QRS complex is a PVC). There is no clinical importance to the presence of a bigeminal pattern, except that the PVCs are frequent. No antiarrhythmic therapy (antiarrhythmic drug or implantable cardioverter–defibrillator) is indicated simply based on the presence of ventricular bigeminy. Typically, a defibrillator will be placed for non-ischemic cardiomyopathy only if one of the following criteria is met:

- The ejection fraction is less than 35% and the cardiomyopathy has been present for more than 9 months regardless of any rhythm disturbances. This is based on the Sudden Cardiac Death in Heart Failure Trial (SCD-HeFT).

- The patient has an ejection fraction less than 40%, nonsustained ventricular tachycardia, and inducible ventricular tachycardia on electrophysiology study.

- The patient experiences an episode of sustained ventricular tachycardia or ventricular fibrillation, regardless of ejection fraction.

It is important to remember that such a high frequency of PVCs over a period of months may uncommonly result in a cardiomyopathy. If this occurs, the PVCs should be treated aggressively (*ie*, with a class III antiarrhythmic drug or even radiofrequency ablation) if no other etiology is identified. ■

Notes

A 46-year-old woman with no past medical history presents to your clinic with feelings of extra heartbeats. She denies chest pain, dyspnea, lightheadedness, or syncope. Her physical examination is normal except for a regularly irregular rhythm. The following ECG is obtained.

What is the diagnosis?

What is the underlying mechanism for this rhythm abnormality?

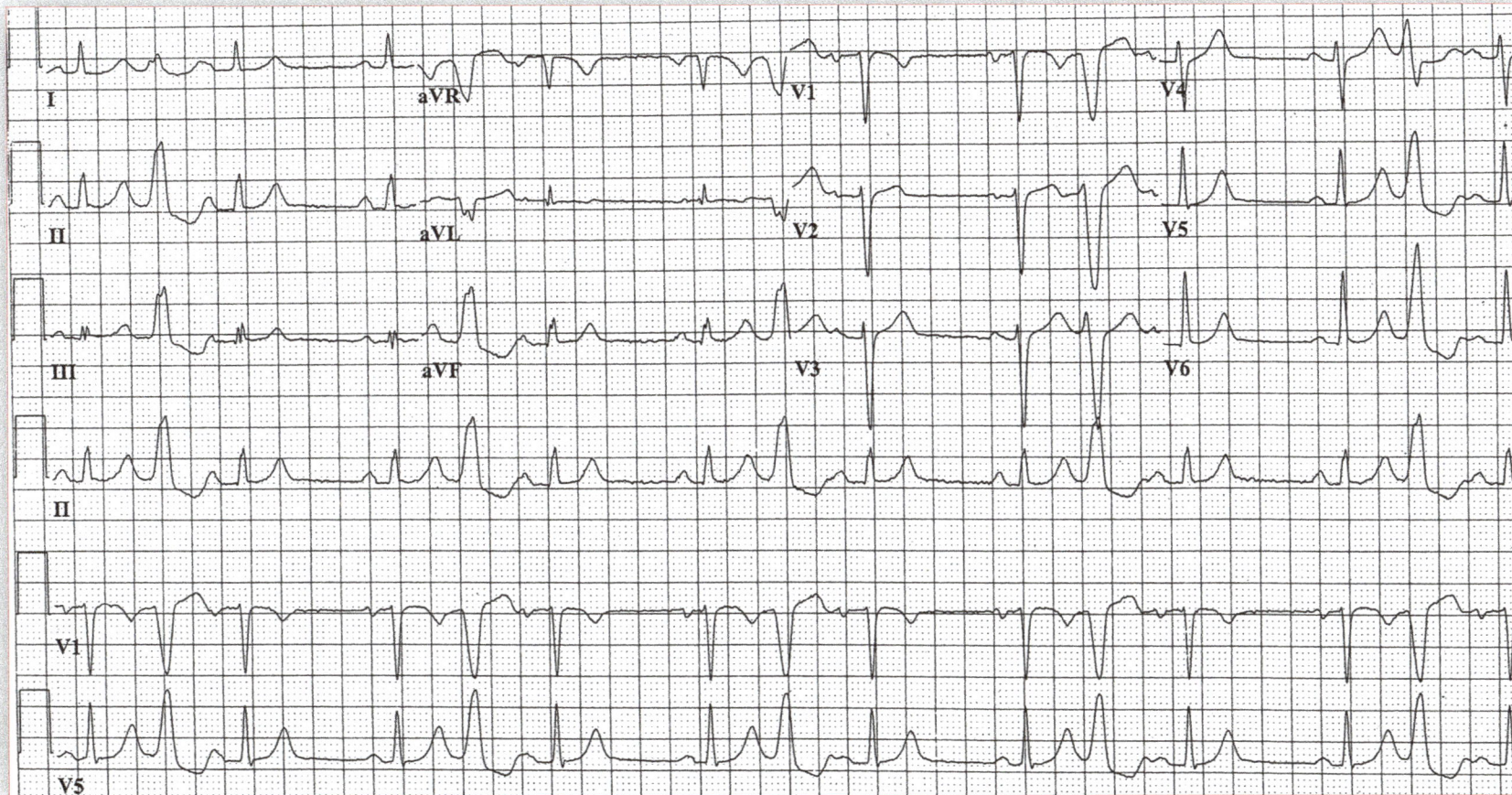

ECG 70 Analysis: Sinus bradycardia, premature ventricular complexes (PVCs) (unifocal, interpolated) in a trigeminal pattern (ventricular trigeminy), retrograde concealed conduction

The ECG shows a regularly irregular rhythm, and there appears to be group beating. All the long intervals (⊔) are the same, the short intervals (⊓) are the same, and the intermediate intervals (⊔⊔) are the same. Noted are two narrow QRS complexes (*), after which there is a wide QRS complex (^) that is early or premature. The narrow QRS complex duration is 0.08 second, and there is a normal morphology and normal axis, between 0° and +90° (positive QRS complex in leads I and aVF). There is low voltage (*ie*, < 5 mm) in each limb lead. The QT/QTc intervals are normal (400/390 msec). There is a P wave before each narrow QRS complex (+), and the P wave is positive in leads I, II, aVF, and V4-V6. Hence there is an underlying stable sinus mechanism, at a rate of 56 bpm (sinus bradycardia), as a P wave is seen before each of the narrow QRS complexes.

There are no P waves before the early, wide QRS complexes, which have an abnormal morphology that resembles a left bundle branch block (broad QS complex in lead V1 [←] and broad R wave in leads I and V5-V6 [→]). These are premature ventricular complexes (PVCs) and they are occurring after every second sinus complex; hence this is ventricular trigeminy. As with a bigeminy, trigeminy indicates a repeating pattern. There is no clinical importance to the presence of trigeminy except that the PVCs are frequent. Each PVC has the same morphology, so they are unifocal. The interval between the sinus complex and the PVC (⊓) is the same each time (*ie*, there is a fixed coupling interval). This indicates that the etiology for the PVC is a reentrant circuit that is activated and generates only a single premature impulse.

The PVCs are not followed by a pause and they do not affect the underlying PP interval (↔), which is stable. Hence the PP interval around the PVC is identical to the PP interval without the PVC. Therefore, these PVCs are called interpolated. However, the PR intervals of the sinus complexes before and after the PVC are different. The sinus complex following the PVC has a PR interval that is longer (0.20 sec) than the PR interval of the sinus complex before the PVC (0.16 sec). This is the result of concealed retrograde (ventriculoatrial) conduction. The PVC partially penetrates the AV node in a retrograde direction but does not completely depolarize this structure. Hence it is concealed within the AV node. However, the AV node becomes partially depolarized and hence the next on-time sinus impulse conducts through the AV node but with a slower conduction velocity, accounting for the longer PR interval. ■

A 32-year-old black man presents with palpitations and dyspnea. He has noted the dyspnea for many months now, ever since he lost 30 pounds. His only past medical history is that of uveitis treated with steroid drops 6 months ago. On physical examination, his jugular venous pressure is elevated, lower extremity edema and hepatomegaly are present, and his heart is dilated on palpation with an audible S3. There is also cervical lymphadenopathy. Chest imaging reveals bilateral hilar lymphadenopathy with pulmonary reticular opacities. An ECG is obtained because of the palpitations.

What is the diagnosis on ECG?

What is the most likely overall clinical diagnosis?

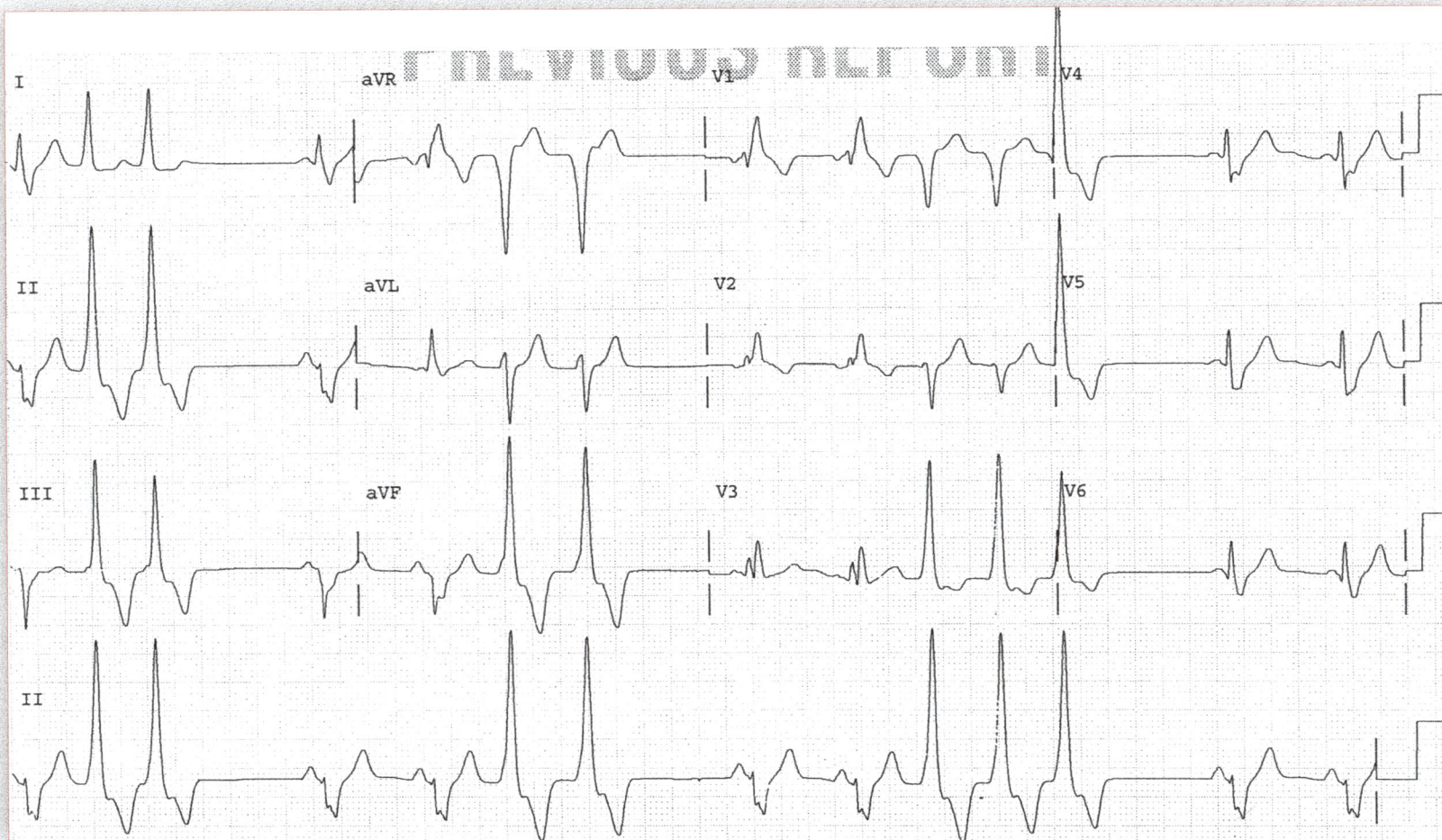

ECG 71 Analysis: Sinus rhythm, right bundle branch block (RBBB), left anterior fascicular block (LAFB), bifascicular disease, ventricular couplet (unifocal), ventricular triplet (nonsustained ventricular tachycardia [NSVT], monomorphic)

The ECG shows a regularly irregular rhythm. There are two different QRS complex morphologies. Complexes 1, 4, 5, 8, 9, 13, and 14 (^) are wide (0.14 sec) and have a right bundle branch block (RBBB) morphology (RSR′ in lead V1 [→] and broad S waves in leads I and V4-V6 [←]). The broad R′ in lead V1 and terminal broad S waves in leads I and V4-V6 result from terminal forces going from left to right. There is a P wave (+) before each of these QRS complexes with a stable PR interval (0.16 sec). The P wave is positive in leads I, II, aVF, and V4-V6. Hence these are sinus complexes and the sinus rate is 80 bpm. The axis is extremely leftward, between −30° and −90° (positive QRS complex in lead I and negative QRS complex in leads II and aVF with an rS morphology). This is a left anterior fascicular block (LAFB), which, along with the RBBB, indicates bifascicular disease (*ie*, disease of two of the three major fascicles innervating the ventricles). The QT/QTc intervals are normal (380/440 msec and 320/370 msec when corrected for the prolonged QRS complex duration).

After the first and fifth complexes (both of which are sinus), there are two sequential wide (0.18 sec) and early QRS complexes (↓) that are not preceded by a P wave. These QRS complexes have a left bundle branch block morphology (wide and deep QS complex in lead V1 [▼] and broad R waves in leads I and V5-V6 [↑]). These are premature ventricular complexes (PVCs). Two sequential PVCs is termed a ventricular couplet (⊓). After the ninth QRS complex (which is sinus) there is one episode of three sequential PVCs (▲); this is called a ventricular triplet (⊔). By definition, three or more sequential PVCs lasting up to 30 seconds has also been called nonsustained ventricular tachycardia (NSVT). The term ventricular triplet or NSVT can be used in this situation. As all of the ventricular complexes have the same morphology, the couplets are unifocal and the NSVT is termed monomorphic.

This patient's overall clinical presentation includes evidence of biventricular heart failure, conduction abnormalities, uveitis, lymphadenopathy, and pulmonary reticular opacities. These are the characteristic findings of sarcoidosis, which typically presents between the ages of 10 and 40 years and is much more common among blacks than other races. Cardiac sarcoidosis typically presents with heart failure or rhythm disturbances such as AV nodal block, intraventricular conduction delay, or ventricular arrhythmias, which are due to direct granulomatous inflammation and infiltration of the myocardium. ■

A 73-year-old man with an idiopathic dilated cardiomyopathy and a known ejection fraction of 30% presents with palpitations and dizziness. An implantable cardioverter–defibrillator was placed 2 years ago for primary prevention of sudden cardiac death. The following ECG is obtained while the patient is symptomatic.

What is the diagnosis?

Would any additional treatment be necessary?

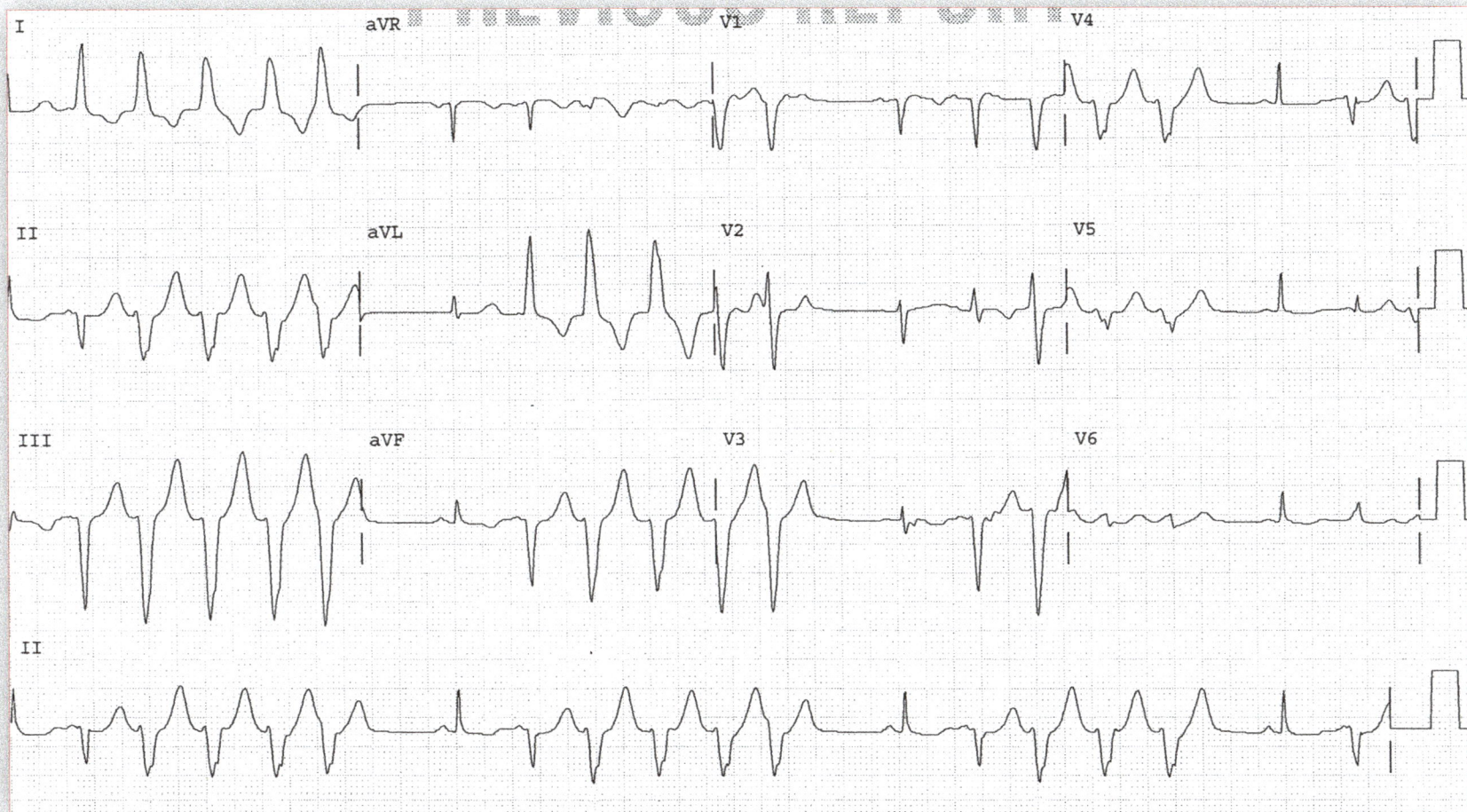

ECG 72 Analysis: Sinus tachycardia, nonsustained ventricular tachycardia (NSVT) (monomorphic), fusion complexes

The ECG shows a regularly irregular rhythm with wide (^) and narrow (*) QRS complexes. There are three narrow QRS complexes (*) (duration 0.08 sec), which are preceded by a P wave (+) with a stable PR interval (0.14 sec). The P wave is positive in leads II, aVF, and V4-V6; hence these are sinus complexes. These QRS complexes have a normal axis, between 0° and +90° (positive QRS complex in leads I and aVF). The QT/QTc intervals are slightly prolonged (360/460 msec). Following each of the sinus complexes is a four- to five-beat run (⊓) of a wide complex rhythm (QRS complex duration = 0.16 sec) at a rate of 134 bpm. The first QRS complex of these runs is premature. These QRS complexes do not have any apparent P wave before them. Therefore, these are ventricular complexes, or nonsustained ventricular tachycardia (NSVT), which is defined as a ventricular rhythm of three or more sequential premature ventricular complexes lasting up to 30 seconds at a rate higher than 100 bpm. The morphologies of the ventricular complexes are similar, with very subtle differences; hence this is monomorphic NSVT.

There does appear to be a P wave (•) before the first QRS complex of the NSVT run (▲). It should be noted that the PR interval before this complex is much shorter (‖) (0.10 sec) than the PR interval of the sinus complexes. In addition, the width of the first QRS complex of the run of NSVT (▲) is slightly wider (0.10 sec) than the sinus complexes but narrower than the subsequent ventricular complexes. Hence this is termed a fusion complex (*ie*, the QRS complex of this first complex of the run is the result of ventricular activation via both the normal AV node–His-Purkinje system and the ventricular pathway that is responsible for the NSVT). Hence, the complex represents fusion of activation by these two pathways. The presence of fusion is a feature of AV dissociation, which is commonly seen during a ventricular tachyarrhythmia (either NSVT or sustained ventricular tachycardia). Hence there is an independent atrial and ventricular rhythm; the ventricular rate is faster than the atrial rate. If the PP interval observed on the ECG is measured (*ie*, between the sinus P wave and the P wave just prior to the first QRS complex of the NSVT), it can be seen that the P waves thereafter occur on time and "march through" the NSVT; that is, there is a stable PP interval or atrial rate. Thus, the interval between the P wave of the sinus complex and the P wave before the first complex of the run is at a rate 100 bpm. By using this atrial rate, it can be seen that although the next P wave is within the second QRS complex of the run, the following on-time P wave is seen as a waveform at the very end of the third QRS complex of the run. By continuing to march out the P waves, it can be seen that the sinus P wave is on time.

continues

Ventricular rhythms can be identified by the following characteristics:

- QRS complexes are wide (> 0.12 sec) and have an abnormal morphology that resembles neither a typical right nor left bundle branch block.

- P waves (if seen) are usually unrelated to the QRS complexes (*ie*, AV dissociation is identified by a variable PR interval), and the ventricular rate is higher than the atrial rate. Often no P waves can be identified, especially if the ventricular rate is rapid.

- A negative P wave may be seen after the QRS complex if ventriculoatrial (VA) conduction is present. This usually occurs when the ventricular rate is slower and hence allows for VA conduction.

- Often the QRS complexes and ST-T waves demonstrate non–rate-related variability in morphology. This may be the result of subtle changes in ventricular depolarization and repolarization due to the fact that direct myocardial activation originates from a ventricular circuit that bypasses the normal His-Purkinje system. Hence there may be changes in the direction of the ventricular activation sequence. The changes in ST-T waves may also represent P waves that are superimposed on these waveforms.

- Fusion beats or completely captured (Dressler) beats may be seen. Fusion beats result from activation via two different pathways (the normal His-Purkinje system and the ventricular reentrant circuit). There is a P wave before the QRS complex, and the PR interval is shorter than that of the sinus complex. The QRS complex does not resemble either the sinus or the ventricular QRS complex but has features of both. Complete capture (Dressler complex) is more commonly seen when the rate of the ventricular rhythm is slower. At a slower rate there is less retrograde conduction into the AV node, thereby allowing more time for a sinus beat to completely penetrate the AV node antegradely and capture the ventricular myocardium. In this situation there is a definable PR interval followed by a QRS complex that has the same morphology as the sinus complex.

NSVT is commonly seen in patients with an idiopathic dilated cardiomyopathy. Although the patient does have an implantable cardioverter–defibrillator (ICD) placed for primary prevention of sudden death as a result of a low ejection fraction, the ICD only terminates sustained arrhythmia; it does not prevent arrhythmia. Hence it will not prevent the episodes of NSVT. If the symptoms do correlate with NSVT, this arrhythmia might need to be suppressed (for symptom relief and not for mortality benefit). In addition, if the runs of NSVT are long, they could impact ICD function and result in multiple ICD therapies and possible shocks. Suppression of the NSVT would require a standard antiarrhythmic drug. In a patient with a dilated cardiomyopathy, the safest agent would be amiodarone, dofetilide, or sotalol. ■

A 40-year-old man with diabetes and a family history of early coronary artery disease presents to the emergency department with acute-onset chest burning, jaw pain, and diaphoresis. When an initial ECG reveals inferior ST-segment elevations, the patient is taken emergently for cardiac catheterization.

Angiography reveals a proximal right coronary artery thrombotic occlusion, which is opened via angioplasty and then stented. He subsequently is admitted to the hospital's coronary care unit. The following ECG is obtained a few hours later when the patient's vital signs are stable.

What is the diagnosis?

How should this be managed?

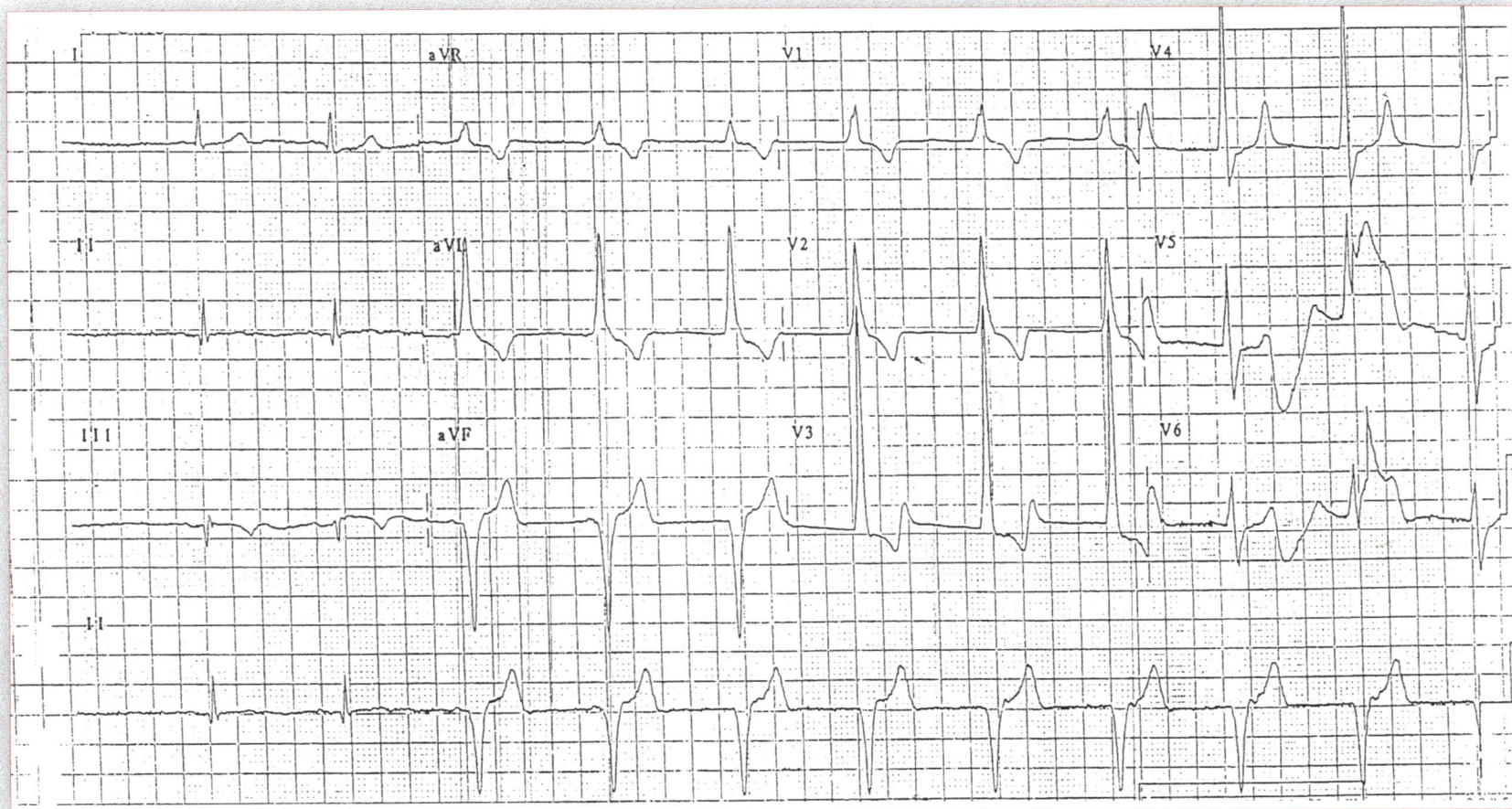

ECG 73 Analysis: Normal sinus rhythm, accelerated idioventricular rhythm (AIVR)

The ECG begins with two narrow QRS complexes (^) (duration = 0.08 sec) that are preceded by P waves (+) (PR interval = 0.16 sec) and are at a rate of 64 bpm. These are sinus complexes. The QT/QTc intervals are normal (400/410 msec). The third QRS complex (*) is wide (0.14 sec) with an abnormal morphology. This QRS complex is early, with a PR interval (‖) that is shorter (0.10 sec) than the baseline PR interval. The fourth QRS complex (▲) is also premature and wide with an abnormal morphology; the PR interval (●) is even shorter (0.08 sec). There are no P waves before the remaining QRS complexes. These are ventricular complexes and there is AV dissociation, as established by the initial variable PR intervals. The QRS complexes have a QS morphology in leads II and aVF, suggesting that they are originating from the inferior wall, likely from the area of the recent myocardial infarction (MI). The wide QRS complexes occur at a rate that is slightly faster (ie, 68 bpm) than the sinus rate. Hence this is an accelerated idioventricular rhythm (AIVR), which has also been termed slow ventricular tachycardia. The QRS complexes of the AIVR have a right bundle branch block pattern, with positive concordance (ie, there are tall R waves across the precordium). In addition, P waves can be seen following the fifth ventricular complex [↓] and the QRS complexes thereafter (note notching [▼] of the ST segment), with a fixed RP interval (↔). These are retrograde P waves as a result of intact ventriculoatrial conduction.

An AIVR arises below the AV node and has, by definition, a rate between 60 and 100 bpm. Although it may be the result of pacemaker failure, and therefore an escape rhythm, AIVR most often represents an abnormal ectopic focus in the ventricle that is accelerated by sympathetic stimulation and circulating catecholamines. It may be seen in up to 50% of patients with an acute MI. AIVR is often observed in the setting of coronary artery reperfusion, especially with thrombolytics. It is believed to be a reperfusion arrhythmia, although its mechanism is not clear. It may be related to rapid reperfusion with the washout of various substances that are released by the damaged myocardium, including potassium and other electrolytes. AIVR is usually transient and asymptomatic.

No specific treatment is necessary unless the rate is rapid and it is associated with symptoms or evidence of hemodynamic impairment. In this situation, a standard antiarrhythmic drug may be effective for its suppression. However, before therapy is initiated it is important to make certain that the ventricular rhythm is not an escape rhythm as a result of complete heart block. In this situation a pacemaker may be required before suppression of the ventricular rhythm as the ventricular arrhythmia is escape and its suppression would result in asystole. If the onset of the arrhythmia can be seen, a ventricular rate that is faster than the sinus rate is characteristic of AIVR. Observing AV dissociation during the ventricular rhythm with an atrial rate slower than the ventricular rate is also characteristic of an accelerated ventricular focus. In contrast, a long pause and often a nonconducted P wave after which the ventricular rhythm occurs is characteristic of complete heart block and an escape ventricular rhythm. If AV dissociation is seen in this situation, the atrial rate is faster than the ventricular rate. ■

Case 74

ECG 74A

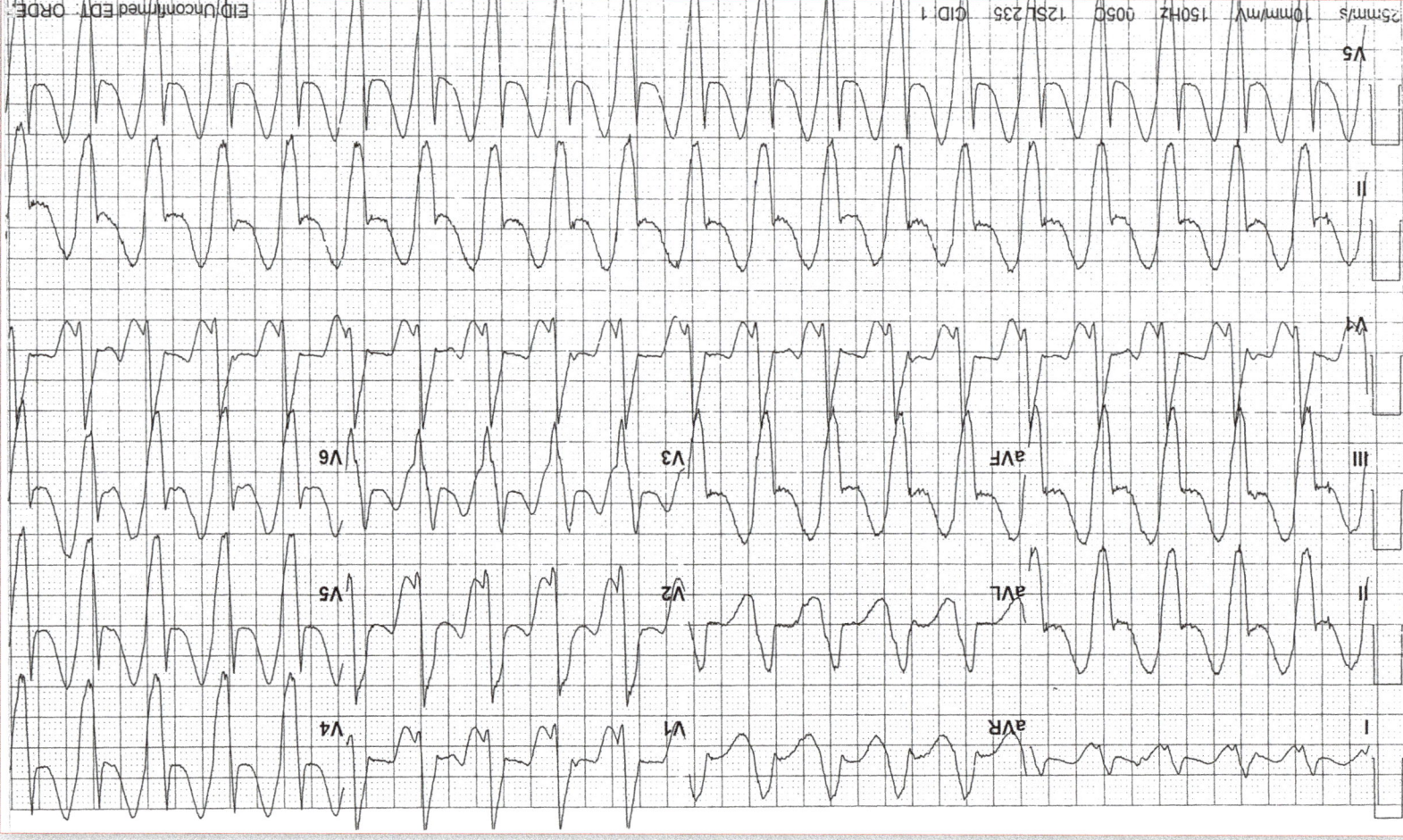

A 59-year-old man who had a myocardial infarction 5 months previously presents to the emergency department with a history of palpitations, presyncope, and one syncopal episode. While in the emergency department, his symptoms return. ECG 74A is obtained while the patient is symptomatic; ECG 74B is the baseline ECG obtained when he first presented and before the onset of symptoms.

What is the diagnosis?

What therapy would be indicated for this patient?

ECG 74B

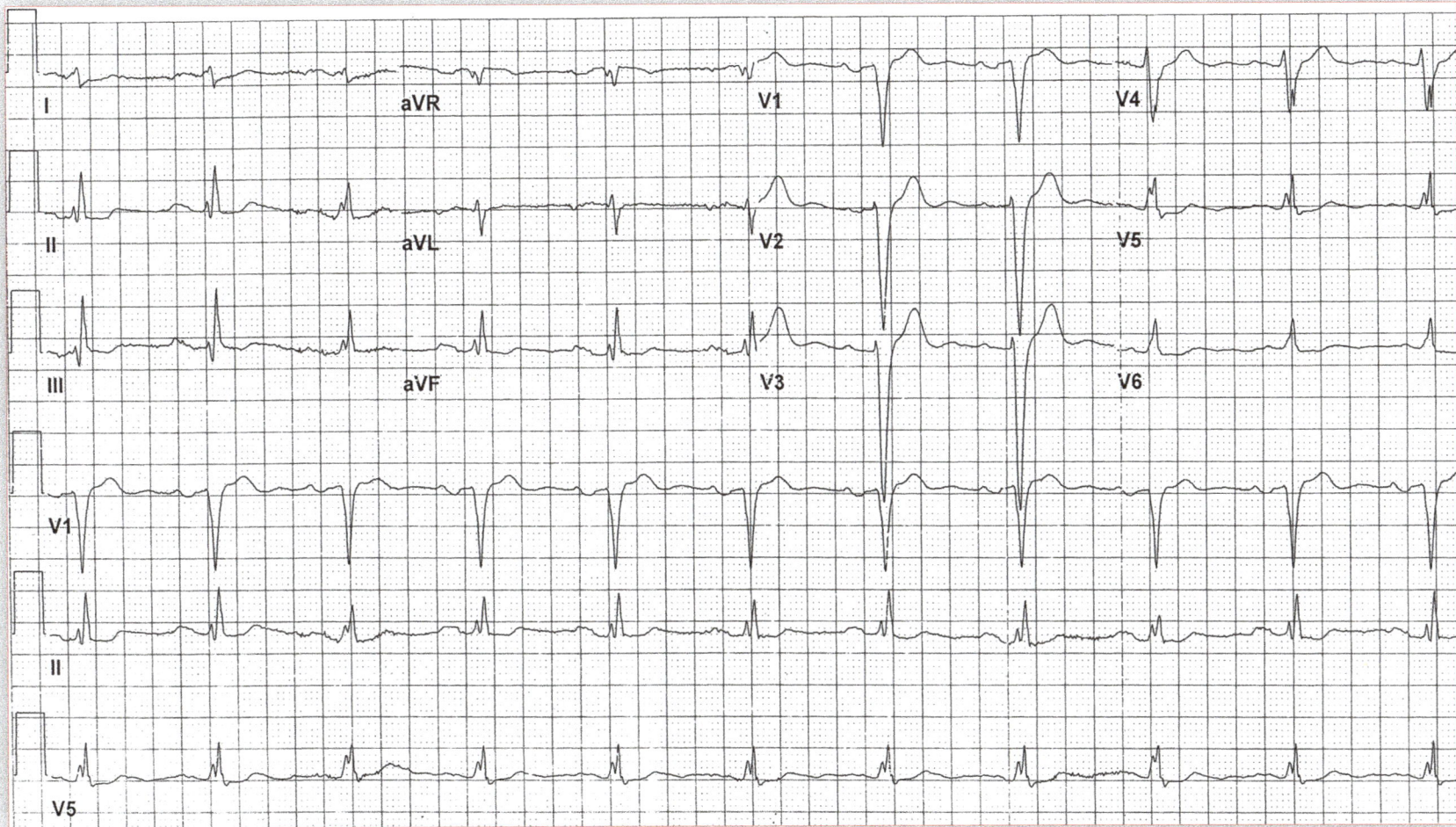

ECG 74A Analysis: Sustained monomorphic ventricular tachycardia

ECG 74A shows a wide complex tachycardia (QRS width = 0.18 sec) at a rate of 130 bpm. No obvious P waves are seen before or after the QRS complexes. However, there appears to be a P wave (*) in front of the second, seventh, and 12th QRS complexes in lead V1. In addition, the T waves after the third, eighth, 13th, and 18th QRS complexes in lead V1 have a different morphology (+) compared with the other T waves; they have a positive deflection at the very end of the waveform (+), suggesting a superimposed P wave. Lead I shows a notching of the T wave (↓) after the third QRS complex that is not seen after the other QRS complexes in this lead. Thus, there is evidence of AV dissociation. Although the P waves cannot be marched out through the ECG tracing, the fact that there are P waves associated with some but not all of the QRS complexes is indicative of AV dissociation. Moreover, the association between the P wave and QRS complex is variable. The presence of AV dissociation is also indicated by the presence of subtle changes in the morphology of the ST-T waves. Any wide complex arrhythmia with evidence of AV dissociation is ventricular tachycardia.

It should be noted that the positive waveform after the QRS complex in leads V1-V2 is not a P wave but is the terminal part of the QRS complex, which is determined by comparing the QRS width in another lead, such as lead aVF, II, or V3 (‖). The QRS complexes have a uniform morphology that resembles a right bundle branch block (RBBB), but it is not a typical RBBB and there is a marked leftward axis. This is sustained monomorphic ventricular tachycardia. Sustained ventricular tachycardia is defined as a ventricular rhythm at a rate higher than 100 bpm that lasts for more than 30 seconds or is terminated within 30 seconds because of hemodynamic instability. Sustained monomorphic ventricular tachycardia is not an ischemically mediated arrhythmia; it results most often from reentry in myocardium that has been previously damaged by infarction (ischemic heart disease) or inflammation (cardiomyopathy) and has areas of fibrosis adjacent to areas of normal myocardial tissue, allowing for the existence of reentrant circuits. Therefore, in patients with heart disease it is scar related.

An important concern is establishing the etiology for a wide complex tachycardia (*ie*, ventricular tachycardia vs. supraventricular tachyarrhythmia associated with aberrancy). Ventricular tachycardia has the following features:

- QRS complexes are wide (> 0.12 sec) and abnormal in morphology. QRS complexes wider than 0.16 second are usually ventricular.

- P waves (if seen) are dissociated from QRS complexes (AV dissociation; *ie*, the PR interval is variable), and the ventricular rate is faster than the atrial rate.

- On occasion a negative P wave may be seen after the QRS complex, indicating the presence of ventriculoatrial conduction. This is most often seen when the ventricular tachycardia rate is slower.

continues

- Often, QRS complexes and ST-T waves show non–rate-related variability in morphology. This may be the result of subtle changes in ventricular depolarization and repolarization due to the fact that there is direct myocardial activation originating from a ventricular circuit that bypasses the normal His-Purkinje system. Hence there may be changes in the direction of the ventricular activation sequence. The changes in ST-T waves may also represent P waves that are superimposed on these waveforms.

- Fusion or captured (Dressler) beats may be seen. Fusion beats result from myocardial activation via two different pathways that "fuses" (*ie*, the normal His-Purkinje system and the ventricular reentrant circuit). There is a P wave before the QRS complex, and the PR interval of the QRS complex is shorter than that of the sinus complex. The QRS complex does not resemble either the sinus or the ventricular QRS complex but has features of both. Complete capture is more commonly seen when the rate of the ventricular rhythm is slower, allowing more time for a sinus beat to completely penetrate the AV node and capture the ventricular myocardium in an antegrade direction. In this situation there is a definable PR interval (similar to or longer than that of the sinus PR interval) followed by a QRS complex that is the same as the sinus complex.

Other important features that also suggest ventricular tachycardia as the etiology for a wide complex tachycardia include:

- Indeterminate axis (*ie*, a QRS complex that is negative in leads I and aVF). An indeterminate axis may also be seen when there is direct myocardial activation, such as with arrhythmias associated with a Wolff-Parkinson-White (WPW) pattern or in paced rhythms. A significant shift in axis compared with sinus rhythm is also seen with ventricular tachycardia.

- Positive concordance (tall R waves) across the precordium. This may also be seen in situations in which there is direct myocardial activation, such as WPW or a paced rhythm. Negative concordance is less useful as this pattern may be seen with a left bundle branch block.

- QRS complex width longer than 0.16 second

- If R/S morphology is seen in any precordial lead, an R wave that is wider than the S wave (R/S >1) or an R wave longer than 100 msec is strongly correlated with a ventricular complex. With a ventricular complex the initial ventricular activation is directly through the ventricular myocardium and hence it is slow, resulting in a QRS complex that has an initial waveform (*ie*, the R wave) that is widened. Indeed, the entire QRS complex is abnormal. In contrast, when there is a supraventricular complex that is aberrated, the widened QRS complex is a result of terminal delay in activation (*ie*, the terminal portion of the QRS complex is widened as a result of conduction block in the right or left bundle branch). In this situation, the R wave is narrower than the S wave and less than 100 msec because the initial forces and waveform of the QRS complex are normal as a result of normal ventricular conduction through the normal functional bundle, while the terminal portion of the QRS complex is due to abnormal and slow conduction through the ventricle served by the bundle that is not functional.

- Other morphologic features of the QRS complex that may be useful include the following:

  – A monophasic R or biphasic qR complex in lead V1 favors ventricular tachycardia; this represents the lack of an RSR′ pattern.

  – A triphasic RSR′ or RsR′ complex (the so-called "rabbit-ear" sign) in lead V1 usually favors a supraventricular tachyarrhythmia. As an exception, if the R wave (initial positive waveform) of the RsR′ complex is taller than the R′ (terminal positive deflection), ventricular tachycardia is suggested.

– An rS complex (R wave smaller than S wave) in lead V6 favors ventricular tachycardia. In contrast, an Rs complex (R wave larger than S wave) in lead V6 favors a supraventricular tachyarrhythmia.

– A broad initial R wave 40 msec in duration or longer in lead V1 or V2 favors ventricular tachycardia. In contrast, the absence of an initial R wave or a small initial R wave of less than 40 msec in lead V1 or V2 favors supraventricular tachyarrhythmia.

– A slurred or notched downstroke of the S wave in lead V1 or V2 and a duration from the onset of the QRS complex to the nadir of the QS or S wave of 60 msec or longer in lead V1 or V2 favors ventricular tachycardia. In contrast, a swift, smooth downstroke of the S wave in lead V1 or V2 with a duration of less than 60 msec favors a supraventricular complex.

– The presence of any significant Q wave or a QS complex in lead V6 is suggestive of ventricular tachycardia. In contrast, the absence of a Q wave in lead V6 favors a supraventricular complex.

continues

ECG 74B Analysis: Normal sinus rhythm, intraventricular conduction delay, first-degree AV block

ECG **74B**, from the same patient, is the baseline ECG. There is a regular rhythm at a rate of 64 bpm. There is a P wave (+) before each QRS complex with a stable PR interval of 0.24 second (first-degree AV block). The P wave is positive in leads I, II, aVF, and V4-V6. Hence this is a normal sinus rhythm. The QRS complex duration is increased (0.14 sec) without any specific pattern of a bundle branch block. Therefore, this is an intraventricular conduction delay. The axis is normal, between 0° and +90° (positive QRS complex in leads I and aVF). The QT/QTc intervals are normal (380/390 msec and 320/330 msec when corrected for the prolonged QRS complex duration). When compared with the QRS complexes seen in **ECG 74A**, it can be seen that the morphology and axis of the QRS complexes during the tachycardia are unlike those during sinus rhythm. Along with the presence of AV dissociation, it is clear that the rhythm in **ECG 74A** is ventricular tachycardia. ■

The following ECG was obtained during an exercise tolerance test in a 32-year-old man who collapsed after 3 minutes of exercise. He had initially presented with progressive dyspnea on exertion. On physical examination prior to the test, a grade III/VI systolic murmur was audible, best heard at the left lower sternal border and increased with Valsalva. The patient reported having an uncle who died suddenly in his 30s. Of note, his resting blood pressure was 140/90 mm Hg, but within 2 minutes of exercise it had dropped to 90/50 mm Hg.

What is the rhythm diagnosis?

What is the overall likely clinical diagnosis?

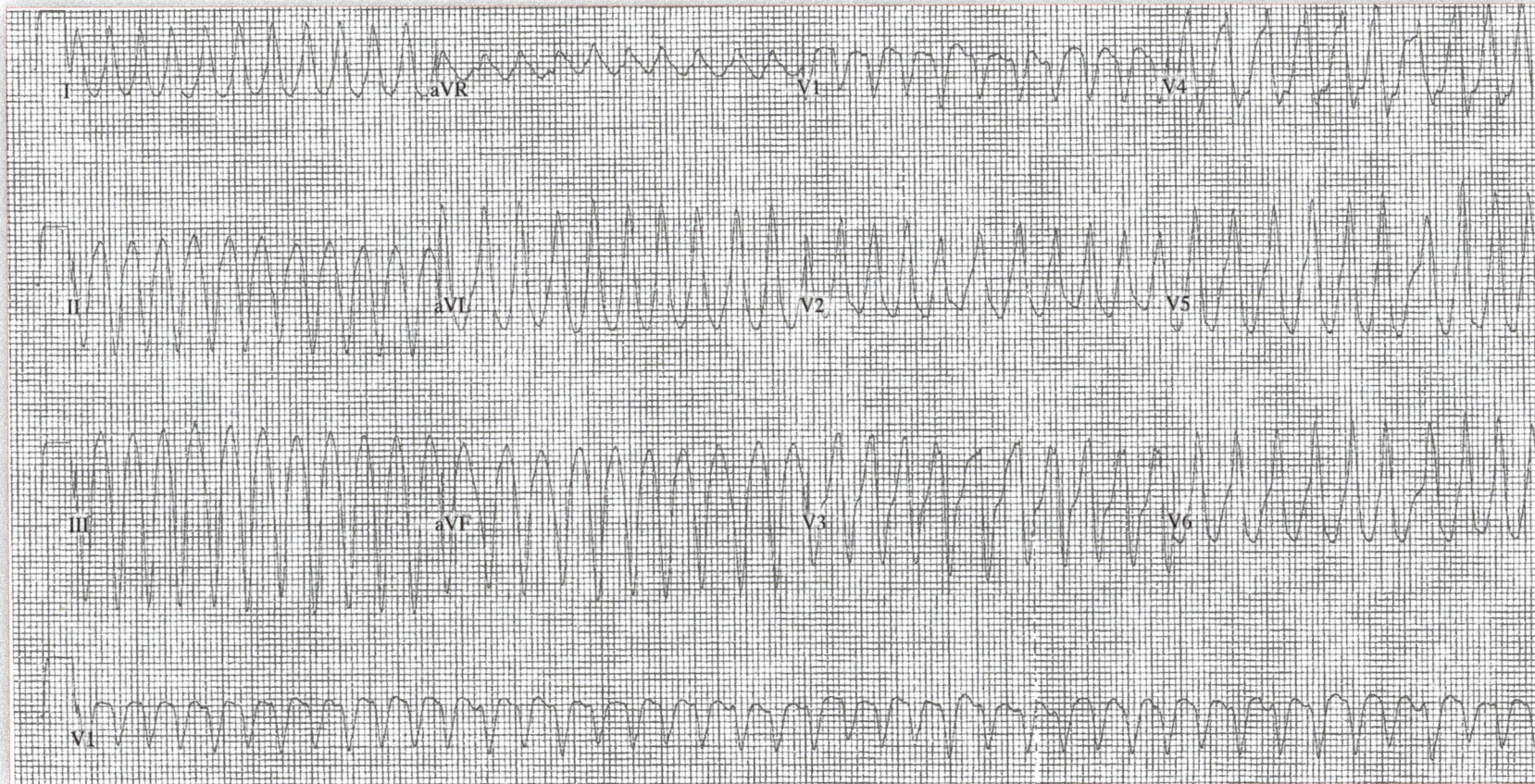

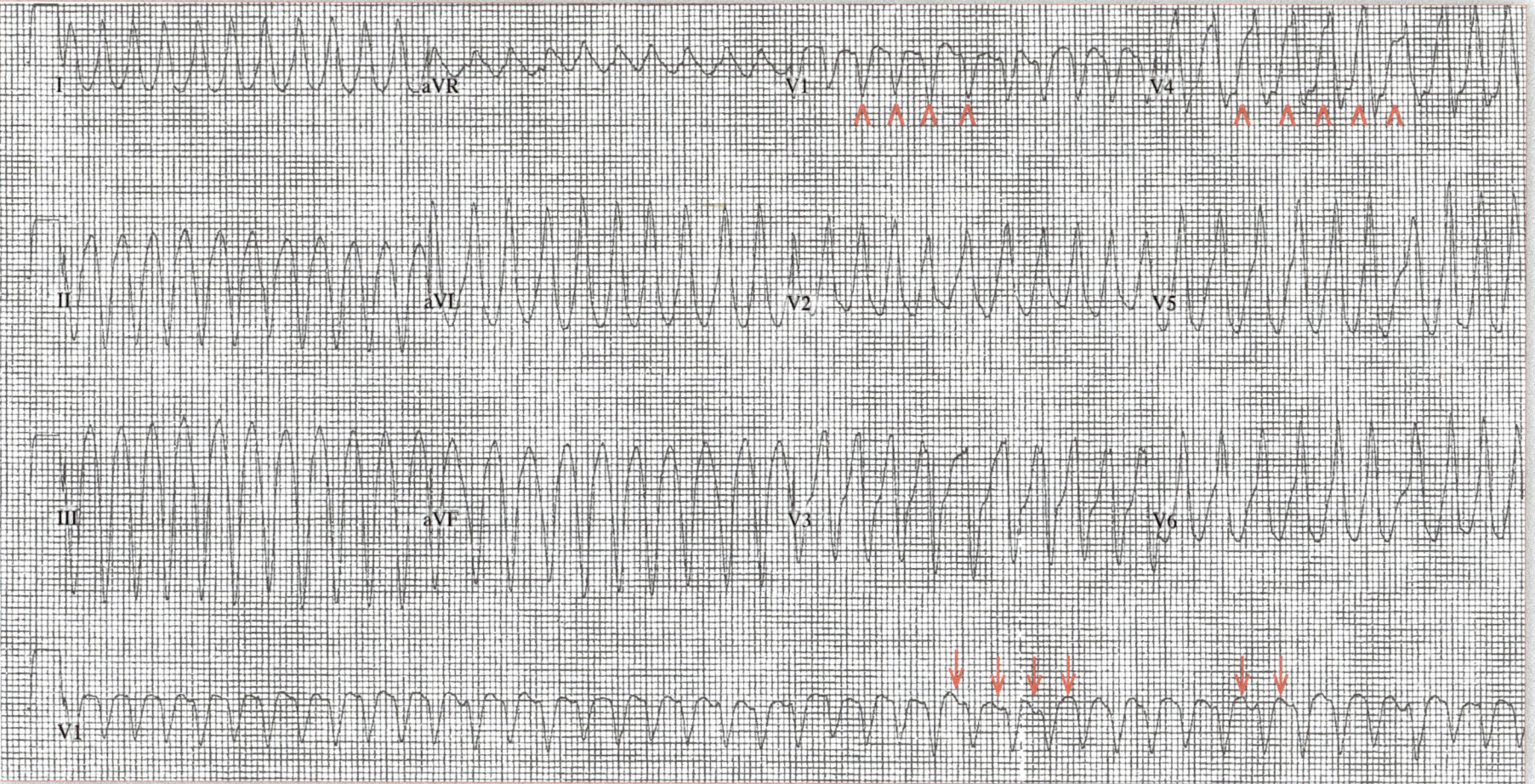

ECG 75 Analysis: Sustained monomorphic
ventricular tachycardia (ventricular flutter)

The ECG shows a wide QRS complex (0.20 sec) tachycardia at a rate of 270 bpm. There are only two rhythms that present with rates higher than 260 bpm: atrial flutter with 1:1 AV conduction and ventricular tachycardia. Changes can be seen in the QRS morphology (^) as well as in the ST-T waves (↓), most apparent in the precordial leads. These changes would not be seen with any supraventricular tachyarrhythmia because impulse conduction to the ventricles always follows the same conduction pathway and hence there is uniformity of the QRS complexes and ST-T waves. Therefore, this is sustained monomorphic ventricular tachycardia. When ventricular tachycardia occurs at a rate exceeding 260 bpm, it is often termed ventricular flutter.

Typically, 12-lead ECGs are not obtained in the setting of ventricular tachycardia arrest as this would delay time to appropriate therapy (*ie*, defibrillation). However, as the arrest occurred during an exercise test, the patient was already wearing the leads. Based on the history and results from the exercise test, the overall clinical diagnosis is likely hypertrophic (obstructive) cardiomyopathy, a genetic disorder that classically presents with a systolic murmur audible at the left lower sternal border that increases with Valsalva. This aortic stenosis–type murmur represents turbulent flow through an obstructed left ventricular outflow tract (*ie*, subvalvular stenosis). The obstruction is due to a hypertrophic but hypokinetic septum. As a result the pressure is less along the septum compared with the rest of the posterior ventricular wall, resulting in a Venturi effect that "sucks" the anterior leaflet of the mitral valve to the septum (*ie*, systolic anterior movement of the mitral valve), which results in a midsystolic gradient within the left ventricular chamber.

The clinical finding of a systolic murmur that gets louder with Valsalva is due to the decrease in venous return, the decreased filling of the left ventricle, and hence a reduction in the dimension of the outflow tract, causing an increase in the obstruction and in the intensity of the murmur. Patients with hypertrophic cardiomyopathy are at increased risk for sudden cardiac death, particularly those who experience blood pressure drops with exercise, have marked left ventricular hypertrophy (> 30 mm), have a family history of sudden cardiac death, experience syncope or a documented sustained ventricular tachyarrhythmia (ventricular tachycardia or ventricular fibrillation), or have episodes of nonsustained ventricular tachycardia. Therapy for these patient is generally an implantable cardioverter–defibrillator. ■

A 70-year-old man with no known prior cardiac history presents with 3 days of intermittent chest pressure along with episodes of dizziness occurring at rest. The following lead II ECGs are obtained during an episode of chest discomfort.

What is the diagnosis?

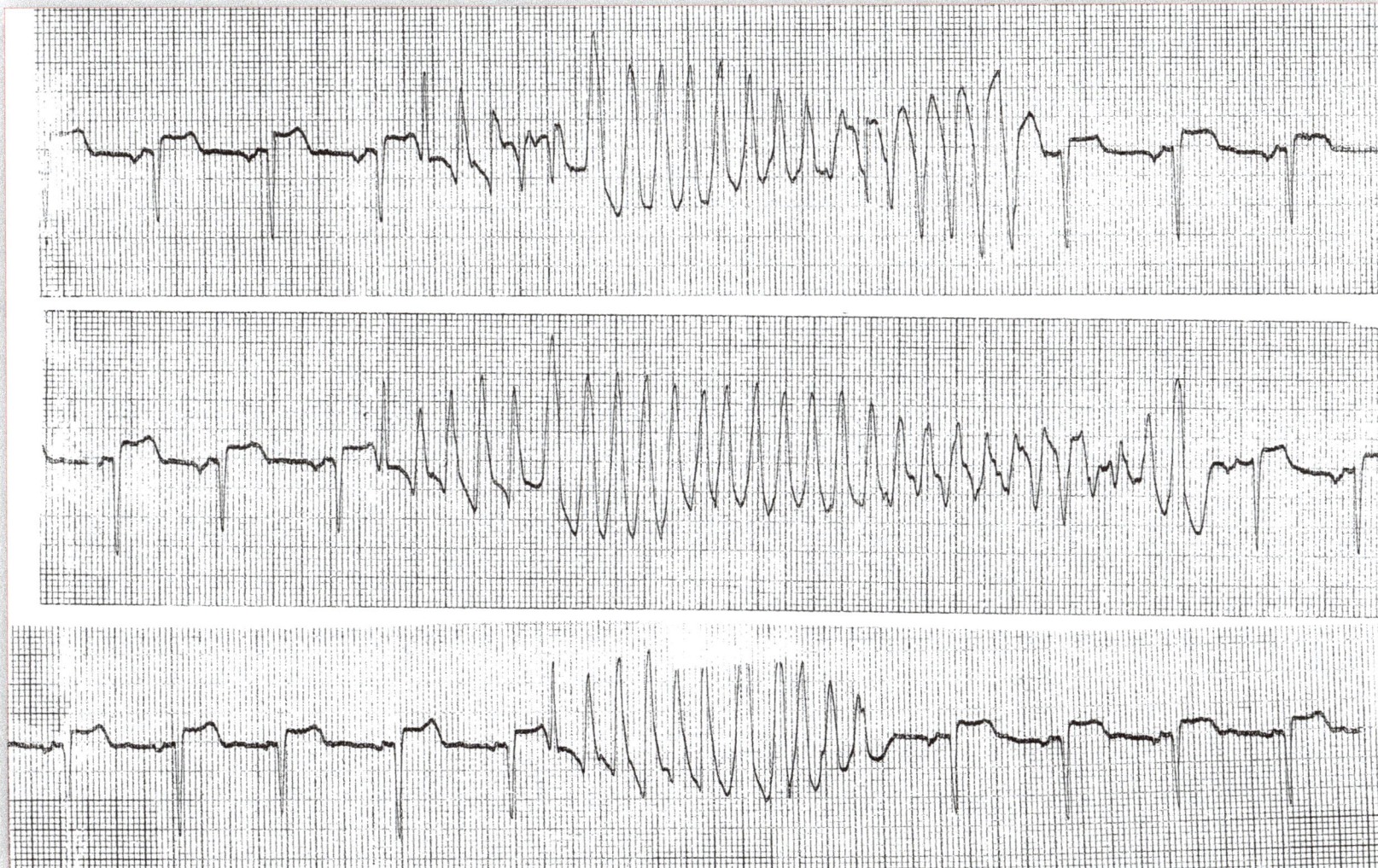

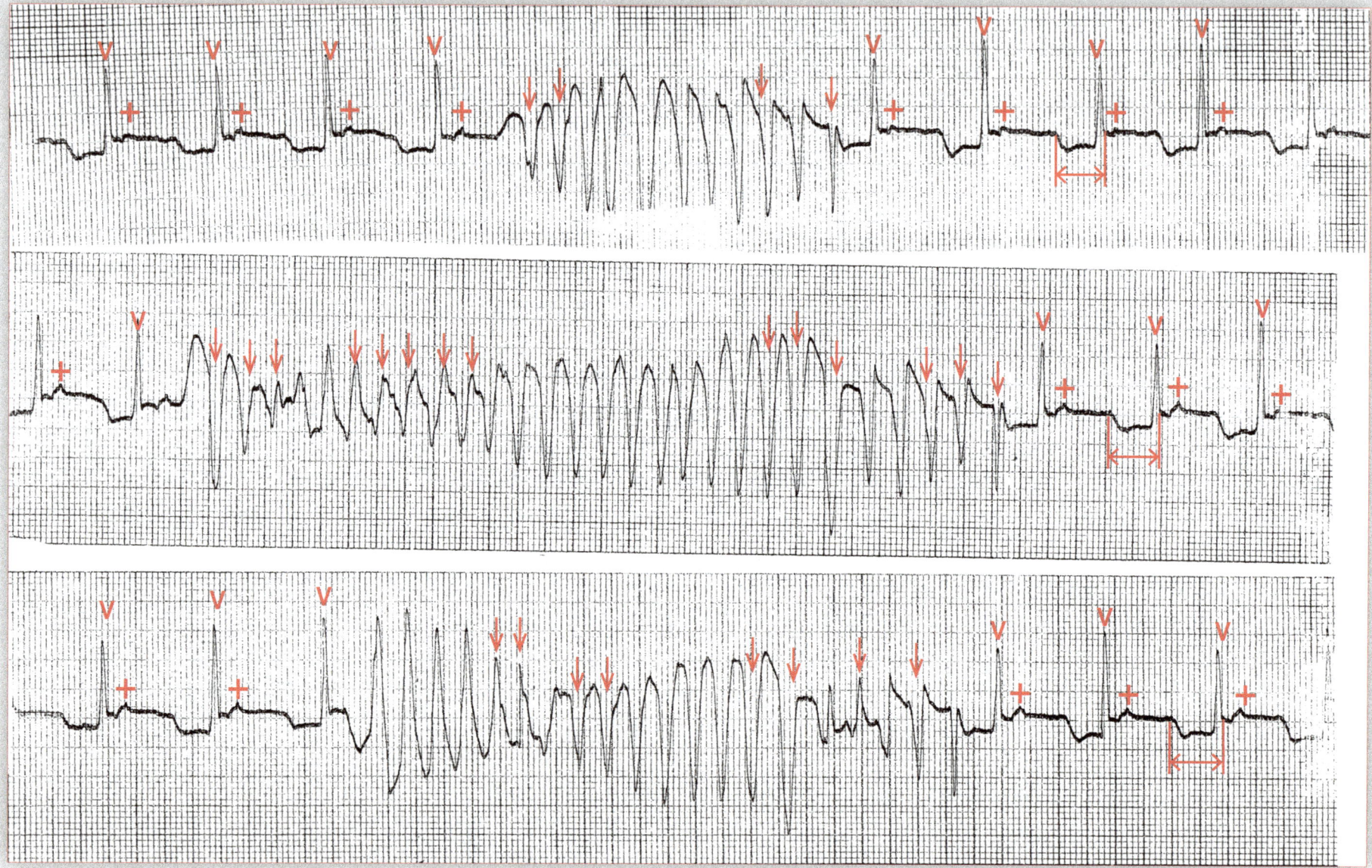

This series of rhythm strips shows narrow QRS complexes (^), preceded by P waves (+) with a stable PR interval (0.16 sec); this is sinus rhythm at a rate of 75 bpm. Each strip shows a nonsustained episode of a rapid wide complex tachycardia that is ventricular in origin. Each episode terminates spontaneously after a few seconds; therefore, this is nonsustained ventricular tachycardia. However, there are marked changes in QRS morphology and QRS axis (↑); therefore, this is polymorphic ventricular tachycardia. The rate of the ventricular tachycardia is about 300 bpm. It should be noted that the QT interval (↔) of the sinus beats is normal at 360 msec. In the presence of a normal QT interval this is termed polymorphic ventricular tachycardia, and the most common etiology is active ischemia. The only three arrhythmias provoked by active ischemia are polymorphic ventricular tachycardia, ventricular flutter (ventricular tachycardia with a rate > 260 bpm), and ventricular fibrillation.

Another less common cause for polymorphic ventricular tachycardia is familial catecholaminergic polymorphic ventricular tachycardia, which is the result of a genetic abnormality affecting the ryanodine or calsequestrin 2 gene. ■

A 54-year-old woman with hypertension, treated with hydrochlorthiazide, and chronic back pain, for which she takes methadone, presents to the emergency department with a severe cough. She is diagnosed with bronchitis, and levofloxacin is prescribed. Three days later she again presents to the emergency department with complaints of severe nausea and vomiting as well as diarrhea. She has attempted to stay hydrated and to eat but has been unable to due to severe emesis with intake. She was prescribed ondansetron for her nausea and ciprofloxacin for her diarrhea at an outpatient clinic. However, her symptoms did not improve. While in the emergency department, the patient has a syncopal episode that is captured on the telemetry strip below.

What is the diagnosis?

What is contributing to her rhythm disturbance?

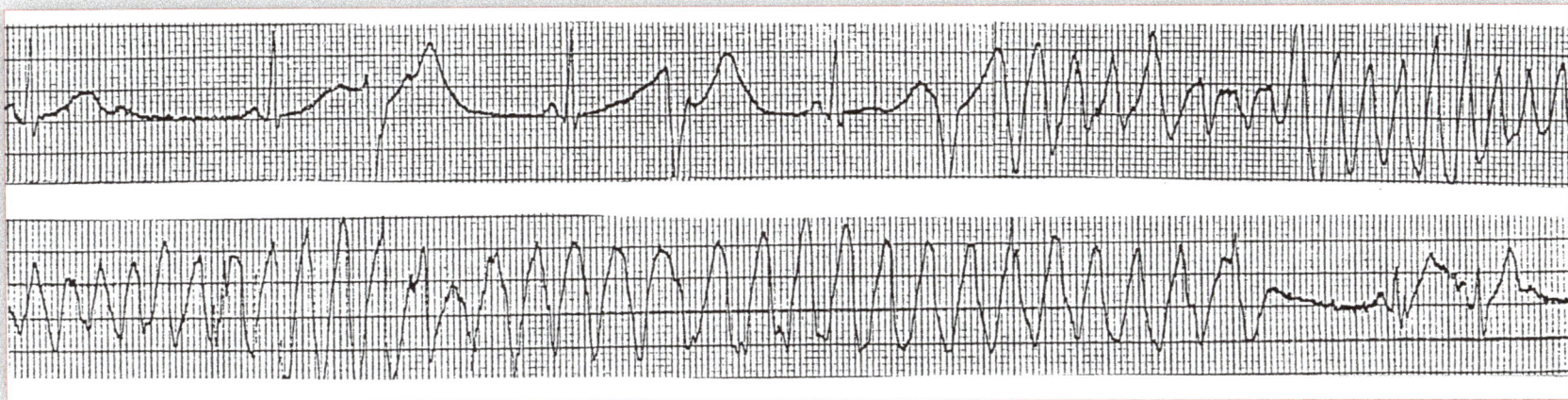

ECG 77 Analysis: Nonsustained polymorphic ventricular tachycardia, torsade de pointes

This continuous lead II rhythm strip shows three narrow QRS complexes (▼) that are preceded by P waves (+). These are likely sinus beats. The third and fifth QRS complexes (*) are premature ventricular complexes (PVCs) that occur slightly after the apex of the T wave (↓) (R on T). After the sixth QRS complex there is an episode of a rapid wide complex tachycardia with QRS complexes that are changing in morphology and axis. The rate of the episode approaches 300 bpm. This is polymorphic ventricular tachycardia.

Although the T waves are interrupted by the PVC, it can be noted that the sinus complexes have a prolonged QT interval (↔), as what can be measured shows a QT interval of at least 600 msec, which is very prolonged. The episode of polymorphic ventricular tachycardia in this case is called "torsade de pointes" or twisting of points, which is defined as polymorphic ventricular tachycardia associated with QT prolongation.

QT prolongation may be congenital or acquired as the result of a medication. In this case, the QT prolongation is most likely acquired. Given her severe diarrhea and emesis with poor oral intake, she is likely hypokalemic and hypomagnesemic, which are two major risk factors for acquired QT prolongation and torsade de pointes. In addition, she has been taking two known QT prolonging agents: a quinolone and methadone. Other commonly known QT prolonging agents include class IA and III antiarrhythmics, psychotropic agents such as haloperidol, macrolides, and antifungal agents such as voriconazole. ■

An 81-year-old man with diabetes but no known cardiac disease and plans for below-the-knee amputation of his right leg for severe osteomyelitis and unhealed skin ulcers develops profound hypotension and altered mental status requiring vasopressor therapy. He is intubated and admitted to the intensive care unit.

Initial laboratory assessment reveals acute renal insufficiency, hyperkalemia, lactic acidosis, and a blood pH of 7.10. Blood cultures grow methicillin-resistant *Staphylococcus aureus*. Despite antibiotic therapy, his clinical situation worsens. Overnight, he acutely loses blood pressure and the following ECG is captured on telemetry.

What is the diagnosis?

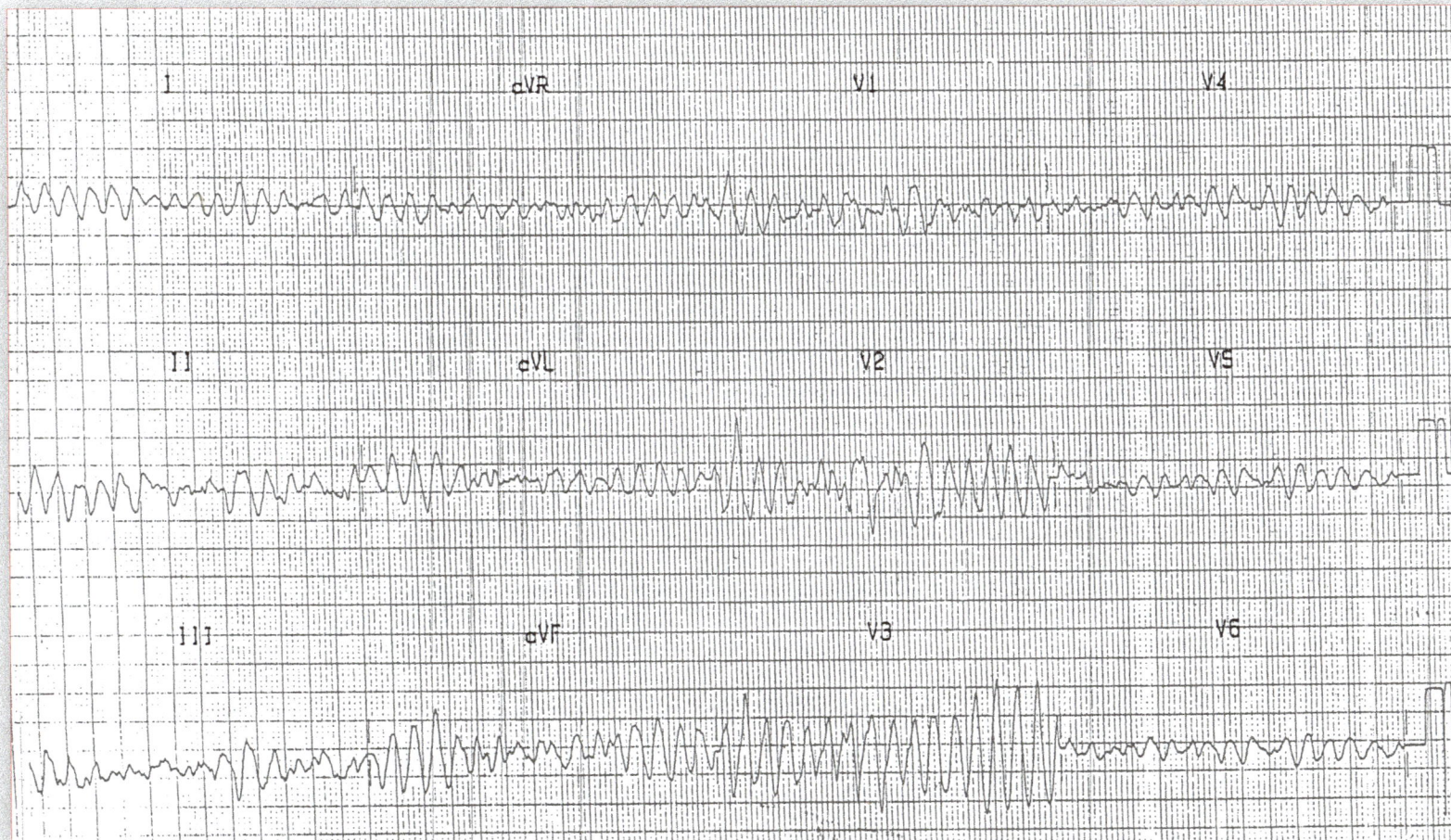

I   aVR   V1   V4

II   aVL   V2   V5

III   aVF   V3   V6

ECG 78 Analysis: Ventricular fibrillation

No organized QRS complexes can be seen on this ECG. Rather, there are rapid and irregular waveforms that are completely disorganized and without any distinct morphology. Therefore, this is ventricular fibrillation. At times the waveforms look more organized (↓), as in lead V3 for example, and resemble polymorphic ventricular tachycardia. However, they fragment thereafter (^).

An arrest due to ventricular fibrillation, which is the most frequent cause of sudden cardiac death, is most commonly associated with active ischemia or an acute coronary syndrome (unstable angina, non–ST-segment elevation myocardial infarction, or ST-segment elevation myocardial infarction) or with significant structural heart disease (ischemic cardiomyopathy, non-ischemic cardiomyopathy, aortic stenosis, aortic dissection, myocarditis, or pericardial tamponade). However, it can also occur in the setting of profound metabolic disturbances such as acidosis and septic shock, as illustrated in this case. Respiratory failure due to aspiration, bronchospasm, sleep apnea, or pulmonary embolism can also result in ventricular fibrillation arrest.

The only effective therapy for ventricular fibrillation is prompt electrical defibrillation. Ventricular fibrillation does not revert spontaneously, nor are antiarrhythmic drugs effective for reversion. ■

An 86-year-old woman with known calcific aortic stenosis and a valve area of 1.0 cm^2 presents with worsening dyspnea on exertion. The following is her ECG.

What are the abnormal findings?

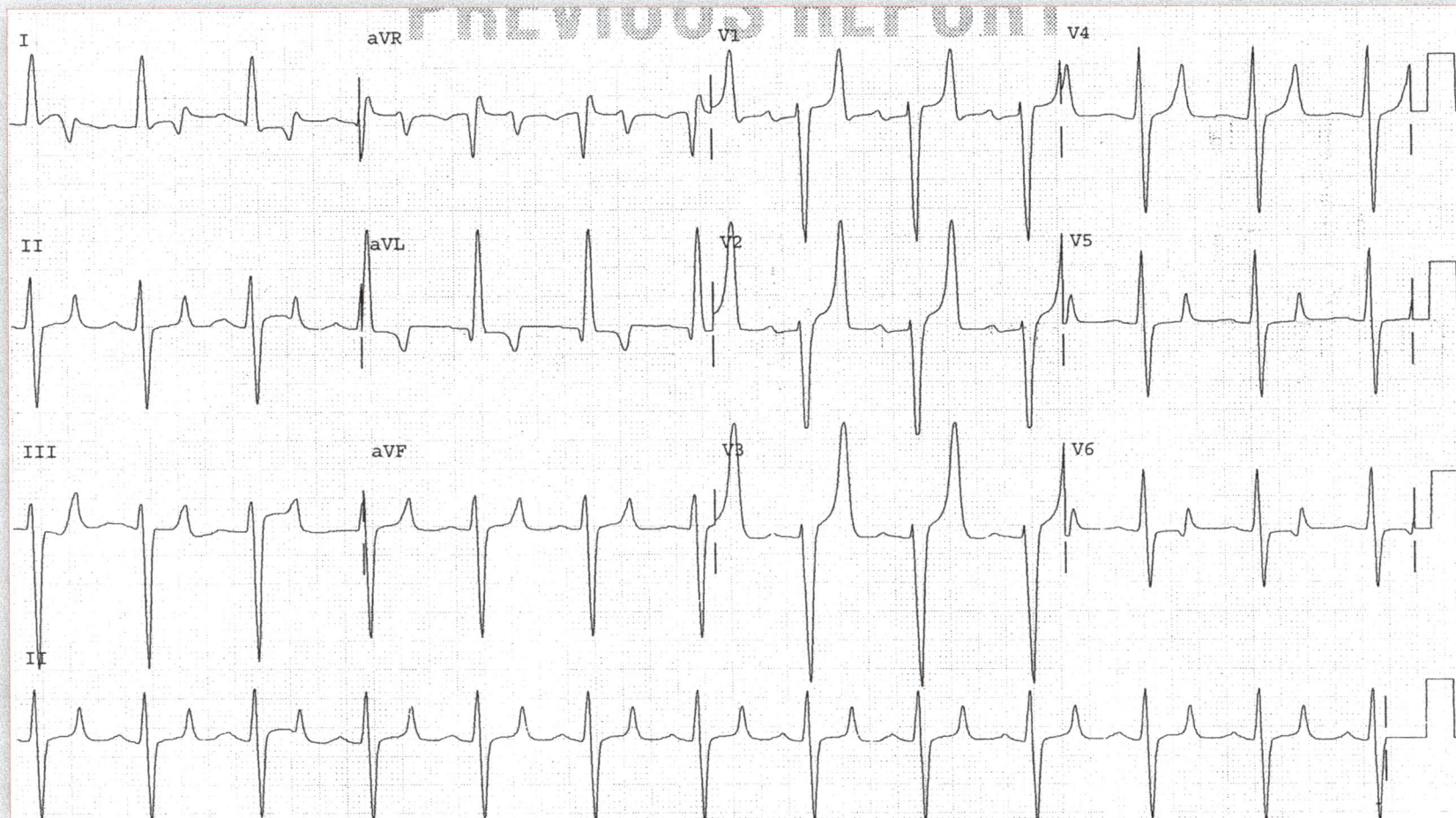

ECG 79 Analysis: Normal sinus rhythm, first-degree AV block, intraventricular
conduction delay (IVCD), left anterior fascicular block, left ventricular hypertrophy (LVH)

The ECG shows a regular rhythm at a rate of 74 bpm. There is a P wave (+) before each QRS complex, with a fixed PR interval (0.24 sec). The P wave is positive in leads I, II, aVF, and V4-V6. Hence this is a normal sinus rhythm with a first-degree AV block.

The QRS duration is increased (0.12 sec). The QRS pattern is not typical for a right bundle branch block and it is not a left bundle branch block, as there is a septal Q wave in lead aVL (▲) and a septal R wave in lead V1 (▼), which cannot be seen with a left bundle branch block as the septal branch innervating the septum is from the left bundle. Hence this is an intraventricular conduction delay (IVCD). The axis is very leftward, between −30° and −90° (the QRS complex is positive in lead I and negative in leads II and aVF) as a result of a left anterior fascicular block. The QRS complexes have a normal morphology, although there is increased amplitude, with an S wave in lead V3 that is 25 mm deep ( ]). This meets a criterion for borderline left ventricular hypertrophy (LVH) (*ie*, S-wave depth or R-wave amplitude in any precordial lead ≥ 25 mm). Along with the IVCD and left axis, LVH is likely present.

The QT/QTc intervals are normal (400/440 msec), but there are very prominent T waves (↓) that are tall and peaked (especially in leads V1-V4). However, the T waves are asymmetric, with an upstroke that is slower than the downstroke. Hence these T waves are normal and are not hyperacute, the result of hyperkalemia. It is likely that they are very prominent as a result of LVH. There are also T-wave inversions in leads I and aVL (^), which are probably repolarization abnormalities due to LVH. ■

A 52-year-old man is started on spironolactone along with an angiotensin-converting enzyme inhibitor for what is thought to be salt-sensitive hypertension. The following ECG is obtained routinely at a clinic visit 4 weeks later.

What is your next step in management?

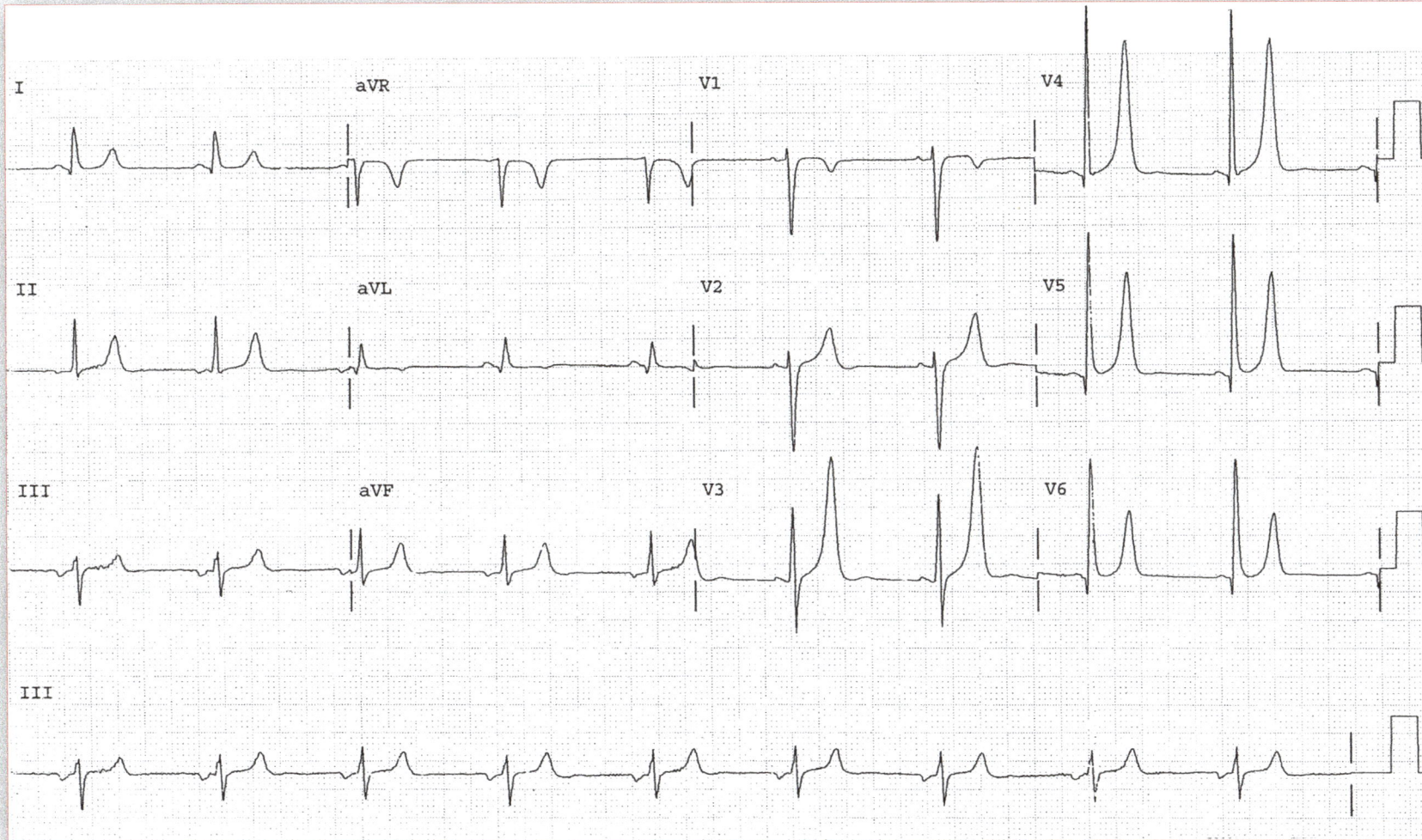

ECG 80 Analysis: Atrial rhythm, left ventricular hypertrophy, hyperacute T waves (hyperkalemia)

The ECG shows a regular rhythm at a rate of 60 bpm. There is a P wave (+) before each QRS complex, with a stable PR interval (0.14 sec). However, the P waves are negative in leads II and aVF. Hence this is not a sinus rhythm; it is an atrial rhythm.

The QRS complex duration is normal (0.08 sec), and the QRS complexes have a normal axis, between 0° and +90° (positive QRS complex in leads I and aVF). The QRS complex morphology is normal, but there is increased voltage with an R wave in lead V4 of 30 mm ([ ), which is diagnostic for left ventricular hypertrophy (ie, S-wave depth or R-wave amplitude in any one precordial lead ≥ 25 mm). The QT/QTc intervals are normal (400/400 msec).

The T waves are tall and peaked and, most importantly, symmetric, or tented (↓). These are termed hyperacute T waves and are seen with hyperkalemia (systemic or local as in an acute myocardial infarction). The patient's potassium level should be checked urgently, and the patient should be maintained on telemetry in a monitored setting with routine vital sign assessment.

Hyperkalemia can cause serious ventricular arrhythmias and conduction abnormalities, particularly if hyperacute T waves and QRS widening are seen on the ECG. QRS complex widening associated with elevated serum potassium levels should be treated in the short-term with intravenous administration of regular insulin with dextrose (for an acute decrease in potassium levels by shifting potassium into cells) and sodium bicarbonate. This treatment should be preceded by calcium infusion to stabilize the cardiac membrane potential in all settings except when digitalis toxicity is also present. Kayexalate (sodium polystyrene sulfonate) is also given for elimination of excess potassium from the body via the gastrointestinal tract.

Spironolactone is a potassium-sparing diuretic that is often used in hypertension and in patients with class IV heart failure. It can cause life-threatening hyperkalemia, particularly in patients with renal dysfunction or in patients also receiving an angiotensin-converting enzyme inhibitor. For this reason potassium levels should be monitored routinely in anyone taking this medication. ■

A 68-year-old woman with end-stage renal disease due to diabetic and hypertensive nephropathy develops an infection as a result of cellulitis at a newly placed arteriovenous fistula. Her blood cultures are positive for staphylococcal bacteremia, and intravenous antibiotics are prescribed. Two days later her blood urea nitrogen and creatinine levels increase, and she develops nausea. An ECG is obtained.

What is the diagnosis?

What is the next step in management?

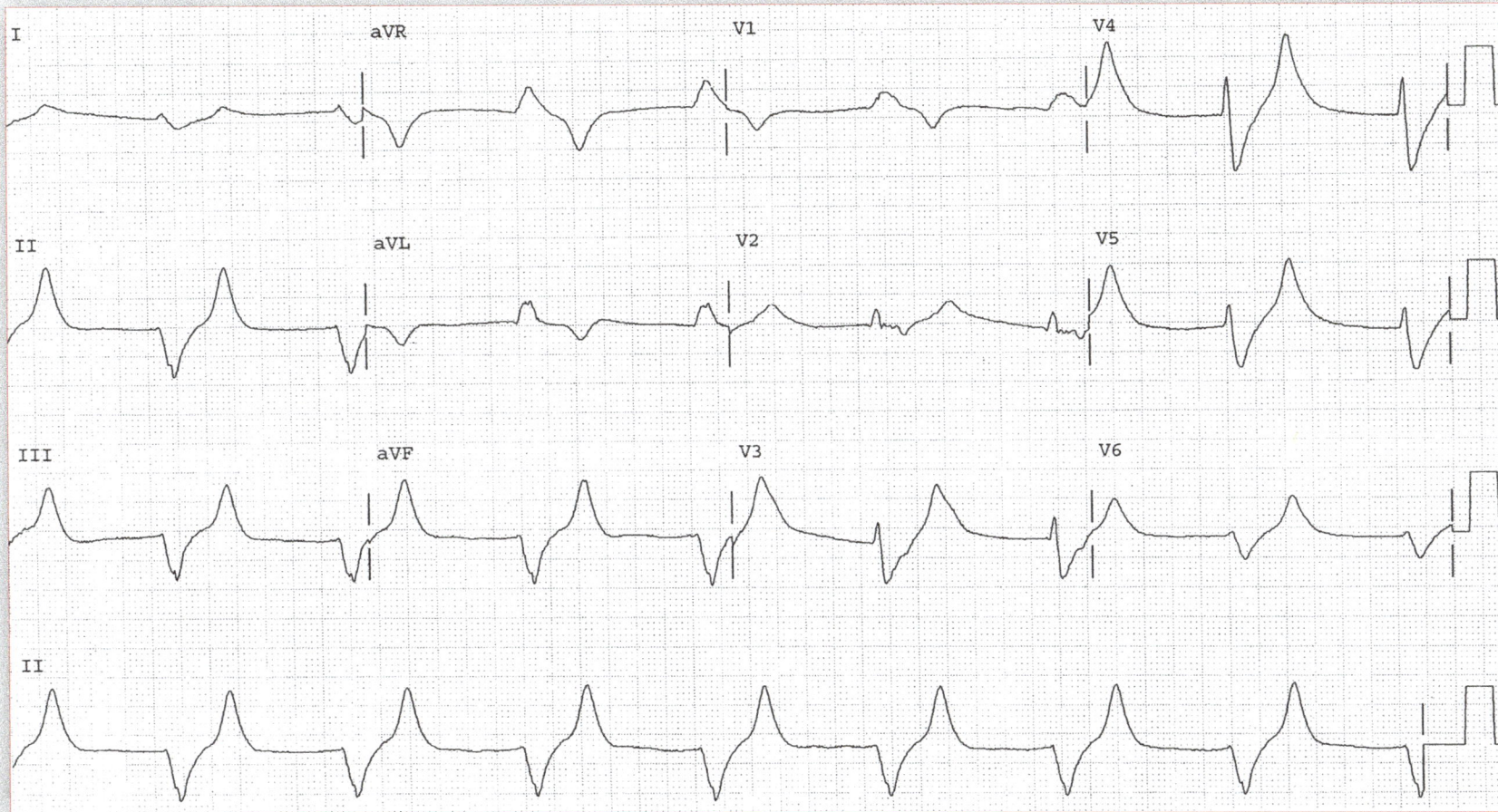

ECG 81 Analysis: Hyperkalemia

The ECG shows a regular wide QRS complex rhythm at a rate of 48 bpm. There is no evidence of atrial activity; therefore, this may be a junctional or ventricular rhythm. The QRS width (↔) is 0.28 second. The only etiology for a QRS that is this wide is hyperkalemia, which causes the resting membrane potential of the ventricular myocardium to become less negative. The normal resting membrane potential is −90 mV, which is maintained by an intracellular potassium level that is higher than the extracellular potassium level. When extracellular hyperkalemia is present, the balance is abnormal and the resting membrane potential becomes less negative. As the resting membrane potential approaches the threshold membrane potential (−60 mV), there is a decrease in the rate of the upstroke velocity of phase 0, which determines the impulse conduction velocity. This decrease in the velocity of impulse conduction through the ventricular myocardium results in a widening of the QRS complex. Hyperkalemia is the only condition that will result in a QRS width of 0.24 second or longer.

Also seen on this ECG are T waves that are very symmetric (+). Although no P waves are seen, this could still be a sinus rhythm, as the atrial myocardium is more sensitive to hyperkalemia than the ventricular myocardium. Atrial asystole can develop before there is QRS widening. This results in a continued sinus rhythm but no obvious P waves since the atrial myocardium is nonresponsive to electrical activity. This has been termed a sinoventricular rhythm.

In addition to the treatment described for Case 80, this patient may need urgent dialysis to treat the hyperkalemia. ■

A 56-year-old man is diagnosed with essential hypertension and is started on hydrochlorothiazide. He has no other medical problems and is otherwise healthy. This ECG is obtained on routine follow-up.

What is the abnormality?

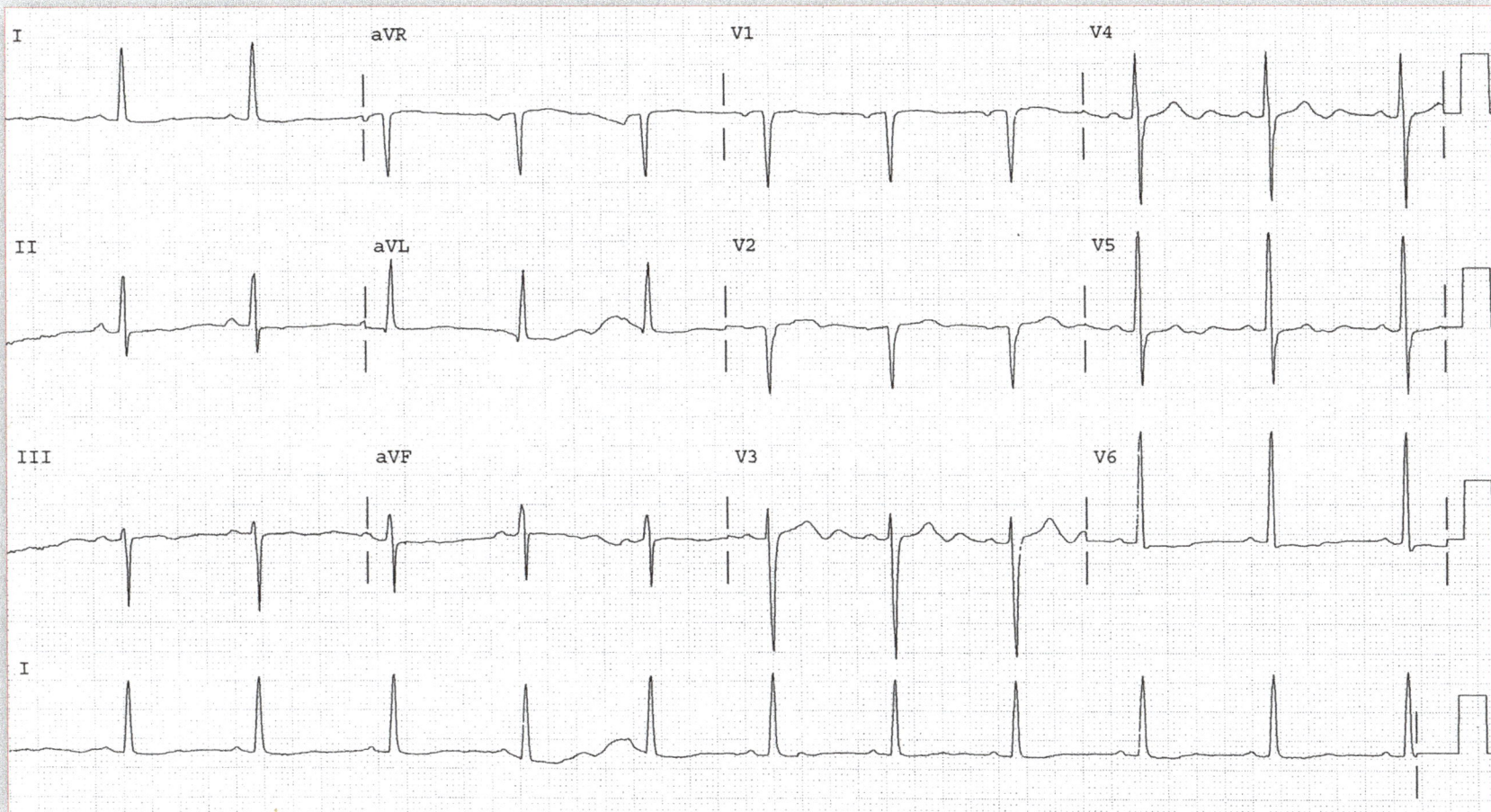

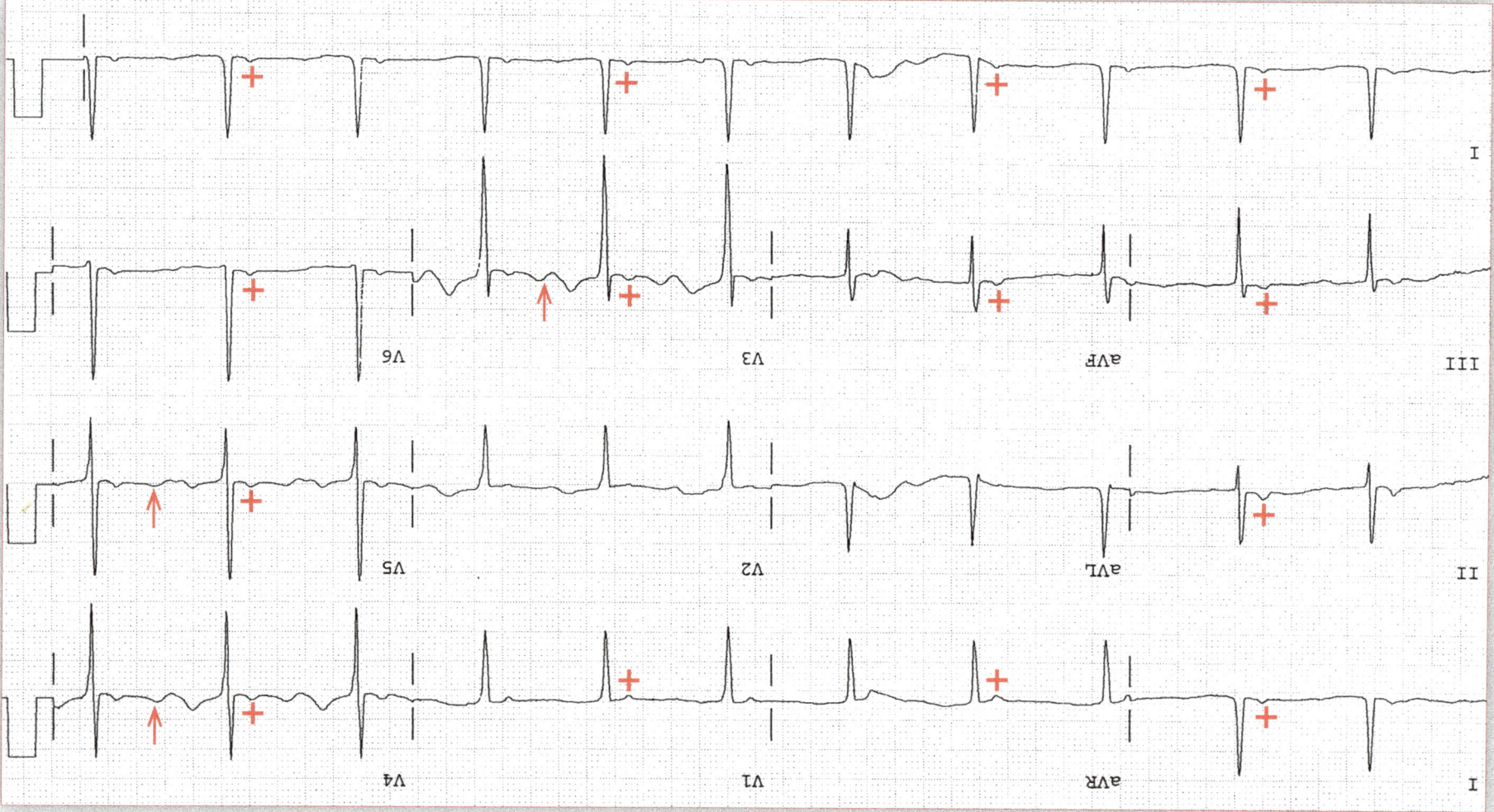

ECG 82 Analysis: Normal sinus rhythm, physiologic left axis,
prominent U wave (hypokalemia)

The ECG shows a regular rhythm at a rate of 64 bpm. There are P waves (+) before each QRS complex with a stable PR interval (0.16 sec). The P wave is positive in leads I, II, aVF, and V4-V6. Hence this is a normal sinus rhythm. The QRS complex duration (0.08 sec) and morphology are normal. The axis is physiologically leftward, between 0° and −30° (positive QRS complex in leads I and II and negative QRS complex in lead aVF). The QT/QTc intervals are slightly prolonged (440/460 sec).

There is a prominent positive waveform after the T wave in leads V3-V5. This is a U wave (↓), which is believed to represent delayed repolarization of the His-Purkinje system (or possibly the papillary muscles). The His-Purkinje system is the first part of the myocardium to depolarize and the last to repolarize. Small U waves are frequently seen in the right precordial leads (V1-V3). However, U waves that become very prominent and extend to the left precordial leads suggest the presence of hypokalemia. Loop diuretics and thiazides can often cause hypokalemia; therefore, serum potassium levels should be checked routinely while patients are taking these medications. Severe hypokalemia (usually < 2.0 mEq/L) can result in serious ventricular tachyarrhythmias, including cardiac arrest due to ventricular fibrillation. Potassium supplementation is necessary for short-term treatment, and either discontinuation of the offending agent or daily potassium supplementation is a reasonable long-term management strategy. ■

A 37-year-old man with an underlying manic disorder has been taking chlorpromazine for mood stabilization. He presents to a walk-in clinic with complaints of lightheadedness and pre-syncope. He states that he mistakenly took several extra chlorpromazine pills. An ECG is obtained.

What are the abnormal findings?

What is the appropriate treatment?

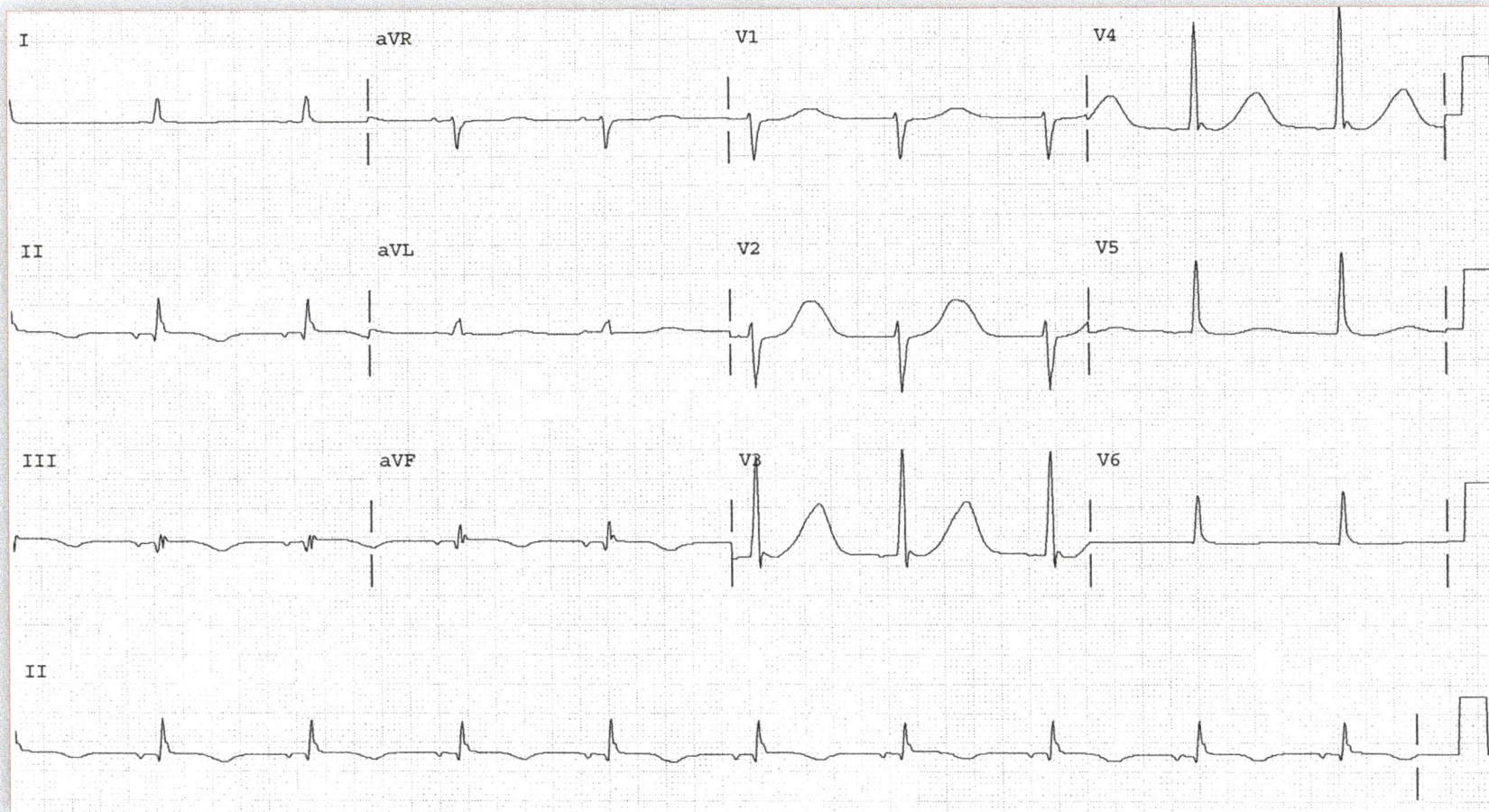

ECG 83 Analysis: Ectopic atrial rhythm, long QT interval, long QT syndrome

The ECG shows a regular rhythm at a rate of 48 bpm. There are P waves (+) before each QRS complex. They are inverted in leads II, aVF, and V3-V5, indicating an ectopic atrial (not sinus) rhythm.

The QRS complex duration is normal (0.08 sec), and there is a normal axis, between 0 and +90° (positive QRS complex in leads I and aVF). Noted is marked prolongation of the QT interval (↔), which measures 680 msec (QTc = 640 msec). The long QT interval is the result of a very prolonged T-wave duration, which represents prolonged repolarization. A long QT interval may be congenital or acquired. QT prolongation (either congenital or acquired) is associated with polymorphic ventricular tachycardia, called torsade de pointes. In this case, the long QT syndrome is possibly related to the use of the antipsychotic agent chlorpromazine, which is known to prolong the QT interval.

The treatment for an acquired QT prolongation is withdrawal of the implicated medication and observation. The occurrence of torsade de pointes is generally bradycardic or pause dependent in acquired QT prolongation. It can be suppressed by increasing the heart rate, as with overdrive pacing or the use of isoproterenol. Magnesium may also be beneficial. In contrast, torsade de pointes in association with congenital QT prolongation is provoked during tachycardia. Initial treatment is β-blockade to interfere with sympathetic stimulation of the heart, which can provoke torsade de pointes in the congenital QT syndrome. ■

A 52-year-old woman develops diffuse muscle cramps 2 days after undergoing thyroidectomy for papillary thyroid cancer. Physical examination is notable for facial muscle twitching upon tapping of the ipsilateral peri-auricular area. The following ECG is obtained.

What is the abnormality?

What is the overall clinical diagnosis?

What treatment is indicated?

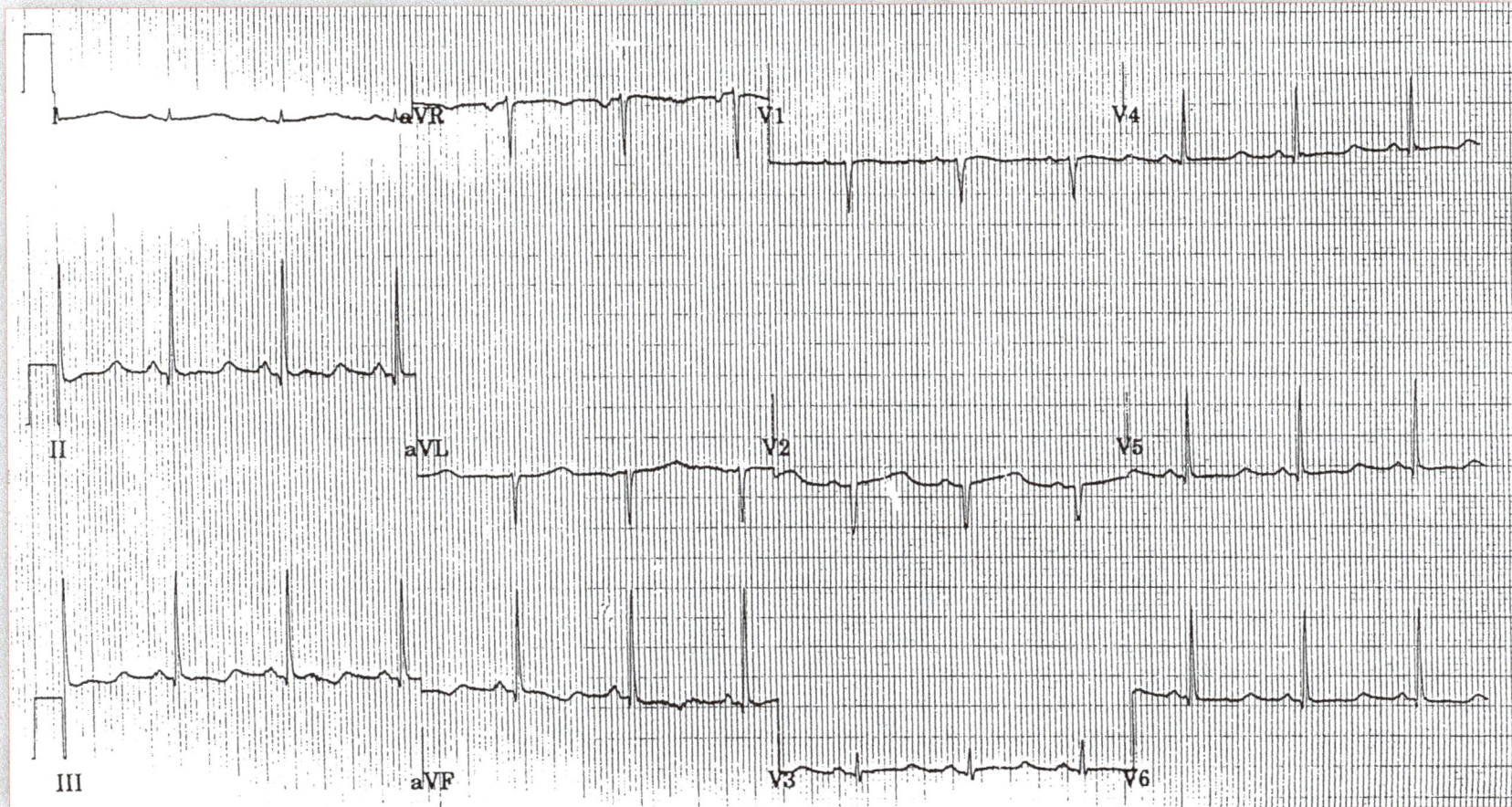

ECG 84 Analysis: Normal sinus rhythm, long QT interval (hypocalcemia)

The ECG shows a regular rhythm at a rate of 76 bpm. There is a P wave (+) before each QRS complex, with a stable PR interval (0.16 sec). The P waves are positive in leads I, II, aVF, and V4-V6, indicating a normal sinus rhythm.

The QRS complex duration is normal (0.08 sec), with a normal morphology and axis, between 0° and +90° (positive QRS complex in leads I and aVF). Notable is a prolonged QT interval (↔) of 560 msec (QTc = 590 msec). The QT prolongation is the result of a long ST segment (↑); the T wave itself is normal in duration. This is termed delayed repolarization and is seen with metabolic abnormalities, primarily hypocalcemia or hypomagnesemia. QT prolongation due to delayed repolarization (a long ST segment) is not associated with arrhythmia, particularly torsade de pointes.

This patient has hypocalcemia due to thyroidectomy, which has resulted in hypoparathyroidism. Hypocalcemia is typically transient in this setting but can be permanent in roughly 1% of patients undergoing thyroidectomy. Chvostek's sign, in which tapping of the facial nerve results in contraction of the facial muscles, is a sensitive sign for hypocalcemia. When QT prolongation is seen, treatment consists of urgent intravenous calcium supplementation.

Case 85

A 56-year-old man with 2 days of epigastric pain   and nausea is found to have evidence of cholecystitis on abdominal ultrasound. He undergoes laparoscopic cholecystectomy without complication.

ECG 85A

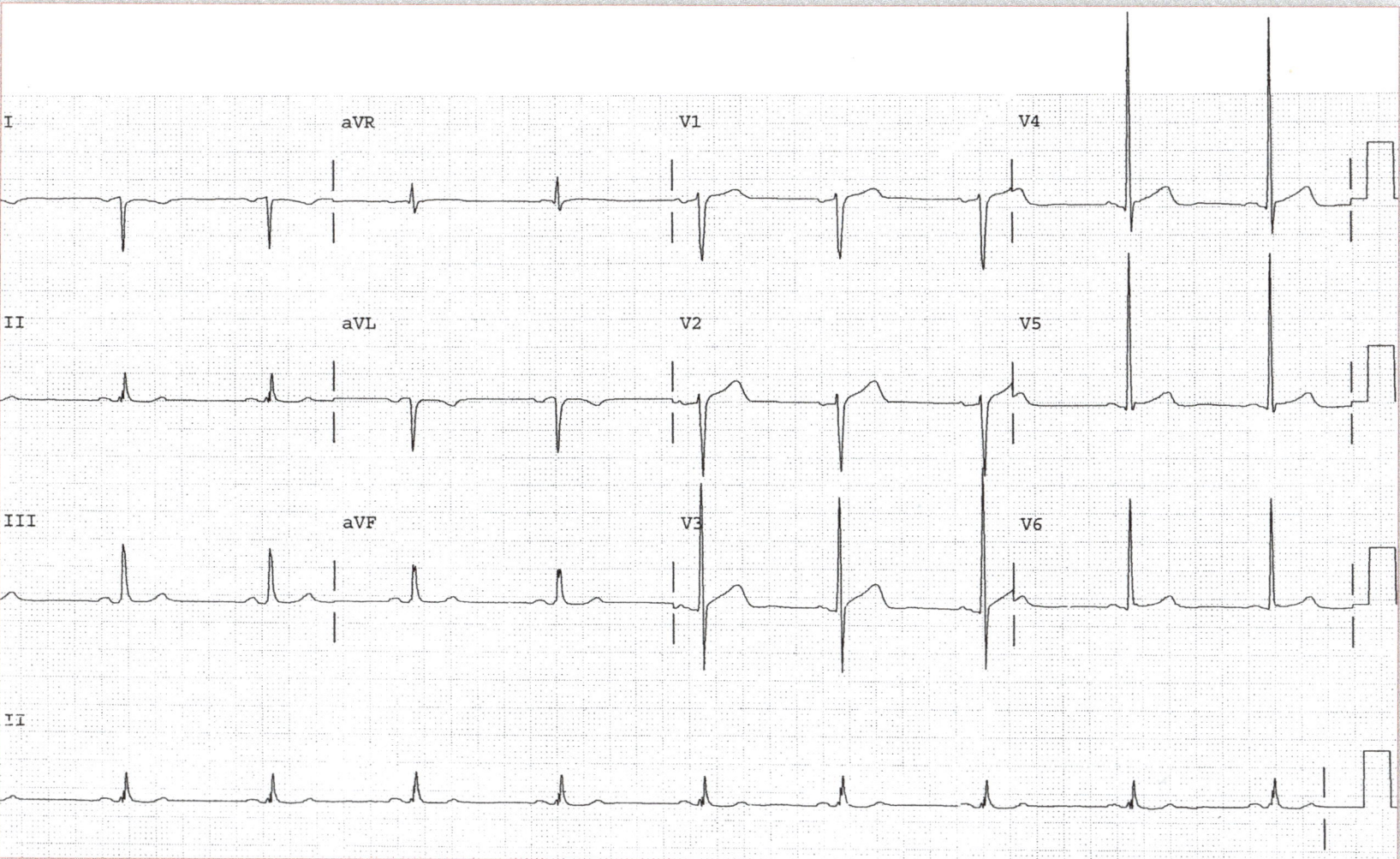

On postoperative day 1, a routine ECG (85A) is obtained.
The patient is otherwise asymptomatic and stable.
The preoperative ECG (85B) is also shown.

Has this patient had a perioperative myocardial infarction?

If so, where would you localize the infarct?

ECG 85B

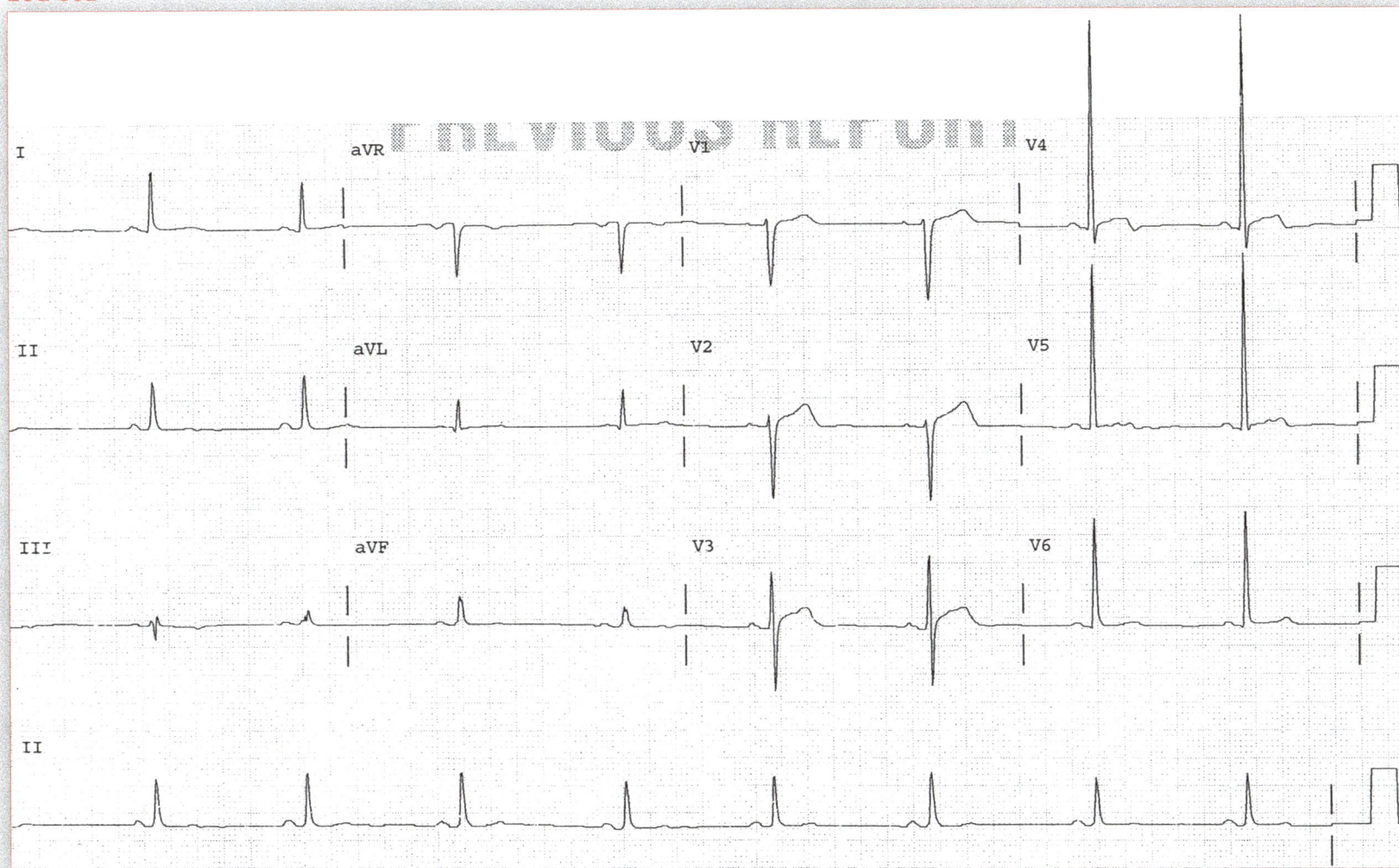

I   aVR   V1   V4

II   aVL   V2   V5

III   aVF   V3   V6

II

ECG 85A Analysis: Sinus bradycardia, right-to-left arm lead switch, left ventricular hypertrophy (LVH), early repolarization

ECG 85A shows a regular rhythm at a rate of 56 bpm. There is a P wave (+) before each QRS complex, with a stable PR interval (0.16 sec). The P waves are upright in leads II, aVF, aVR, and V4-V6; they are inverted in leads I and aVL (^). In addition, the QRS complex is negative in these leads, giving the appearance of a rightward axis, between +90° and +180° (negative QRS complex in lead I and positive QRS complex in lead aVF), from either a lateral myocardial infarction (MI) or a left posterior fascicular block.

The QRS complex duration is normal (0.08 sec), and the QT/QTc intervals are normal (380/370 msec). The QRS complex has a QS morphology in leads I and aVL (↓), which suggests a lateral wall MI. There is a tall R wave in lead aVR (▼), which is abnormal. The T waves are also inverted in leads I and aVL (*) and upright in lead aVR. Although a lateral wall MI is strongly suggested by the Q waves and T-wave inversions, the negative P wave (^), QRS complex (↓), and T wave (*) in leads I and aVL and the positive P wave and QRS complex in lead aVR are characteristic of a right-to-left arm lead switch, which is a very common error. Although the activation sequence of the atria and ventricles is normal, going from right to left, the impulse is going toward the right arm lead (rather than away from the right arm lead) and away from the left arm lead (rather than toward the left arm lead), accounting for the negative waveforms. Thus, the patient has not suffered from a lateral MI.

Also noted is an R wave in leads V4-V5 ([ ) that is increased in amplitude (27 to 33 mm), which is diagnostic for left ventricular hypertrophy (LVH) (*ie*, S-wave depth or R-wave amplitude in any one precordial lead ≥ 25 mm). A minimal amount of early repolarization (↑) (slight J-point and ST-segment elevation) can also be seen in leads V2-V4.

continues

I aVR V1 V4

II aVL V2 V5

III aVF V3 V6

II

ECG 85B Analysis: Sinus bradycardia, LVH

In ECG 85B, the leads have been placed on the correct arms. The rate is 50 bpm, and the PR interval is normal (0.16 sec). This is a normal sinus rhythm. The P waves (+), QRS complex, and T waves (^) are now upright and normal in appearance in leads I and aVL. The P wave (*), QRS complex (↑), and T wave (▲) are negative in lead aVR, which is normal. The axis is normal, between 0° and +90° (positive QRS complex in leads I and aVF). LVH is present as previously noted.

Deciphering whether an ECG has limb lead reversal is easiest done by first looking at the unipolar leads (aVR, aVL, and aVF). In a right-to-left arm lead switch, the QRS complex in lead aVR (which should be negative) and lead aVL (which should be positive) will be inverted (positive and negative, respectively) on the ECG and lead aVF will be unchanged. Additionally, in a right-to-left arm lead reversal, lead I—which is a bipolar lead that looks at the impulse as it goes from right to left and should always have positive P, QRS, and T waveforms—will have negative P, QRS, and T waveforms. ■

A 67-year-old man with a history of obesity, obstructive sleep apnea, hypertension, and diastolic dysfunction presents to your office with complaints of shortness of breath. He tells you that he has been smoking two packs of cigarettes per day for about 50 years.

ECG 86A

04 2:30:

I   aVR   V1   V4

II   aVL   V2   V5

III   aVF   V3   V6

II

On physical examination, he has rhonchous sounds
in both lung fields and 2+ peripheral edema in both legs.
An ECG is obtained (86A) and is compared with the
baseline ECG (86B).

**Does this patient have
right ventricular hypertrophy?**

ECG 86B

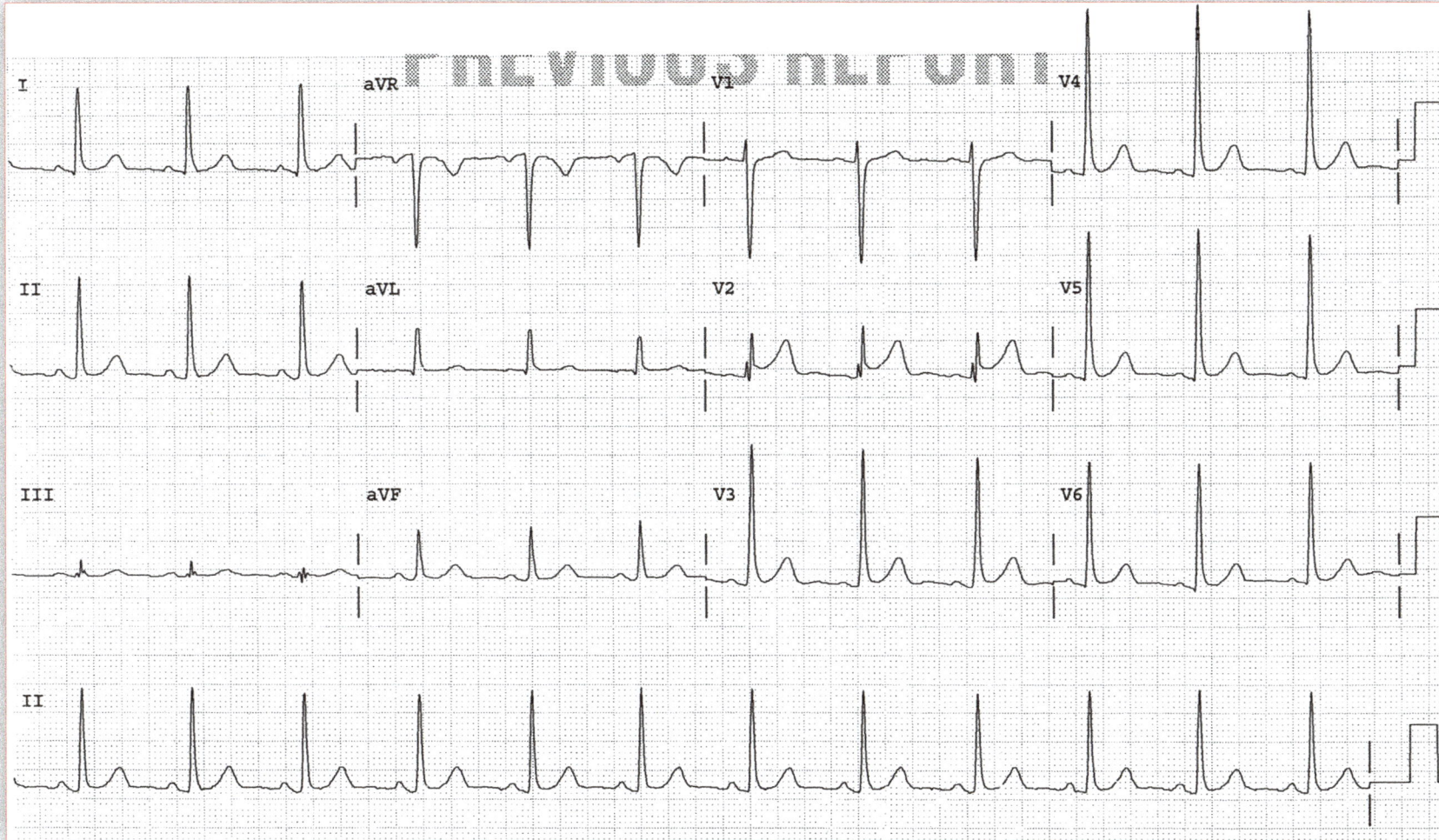

ECG 86A Analysis: Normal sinus rhythm, V1-V3 lead switch,
left ventricular hypertrophy (LVH)

ECG 86A shows a regular rhythm at a rate of 66 bpm. The P waves (+) are upright in leads I, II, aVF, and V4-V6. Hence this is a sinus rhythm. The QRS complex duration is normal (0.08 sec), and there is a normal morphology. The axis is normal, between 0° and +90° (positive QRS complex in leads I and aVF). The QT/QTc intervals are normal (400/420 msec). However, lead V1 has a very tall R wave (←), which is characteristic of right ventricular hypertrophy or a posterior wall myocardial infarction. The R-wave amplitude in lead V2 is smaller (→); it is even smaller in lead V3 (↓). The R-wave amplitudes in leads V4-V6 are normal. Hence leads V1-V3 show reverse R-wave progression. This is the result of a V1-V3 lead switch, which is a very common error.

In addition, there are voltage criteria for left ventricular hypertrophy (LVH), with R waves in leads V4-V5 ( ]) of 30 to 37 mm (S-wave depth or R-wave amplitude in any one precordial lead ≥ 25 mm is one of the criteria for LVH).

continues

PREVIOUS REPORT

ECG 86B Analysis: Normal sinus rhythm, LVH

In **ECG 86B**, the precordial leads have been placed in the correct position. The R-wave progression in leads V1-V3 is now normal. By comparison, lead V1 in **ECG 86A** is actually lead V3, V2 is actually V1, and V3 is actually V2. The rate is 72 bpm, and the P waves; PR interval; QRS complex morphology, axis, and duration; and QT/QTc intervals are the same as in **ECG 86B**. ■

Notes

A 47-year-old man with HIV and a new diagnosis of B-cell lymphoma presents with progressive lightheadedness and dizziness as well as the sensation of a racing heartbeat. On physical examination, his blood pressure is 72/palp, his jugular venous pressure is elevated, and his lung fields are clear. An arterial line is placed for precise blood pressure monitoring, and there is significant respiratory variation in the tracing with a decrease occurring on inspiration. The following ECG is obtained.

What is the ECG abnormality?

What is the overall clinical diagnosis?

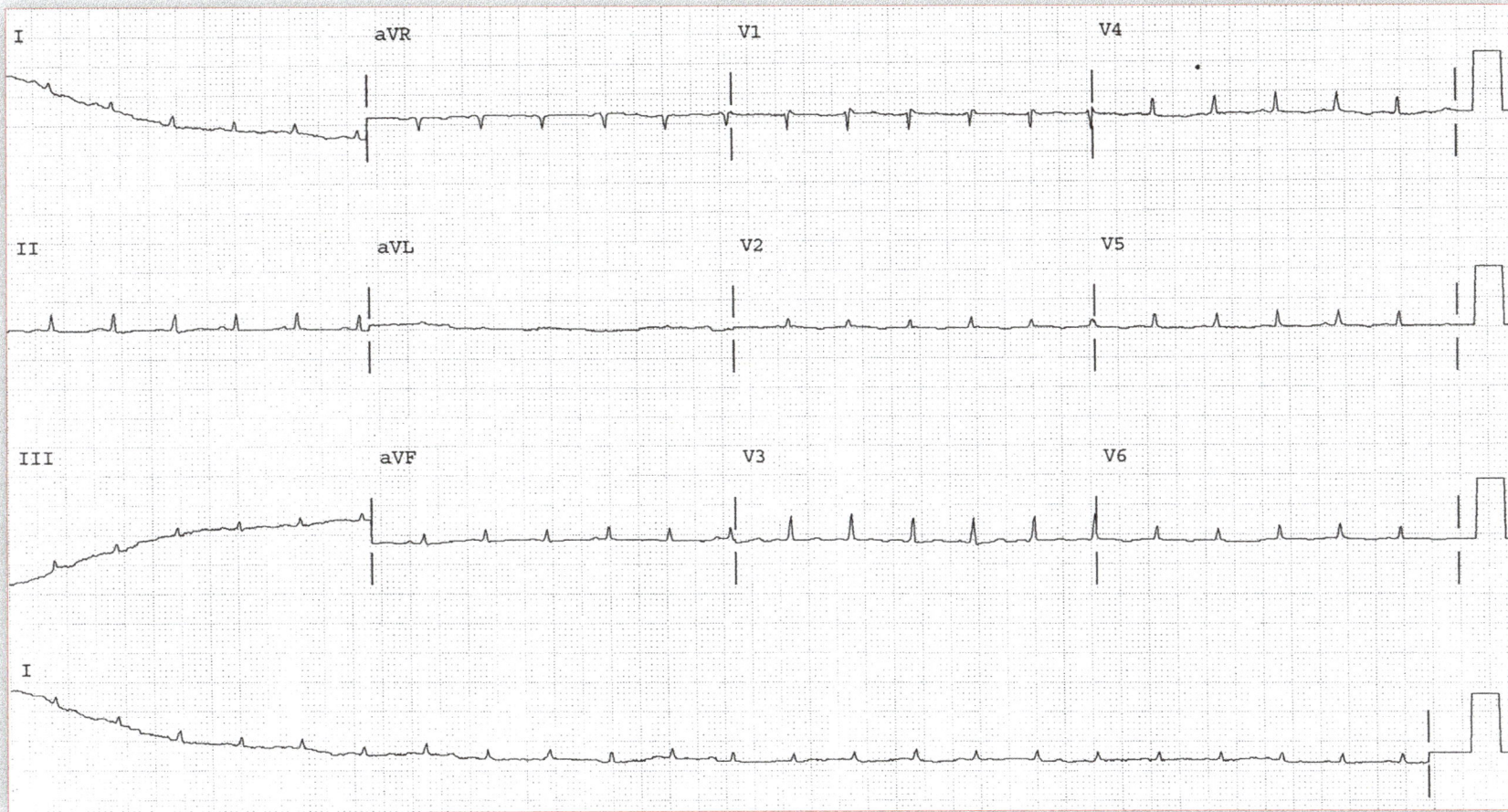

ECG 87 Analysis: Sinus tachycardia, low voltage

The ECG shows a regular rhythm at a rate of 140 bpm. P waves (+) are noted before each QRS complex, with a fixed PR interval (0.10 sec), and the P waves are upright in leads I, II, aVF, and V4-V6. Hence this is a sinus tachycardia. The PR interval (‖) is short as the result of increased sympathetic stimulation, which accounts for the sinus tachycardia as well as increased AV nodal conduction velocity and hence the shorter PR interval.

The QRS complex duration is normal (0.06 sec), and the axis is normal, between 0° and +90° (positive QRS complex in leads I and aVF). The QT/QTc intervals are normal (260/400 msec). However, the R-wave voltage in all the leads is very reduced, although it should be noted that the ECG is recorded at normal standardization (^) (ie, 1 mV = 10 mm or 10 small boxes in height). Therefore, this demonstrates low voltage in all leads.

The definition of low voltage is less than 5 mm of amplitude in each of the limb leads and less than 10 mm of amplitude in each of the precordial leads (when the ECG is recorded at normal standard). Low voltage may be seen in the limb leads, precordial leads, or all leads. The presence of low voltage indicates that there is less electrical activity from the heart reaching the surface of the body to be recorded. This may be the result of body habitus (ie, obesity), significant lung disease (particularly chronic obstructive pulmonary disease), a pericardial effusion or thickened pericardium, or loss of myocardial muscle mass (eg, as in amyloidosis).

In this case, based on the history and physical examination, the patient has a pericardial effusion with tamponade physiology. Beck's classic triad for a pericardial effusion consists of elevated jugular venous pressure, muffled heart sounds, and hypotension. A drop of more than 10 points in systolic arterial blood pressure during inspiration is a classic finding in tamponade known as pulsus paradoxus and is related to the interventricular dependence that occurs with a substantial pericardial effusion. With inspiration and an increase in venous return to the right ventricle, there is reduced filling of the left ventricle and hence a reduction in stroke volume and blood pressure. With expiration, there is a reduction of venous return and right ventricular filling during inspiration, and hence left ventricular filling, stroke volume, and blood pressure increase. Treatment consists of intravenous fluids and pericardiocentesis. The most common ECG findings are sinus tachycardia and low voltage. Diagnostic for tamponade, but not always seen, is electrical (QRS) alternans (beat-to-beat variation in the QRS amplitude). If pericarditis is also present, then one might also see diffuse concave ST-segment elevations with PR depression. In this patient with B-cell lymphoma, a malignant pericardial effusion is high on the differential diagnosis. ■

A 65-year-old man with known coronary artery disease and chronic hypertension has the following ECG.

Does this ECG meet criteria for left ventricular hypertrophy?

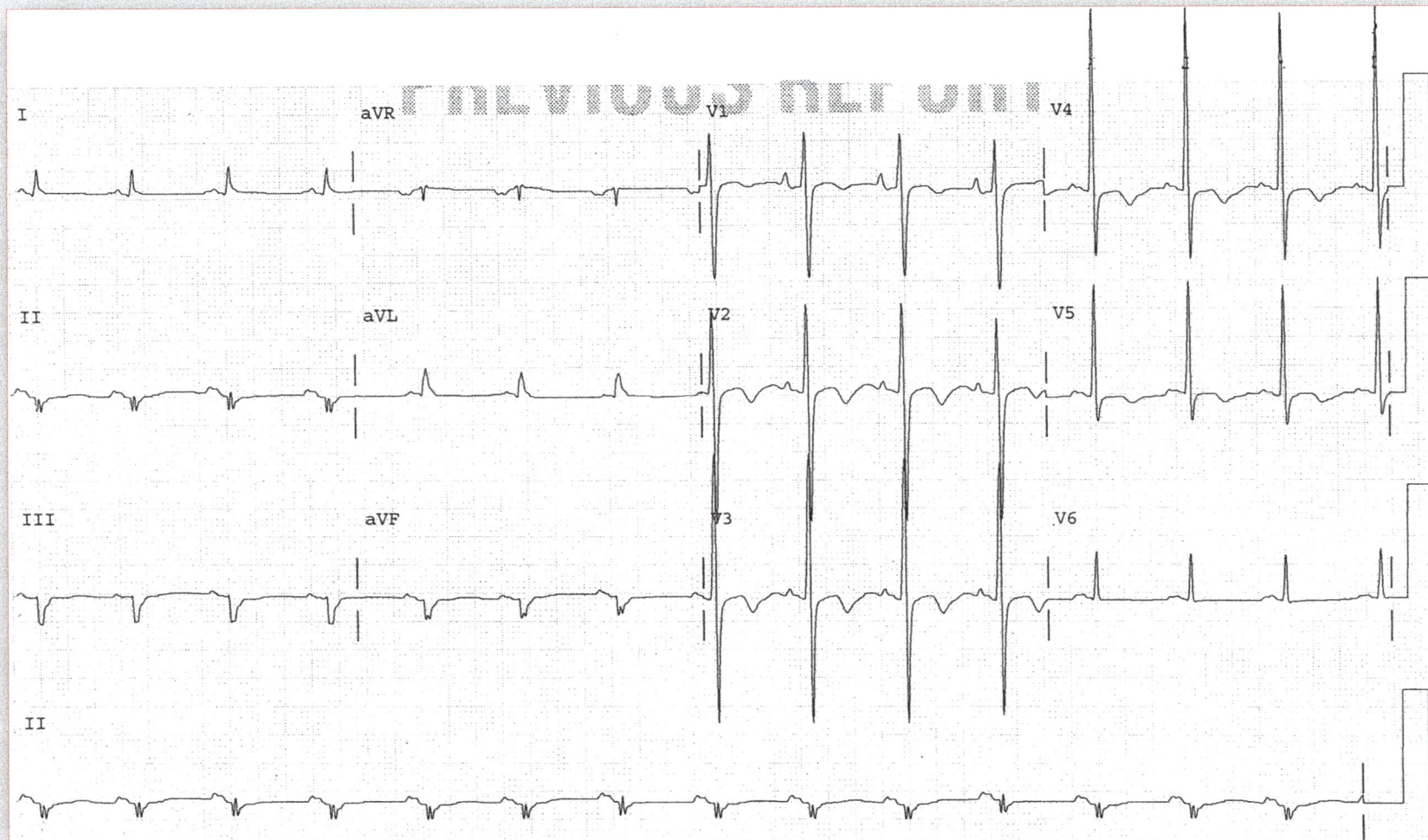

ECG 88 Analysis: Normal sinus rhythm, chronic inferior wall myocardial infarction, low-voltage limb leads, recorded at double standard

The ECG shows a regular rhythm at a rate of 86 bpm. There is a P wave (+) before each QRS complex, with a stable PR interval (0.16 sec). The P waves are upright in leads I, II, aVF, and V4-V6, indicating a normal sinus rhythm. There are Q waves (↑) in leads II, III, and aVF, defining the presence of a chronic inferior wall myocardial infarction (MI). As a result of the inferior wall MI, with negative QRS complexes in leads II and aVF and a positive QRS complex in lead I, the axis is extremely leftward, between −30° and −90°. Because there is an infarction pattern (QS morphology), however, this is not a left anterior fascicular block, which cannot be diagnosed in the presence of an inferior wall MI.

The R-wave voltage in the limb leads is small and is considered low (< 5 mm of amplitude in each limb lead). However, the QRS voltage in the precordial leads is increased, and the S-wave depth in lead V2 ([ ) is 23 mm and the R-wave height in lead V4 ( ]) is 32 mm. This meets one of the criteria for left ventricular hypertrophy (LVH) (S-wave depth + R-wave amplitude in any precordial lead ≥ 35 mm). In addition, there is a very tall R wave in lead V1 (←) (9 mm), which meets a criterion for right ventricular hypertrophy (RVH). There is also a tall P wave (^) in lead V1, which suggests right atrial hypertrophy, and T-wave abnormalities (*) in leads V2-V6, which are often seen in association with ventricular hypertrophy.

However, it should be noted that the ECG was recorded at double standard (↓) (*ie*, 1 mV = 20 mm or 20 small boxes in height). Hence the QRS voltage as measured needs to be reduced by half in all leads. Therefore, the QRS voltage in the precordial leads is normal (S-wave depth in lead V2 = 12 mm; R-wave amplitude in lead V4 = 16 mm; and R-wave amplitude in lead V1 = 4 mm), and LVH and RVH are not present. Despite the fact that the ECG was recorded at double standard, the QRS amplitude in the limb leads is low. If recorded at normal standard the QRS complexes would be barely visible. The limb leads reflect voltages in the frontal plane of the heart, whereas the precordial leads reflect voltages in the horizontal plane. Hence, there can be a marked difference in voltage amplitude between the limb leads and precordial leads. ■

Case 89

The following routine ECGs are obtained from a 32-year-old athletic man with no cardiac history who is undergoing surgery for a torn

ECG 89A

anterior cruciate ligament. He reports being anxious and feeling his heart racing a bit.

What is the diagnosis?

ECG 89B

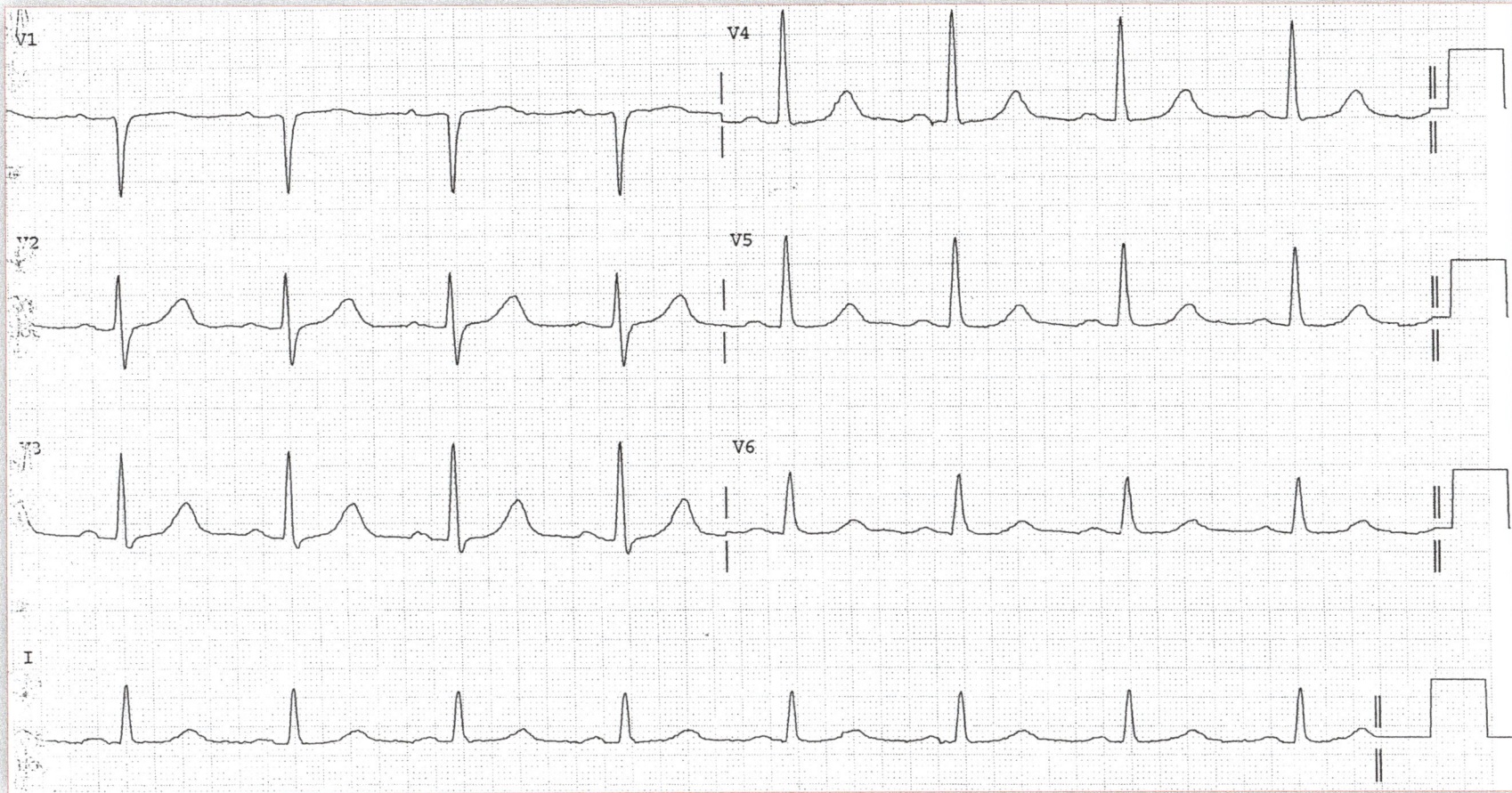

ECG 89A Analysis: ECG recorded at double speed

ECG 89A shows a regular rhythm at a rate of 50 bpm. There is a P wave (+) before each QRS complex, with a stable PR interval (↔) (0.32 sec). The P waves are positive in leads I and aVF, suggesting sinus bradycardia with a first-degree AV block.

The QRS complex duration is prolonged (⊔) (0.18 sec), and the axis is normal, between 0° and +90° (positive QRS complex in leads I and aVF). The QT/QTc intervals (⊓) are 600/550 msec, which are very long. Hence there is a bradycardia and the PR, QRS, and QT intervals are prolonged. Also noted is the fact that there are only six leads present. This ECG was recorded at double speed, or 50 mm/sec, rather than at the normal speed of 25 mm/sec. Hence the actual heart rate is 100 bpm, the PR interval is 0.16 second, the QRS complex duration is 0.09 second, and the QT interval is 0.34 second, or 0.43 second when corrected for heart rate (QTc). Thus the ECG is normal.

continues

ECG 89B Analysis: ECG recorded at double speed

ECG 89B represents the precordial leads of **ECG 89A**, again recorded at 50 mm/sec. As before, the heart rate is twice as fast as measured and the intervals are half of what is measured. Thus the ECG is normal. ▪

You are on call overnight in a hospital's intensive care unit when you are STAT paged for a patient in the telemetry unit who was admitted for chest pain. As you run to the patient's room, a nurse hands you the following ECG printed from the patient's remote telemetry unit. When you enter the room, you are surprised to see the patient standing next to the bathroom sink, brushing her teeth. She is completely asymptomatic and feeling well.

What is the diagnosis?

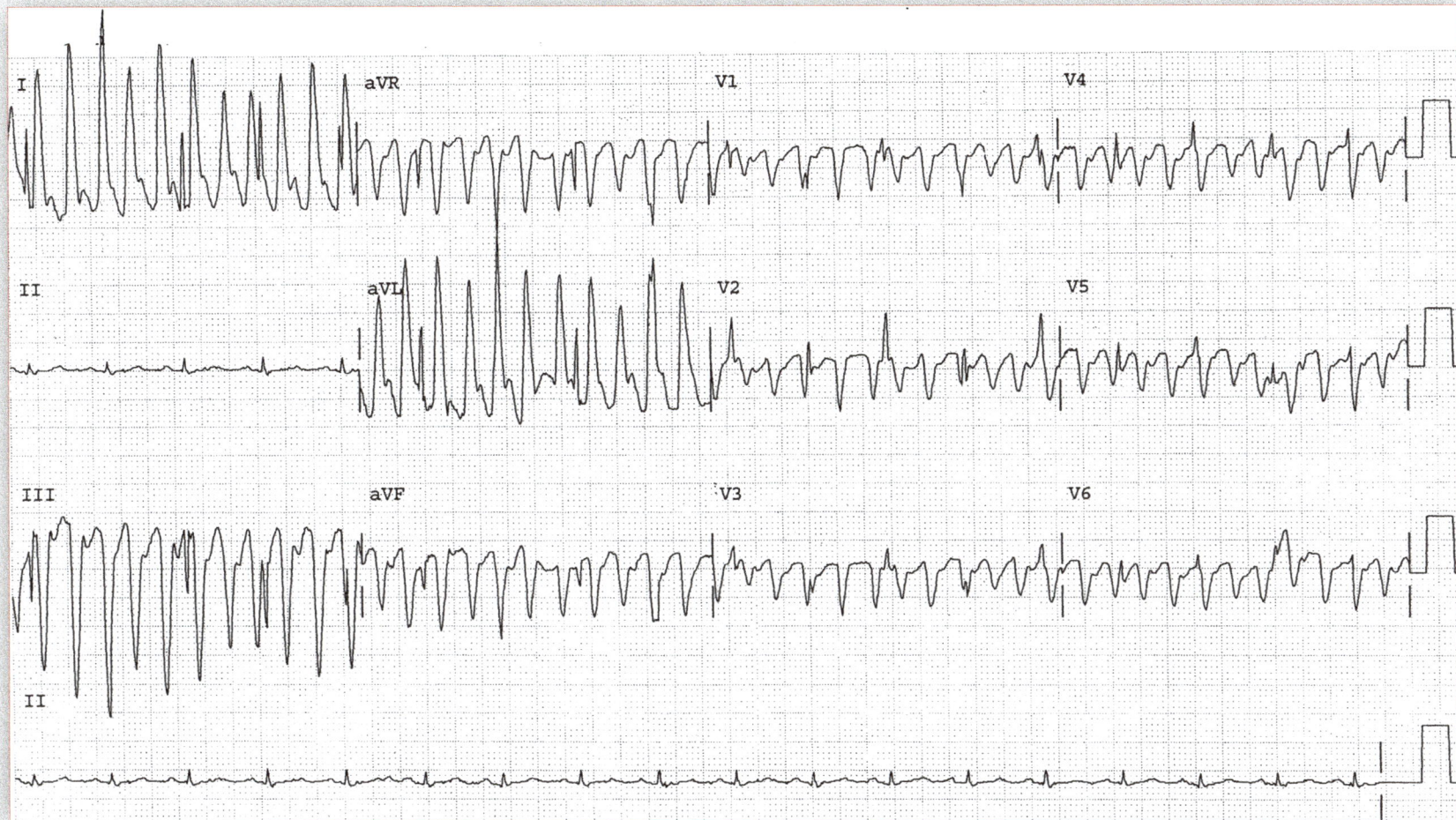

ECG 90 Analysis: Sinus tachycardia, artifact

The ECG appears to show a rapid heart rate of 210 bpm and QRS complexes that are wide, bizarre, and show some variability in morphology, suggesting a sustained ventricular tachycardia. However, lead II shows regular and normal QRS complexes (+). There is a P wave (^) before each QRS complex, with a stable PR interval. The rate is 110 bpm, indicating a sinus tachycardia. Since the leads in each column are simultaneous, the presence of a normal rhythm and QRS complexes in lead II means that the same is present in leads I and III. With closer inspection of most of the leads, organized and narrow QRS complexes (↑) can be seen occurring at a regular interval (⊔) at a rate of 110 bpm. Therefore, this ECG shows sinus tachycardia with artifact being present in all leads except lead II. It is important to recognize the fact that normal narrow QRS complexes can be seen occurring at a regular interval throughout all of the leads. This artifact is likely due to patient motion, often repetitive motion such as tooth brushing. ■

Index

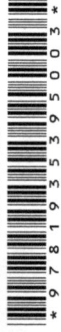